# Cost Control in Hospitals

**health**
**administration**
**press**

*M2240 School of Public Health*
*The University of Michigan*
*Ann Arbor, Michigan 48109*
*(313) 764-1380*

Lewis E. Weeks, Ph.D.
*Editor*

*The Press was founded in 1972 with the support of the W. K. Kellogg Foundation as a joint endeavor of the Association of University Programs in Health Administration and the Cooperative Information Center for Hospital Management Studies.*

# Cost Control in Hospitals

Edited by
John R. Griffith
Walton M. Hancock
Fred C. Munson

Program and Bureau of
Hospital Administration
School of Public Health
The University of Michigan

Health Administration Press
Ann Arbor
1976

**Library of Congress Cataloging in Publication Data**

Main entry under title:

Cost control in hospitals.

Includes bibliographies and index.
1. Hospitals—Cost control. I. Griffith, John R. II. Hancock, Walton M., 1929- III. Munson, Fred C.
RA971.3.C59 658.1'552 75-28579
ISBN 0-914904-12-4

Grateful appreciation is extended to the copyright owners for permission to use the following material:

"Practical Ways to Contain Hospital Costs." *Harvard Business Review*, Vol. 51, No. 6, November-December 1973, pp. 131-139. Copyright 1973 by the President and Fellows of Harvard College.

"Budgeting Process Integral to Effective Cost Control System." *Hospital Financial Management*, Vol. 28, No. 7, July 1974, pp. 12-28. Copyright 1974 by the Hospital Financial Management Association.

"Problems of Implementing Change in Two Hospital Settings." *AIIE Transactions*, Vol. 4, No. 4, December 1972, pp. 258-266. Copyright 1972 by the American Institute of Industrial Engineers, Inc.

"Understanding the Implementing of Change." *Hospital Progress*, Vol. 55, No. 6, June 1974, pp. 54-59. Copyright 1974 by The Catholic Hospital Association.

**Health Administration Press**
**M2240 School of Public Health**
**The University of Michigan**
**Ann Arbor, Michigan 48109**
**(313) 764-1380**

The research upon which this
publication is based was supported by

The National Center for Health Services Research

Health Resources Administration

Department of Health, Education, and Welfare
PHS Grant Number HS00228

John R. Griffith *is Professor and Director of the Program and Bureau of Hospital Administration, The University of Michigan. He received a bachelor's degree in engineering science from The Johns Hopkins University in 1955 and an MBA in Hospital Administration from The University of Chicago in 1957. He joined the faculty at Michigan in 1960. Griffith has written several books and monographs including:* Quantitative Techniques for Hospital Planning and Control; The McPherson Experiment *(with Lewis E. Weeks and James H. Sullivan);* Progressive Patient Care—An Anthology *(editor with Lewis E. Weeks);* Home Care for a Small Community; *and* A Reappraisal of the McPherson Experiment in Progressive Patient Care *(with Lewis E. Weeks and Robert A. DeVries). Professor Griffith served as editor of* Abstracts of Hospital Management Studies, *1964-1971, and has been a member of the editorial advisory board of several scholarly journals including:* Inquiry, Hospital Administration, *and* Medical Care. *He is a Fellow of the American College of Hospital Administrators and of the American Public Health Association. He is a Past President of the Association of University Programs in Health Administration.*

Walton M. Hancock *is Professor of Industrial and Operations Engineering and Professor of Hospital Administration at The University of Michigan. He received his doctorate in engineering from The Johns Hopkins University in 1954. He joined The University of Michigan as Lecturer in Industrial Engineering in 1959, became a full professor in 1962, and served as chairman of the department, 1963-1968. He was appointed Professor of Hospital Administration in 1970. Hancock has written or has been the coauthor of at least fifteen monographs and more than twenty-five published papers. He served as Editor in Chief of* MTM Journal, *1964-1970, and Associate Editor of* TIMS Journal, *1964-1966, and as a member of the Editorial Board of* AIIE Transactions *since 1972.*

Fred C. Munson *is Professor of Hospital Administration and Lecturer in Population Planning, The University of Michigan. He earned a doctorate in economics from Massachusetts Institute of Technology in 1959 after which he joined the faculty of the School of Business Administration, The University of Michigan. He moved to the Program in Hospital Administration at Michigan in 1971. He was a Ford Foundation Consultant for Industrial Relations in India, 1965-1966. Professor Munson is the author of a book titled* Indian Trade Unions: Structure and Functions, *and of a monograph (with Richard Jelinek and Robert Smith) titled* Service Unit Management, *as well as a number of professional papers.*

# Contributors

Richard F. Baum, Ph.D.
Department of Industrial and Operations Engineering
College of Engineering
The University of Michigan

William L. Dowling, Ph.D.
Department of Health Services
School of Public Health and Community Medicine
The University of Washington

M. David Ermann, Ph.D.
Department of Sociology
The University of Delaware

Alan C. Foose, M.P.H.
Applied Management Sciences, Inc.
Silver Spring, Maryland

Paul Fuhs, M.S.
Program and Bureau of Hospital Administration
School of Public Health
and
Department of Industrial and Operations Engineering
College of Engineering
The University of Michigan

John R. Griffith, M.B.A.
Program and Bureau of Hospital Administration
School of Public Health
The University of Michigan

Walton M. Hancock, D. Eng.
Program and Bureau of Hospital Administration
School of Public Health
and
Department of Industrial and Operations Engineering
College of Engineering
The University of Michigan

Shyam Heda, M.S.
Medicus Systems Corporation
Chicago, Illinois

Stephen H. Lipson, M.H.A.
Virginia Hospital Association
Richmond, Virginia

Fred C. Munson, Ph.D.
Program and Bureau of Hospital Administration
School of Public Health
The University of Michigan

Ronald F. Perry, Ph.D.
Department of Industrial Engineering
Northeastern University

Kurt R. Student, Ph.D.
Rohrer, Hibler, and Replogle
Southfield, Michigan

Vandankumar M. Trivedi, Ph.D.
Department of Health Services
School of Public Health and Community Medicine
The University of Washington

Edwin H. Tuller, M.P.H.
Blue Cross Association
Chicago, Illinois

D. Michael Warner, Ph.D.
Department of Health Administration
Duke University

To the people of Able and Baker Hospitals, whose commitment to service and to the control of unnecessary costs made this work possible.

J.R.G.
W.M.H.
F.C.M.

# Contents

# Figures

# Tables

# Section I

# Overview and General Conclusions

# I.1

# Introduction

Concern over the rising cost of hospital care has been widespread since the late 1960s, when increases of fifteen percent per year and higher became routine. As a result, increasing public discussion and reaction have led to a variety of systematic efforts to influence individual institutions toward less costly operation. These efforts were prominent in the Economic Stabilization Program—hospitals were among the limited group of industries where controls were retained after the general relaxation in January 1973[1]—in the Social Security Amendments of 1972,[2] and in the Health Planning and Resources Act of 1974.[3] At the state level, most large states either have passed or are considering passage of laws establishing hospital rate regulatory commissions.

These actions substantially change the operating environment of hospitals from that which prevailed throughout the 1960s. In those days, the mood was expansionistic, and hospitals were frequently encouraged to increase services and facilities. Cost increases, which inevitably accompany such expansion, especially when it is undertaken rapidly, were not strongly resisted, and in some ways were at least tacitly encouraged. Much of the Federal action was aimed either at subsidizing the hospital industry or at providing insurance protection for the people. The Hill-Burton program, for example, was well funded throughout this period and directly subsidized new facility construction. Federal assistance programs were implemented for training of health manpower, including doctors, nurses, public health workers and allied health professionals. Research in health care was heavily funded through the National Institutes of Health Program. Finally, the prevailing payment mechanisms were the hospital's charges, or full cost reimbursement programs. In some cases, including the Medicare program, "cost plus" reimbursement was used.

In such an atmosphere of largesse it is little wonder that hospital costs accelerated as they did. However, each of these programs has been curtailed or reduced.

The result of the reductions in the old programs and the development of the new is to enforce much greater rigor upon hospital management decisions which affect cost. As the legislative programs indicate, these decisions lie in three general areas: the expansion or investment decision, the appropriate utilization of hospital facilities and services, and the efficiency of routine management in staffing, scheduling, and control of supplies.

*Cost Control in Hospitals* attacks these decisions with a variety of technical aids for the management of the individual institution. It follows a format consistent with the legislative thrust and with a general strategy our work indicates to be sound. In this strategy, the starting point is planning an adequate, efficient facility supply, the interim steps involve improvement of day-to-day scheduling and staffing decisions, and the third level establishes reporting and control systems on managerial performance. Obviously nothing as complicated as a hospital is ever managed in neat sequential steps. There are many possibilities which cannot be pursued, projects which are delayed or discontinued, and short run opportunities which must be taken out of sequence. In general, however, following these levels of approach is fruitful, while deviating from them risks failure and setbacks. The book format follows this strategic approach.

Taken as a whole, *Cost Control in Hospitals* can be viewed as a new system of hospital management to meet the new operating environment. It results from an effort at the comprehensive application of systems analysis to the problems of conventional community hospital operations, toward the objective of reduced cost of care without sacrifice of quality. In one sense, this new system of management is an effort to "engineer" the hospital; that is, to apply technical aids to decision making in a manner which makes the decisions more appropriate to social needs, less difficult to make, and more accurate. Like all technological systems, this one starts with elementary applications which become increasingly sophisticated as time goes on. What is described here are initial solutions likely to be viewed as rudimentary and primitive in the future.

In such a venture, a key measure of success is not how well the new systems solve the immediate problems—though they should offer a clear improvement over their predecessors—but how well they stimulate and support later development. The goal is not to offer finished, sophisticated work, but to provide practical, achievable foundations for an evolving development over many years. Good foundations will have three characteristics: centrality, comprehensiveness, and expansibility. They should permit substantial improvement in important central decisions, cover as many of these decisions as possible, and be consistent with further work on less central decisions as well as further improvement of their own processes. That is, they should permit both horizontal and vertical expansion, extension, and improvement.

The systems presented here are reasonably successful in the centrality criterion and somewhat lacking on the comprehensiveness measure. Their expansibility remains to be proven. They cover three major areas of resource allocation: planning of facilities and services, forecasting and control of manpower expenditures, and scheduling of patients and personnel. The most serious omissions are in the areas of professional quality. The systems described here should be supplemented with a fourth major area covering decision aids and control systems for utilization, medical care review, and quality of nursing and other hospital professional services. Some systems already exist in the missing area, however, and many people are working on their improvement. Professional standards review organizations may provide additional assistance both in doctors' resource allocation decisions and in understanding the need for scheduling improvements. The PAS, MAP, and length of stay packages available through the Commission on Professional and Hospital Activities[4] are a well-known example in the medical care area. Many of the hospital services—particularly laboratory and nursing—have workable quality assessment programs. The best available systems in these areas should be a satisfactory complement to the systems presented here.

The technology presented here concentrates on the administrative rather than the medical aspects of cost control decisions, yet we have found the distinction between the two less clear than one might suppose. The statement, "The doctor controls the use of resources in the hospital, because he decides what patients are admitted, how long they stay, and what services they get," is at best overly simplistic. In some important ways, it may be erroneous. We believe the doctor decides who should be admitted based upon the situation he faces. The availability of alternatives to admission, the occupancy level, the delays and inconvenience surrounding admission and service, the payment mechanism, and the attitude of his peers influence that decision as well as the patient's needs and attitudes. Systems which raise hospital occupancy, guarantee admission dates, and encourage preadmission testing affect the length of stay directly and influence the admission decision at least indirectly. We believe these systems facilitate still other actions, such as more effective utilization review and more appropriate response to acute hospital substitutes like home care and ambulatory surgery. The work described in the following chapters does not trace these implications or fully justify our conclusions in this regard, because our time was taken up in the primary task of designing the technology itself. Hopefully further work will document these interrelationships between administrative and clinical decisions.

Most of the other failures of comprehensiveness must also be viewed as opportunities for further work. It will be very useful to add better patient scheduling systems—perhaps an integrated critical path schedule for diagnosis, admission and surgery, for example—budgetary controls for supplies and nonlabor services, and other extensions. The present evidence is that with the exception of quality control, these systems are less central than the ones discussed here, or are natural evolutions of this work. However interesting these omissions may be, they are not the proper starting point for a comprehensive new approach to internal management problems of hospitals. They either deal with less significant components of costs or they depend upon work of the type described here to make them practical.

The findings reported here are the work of a four-year multi-disciplinary investigation. A team composed of teachers of hospital administration, industrial engineering, and organizational behavior worked closely with the administration of community hospitals to devise, install, and evaluate a variety of tools for cost control. All of the techniques reported here (with the exceptions noted) have been field tested in one or more hospitals. Most commonly, these were two 300 bed community general hospitals referred to in the text as "Able" and "Baker." Other institutions were used occasionally and are described as necessary in the detailed reports. The two test hospitals were selected because they were known to have skilled management, as reflected by the credentials of the administrator and the achievement of the hospital. They were convenient to Ann Arbor, Michigan, and large enough to develop important cost control problems. Both are owned by governmental units but have private medical staffs, independent boards of trustees, and are financially self-supporting, in terms of all operating and most capital financing. Neither has internship or residency programs, and both have combinations of specialist and general practitioner medical staffs.

Baker Hospital is part of a group of four hospitals, operated under the Michigan Hospital Authority Act. The hospital has its own administrator, medical staff, and departmental organization. Baker is in the suburbs near Detroit and serves a number of predominantly blue collar suburban cities and towns. Most of these people have a choice of several almost equally convenient institutions, including one, Wayne County General, which has an extensive house staff and full time medical staff and provides tax supported care to the needy. The area around Baker, including all the adjacent counties, is part of both the Greater Detroit Area Hospital Council, an old voluntary planning effort of considerable reputation, and the Comprehensive Health Planning Council of Southeast Michigan, a 314b agency supported under the Comprehensive Health Planning Act, 89-749.

Able Hospital is the largest of three general hospitals which provide essentially all care to a part rural, part urban county of 150,000 and some citizens of surrounding counties. The second, a 200 bed church related voluntary hospital, has a nearly identical medical staff. The third, a small voluntary hospital, serves patients of osteopathic physicians. Cooperative planning in the Able community is at a much less organized level than in the Baker community, and there is no source of tax supported care except that provided by Medicaid. There are many other differences between the two study hospitals and these are brought out where they are important in describing the cost control tools or their implementation.

The authors believe this work is broadly applicable, despite its limited testing. Very small hospitals—those under 100 beds—may find parts of it, particularly the bed control and nursing scheduling models, inapplicable because they can easily solve the problems intuitively. Very large hospitals and those with elaborate medical education commitments will probably find the number of exceptions and special problems so numerous that they must nearly redesign the control systems. For both the very large and the very small institution, section I.2, on the general problem of cost control should be a useful framework, and the approaches to planning, budgeting, patient scheduling, and personnel scheduling should suggest the logic of sound solutions. For the remaining hospitals—of which there are between 2,000 and 3,000 in the U.S.—the approaches here provide a general guide to cost reduction and a considerable body of useful specific procedures.

Some constraints or prior requirements should be noted. The most important prerequisite to a major revision of hospital systems is will—a firm conviction that better cost control is important enough to justify a long, patient, and occasionally painful effort. Even with the prototypes and procedures described here, extensive, repeated work will be required with both the technical systems and their impact on the human organization. Drawing upon Dr. Ermann's conclusion (section IV.2), one could even suspect that any quick, easy success is more likely to be apparent than real. The incentive for this hard work has not been clear for hospitals in the past, but the authors believe it is now and will be in the future.

As a second prerequisite, the discussion presumes a nonprofit community general hospital with conventional medical staff, trustee, and administrative structures. While much of the approach could be translated to proprietary or special hospitals, no effort has been made to do this. The hospital must have a well thought out chart of accounts which parallels the authority delegated in the formal and actual organization. A computerized payroll system, accurately related to the chart of accounts, is necessary. A central admitting office with realistic control over admission and placement of patients is assumed. Also assumed is a functioning medical staff, including a utilization review committee, and a joint conference committee or equivalent means of communicating medical staff viewpoint to the administrator and the board of trustees. The organization as a whole must have a strong committee and communication structure which is capable of identifying points of stress and dissatisfaction and resolving them effectively. Most of these requirements could be stated as the first steps to cost control. The hospital which has not achieved them should set them up. The procedures described in the report will test and strengthen this basic structure.

A major part of the problem of systems improvement is gaining the understanding, acceptance, and cooperation of the hospital people, from the trustees to the first line supervisors. (It turns out that the systems themselves act only indirectly on the workers below managerial and professional levels.) Thus a major consideration in systems design becomes the discovery and elimination of those characteristics of the proposed system which create unnecessary difficulties for the operators. A "cut and fit" process is frequently necessary to do this. For example, raising hospital occupancy tends to raise the number of transfers between nursing units. This creates an unnecessary extra burden on nursing (over the one created by the census increase) which must be resolved by revising transfer policies and "fine tuning" the admissions scheduling. The problem must be solved as it arises, and a mechanism to solve it is as important a part of the system as the scheduling technology itself. It is also necessary to devote substantial energy and thought to the change process, bringing to bear all the known techniques for encouraging and managing change. A major portion of the work was consumed in these two related problems. What frequently began as a simple technical problem ended as a complex interaction of technical, organizational, and human factors.

In presenting the findings, an effort has been made to reflect these realities. As a result, a great deal of attention is placed on the justification for specific tchnology, the criteria for its design, the order of approach to implementation, and the foreseeable implications of the installation. Much of this effort is reflected in descriptions of the technologies themselves. Some technology, however, is generally applicable to all three of the major areas, and has been treated separately.

The first section of *Cost Control in Hospitals* deals with the considerations common to the overall effort. "The Concept of Cost Control in Hospitals" is a justification of the selection of the major components of the system. It also discusses each area's relative potential contribution to cost control, the interactions which may be expected between areas, the order of approach, and the role of hospital trustees. We believe it will be valuable to all members of general management, to trustees, and to those concerned with regulatory, planning, and reimbursement agencies.

The second section develops a methodology for planning bed needs consistent with the requirement we believe is inescapable in practical cost control, namely, that there be no excess beds available for use in the community. The methodology proposed can be used to determine excess, with appropriate safeguards against inadequacy. Also in this section is a procedure for evaluating alternative patterns of centralization for both beds and services, given the usual case that a number of hospitals exist in the community and create a relatively inflexible stock of resources.

The third section opens with a general essay on the development and use of controls in hospitals, contrasting the management styles and activities necessary under formal control systems with more traditional conditions in hospitals. Following that there are a number of tools for day-to-day managerial control. Foremost of these, because it occupies a central and critical role, is the patient admission scheduling model. Other scheduling and control systems for nursing personnel and radiology department operation are also presented. Also in this section are two chapters discussing the use of budgeting, cost accounting, and payroll systems in a cost control program.

The fourth section deals entirely with the problems of implementation. The first essay discusses the appropriate attitudes and performance of line administrators and staff technical specialists working in partnership to develop and install controll systems. The second essay describes the reactions of middle management and the hopsital as a whole when control systems are put in place. Two case studies trace in detail the problems encountered in starting admission control systems, and one reviews the impact on the nursing department of several different implementations undertaken simultaneously. The final essay summarizes the findings and conclusions of the demonstration implementations.

Section V reviews in detail the results of the demonstration at the principal implementation site, in terms of the overall cost performance of the hospital.

The book is arranged with the interests of various readers in mind. In general, trustees and others outside the direct management of hospitals will find section I, section II.1, and the introduction to section III of interest. Administrators will also want to review section IV, especially IV.1,2, and 6. Planners, of course, will be interested in section II. Controllers will have special interest in section III.5, 6, and 7, but they should not overlook the balance of section III, especially the introduction, and section IV. 1, 2, and 6. Technical specialists (industrial and systems engineers) and departmental managers will wish to study the appropriate parts of both sections III and IV.

## NOTES

[1]Executive Order 11695, January 11, 1973. Weekly compilation of Presidential Documents, Volume 9, Number 2, Monday, January 15, 1973, pp. 18-21.

[2]PL 92-603, especially Section 1122, requiring approval of expansion and capital investment. Section 249F establishing PSROs, and Section 223 requiring the Secretary of DHEW to impose ceilings upon Medicare payments to hospitals.

[3]PL 93-641.

[4]Commission on Professional and Hospital Activities, 1968 Green Road, Ann Arbor, Michigan 48105.

# I.2

# The Concept of Cost Control in Hospitals[1]

*by John R. Griffith, Walton M. Hancock, Fred C. Munson*

If every trustee in every hospital in the United States were to judge each expenditure request in terms of one question, "What will happen to the health of my community if I say no?" and then say "No" whenever the answer was "Nobody knows," "Nothing," or "Not much," the result would be a precipitous drop in health care costs. It might be a good beginning to containing hospital costs, but the question oversimplifies and therefore needs to be approached with care. This single question is hardly enough. Cost reduction must frequently be approached through changes quite apart from the direct questions of budgets and expenditures. In fact, the biggest yields for many hospitals appear to lie in more indirect actions.

This section is specifically written to provide hospital trustees, physicians, and general executives with a useful overview of the steps which can be taken to control costs and something about the top management roles in leading the process. As such, it may be of interest to more technically and departmentally oriented people as well.

## Major Areas of Cost Control

In approaching the problem of cost control, one is struck by the wide range of potential payoff. Some activities, such as the use of health maintenance organizations or similiar devices to encourage lower rates of hospital admission have potential of saving up to thirty percent of hospital costs. Others, such as optimal reorder quantities for inventories, might save only one percent. Conventional studies of work simplification and productivity are frequently small in magnitude (say, $100,000 per year in a $10,000,000 annual budget) even though they make relatively large reductions for the units where they are applied.[2] Obtaining the HMO-type savings requires major structural shifts in medical practice and health care prepayment, in addition to changes in the role of hospitals. Desirable as these might be, they will not come quickly or uniformly. On the other hand, the sum total of the smaller savings is insufficient. Recent rates of growth of costs far exceed these small improvements.

The demonstration project sought the middle ground—cost controlling activities with the highest possible potential compatible with conventional medical, hospital, and insurance schemes. The results indicate a hierarchy of activities in four levels: planning of facilities and services; scheduling of patients and patient services; medical control of utilization and quality; and administrative control of manpower and expenditures. It also shows important interrelationships between these areas and a need for a carefully ordered priority of approach.

## Facilities Planning

In general, the largest potential cost reductions appear to be possible through effective planning and control of physical resources. Significant operating cost savings as well as capital investment reductions are often possible. This is particularly true in communities where competition rather than cooperative planning has been the rule. Overbedding of adult medicine and surgery in one community was approximately ten percent, for example. The community had three hospitals. It could reduce operating expenses by $100,000 or more annually by merging obstetrics and had already achieved some savings by merging emergency services. Excess surgery and anesthesia capacity was noted, but efforts to reduce service at one hospital led to an increase at another. Opportunities appeared to exist for profitable sharing or merger of laundry, computer services, pediatrics, and laboratories.

There are two fundamental planning questions. One concerns access or utilization, "How much of a given facility or service will be provided?" The other concerns location or management, "Should we buy, or provide ourselves, or provide with others?" There is room for improvement in both these decisions.

Planning should be based on the community or population served. The project developed improved techniques for identifying, measuring, and forecasting this population. Facility size questions can then be approached in terms of quantities of services demanded per person. Any particular facility size reduces to:

$$\text{Size} = \frac{\text{Forecast use rate x Forecast population}}{\text{Capacity factor x Load factor}}$$

"Capacity factor" is the amount of service supplied by one unit of resource, for example, 365 patient days of care per bed-year. The load factor is "occupancy" of beds or, in general, the expected percentage of capacity utilization. Of these four factors, it appears that the largest cost reduction opportunities currently lie with the "use rate" and "load factor" components, in that order. Trustees in particular should review these factors with care. Use rates of the expensive inpatient facilities should be gradually reduced in most communities, and held constant in most of the rest. Use of outpatient services should generally be allowed to expand. The load factor of the hospital bed can frequently be maintained at ninety percent or more, as described below. Large savings will result in both capital and operating costs.

In planning the bed requirement, use rate is in patient days per thousand population, divided into at least the major services, obstetrics, pediatrics, and adult medical-surgical. Only rarely have hospitals planning new facilities calculated this set of measures. Hospital planning consultants have not suggested it. The problem lies in defining the population base to be used. To estimate this, data must be collected from several hospitals and a moderately complicated analysis performed.[3] Several metropolitan planning agencies have already begun collecting the data for use by all their members. Planning consultants can provide the information for almost any hospital if asked.

The Bureau of Hospital Administration has been using the approach and improving its application for many years. Among several Michigan communities we have found variations of nearly fifty percent in adult medical-surgical patient days per thousand population. Since this element accounts for over eighty percent of inpatient costs, and evidence of public benefit or unusual need is rare, questions are clearly in order for hospitals which exceed the state or regional average. Their decision *not* to expand facilities saves their communities both capital and operating dollars. There has not yet been a community which reduced facilities, although it was worth serious consideration in several areas.

Other hospital planning problems become more clear when expressed in a population ratio. One of our study hospitals was vaguely aware of a doctor shortage but was shocked to discover several parts of their service population with doctor-to-population ratios less than half the U.S. average.

The population-based ratio is also important because it relates directly to the payment mechanism. It is increasingly true that health care is purchased per person or per family, through Blue Cross and other programs. Per person cost calculations for a geographic community permit a rough comparison to premium payments. It has always been possible to make the premium calculation in terms of groups of subscribers, using Blue Cross and similar data, but it is now possible to make at least a crude translation back to the point of control of expenditures, at the hospital board level. It is clear from the limited data available that communities have been unequal in their control. Some have been parsimonious and others lavish, although they often pay the same premium. Until the expenditures are reduced to a per person level, it is difficult to identify this unevenness.

The per person cost calculation is particularly useful in evaluating the number, location, and ownership of each program or service, which is the second planning question. It is possible to say, "If we provide such and such a program (versus purchasing it or arranging for its purchase), what is the impact upon per capita health expenses?" The answer can be judged in terms of how the solution would be viewed by subscribers. Thus, another heart surgery unit may increase costs by so much per capita, and its contribution can be assessed in terms of the people who would not otherwise have been able to obtain treatment. A merger of two facilities might save an estimated dollar amount. The inconvenience which may occur to some doctors and patients can be judged in terms of the price being paid by all. The use of a population base tends to identify the need for large populations to support expensive highly specialized services. In the past, these services have been provided in many situations where they should have been purchased.

Facilities planning decisions are made almost entirely at the trustee level. While administrators, medical staff, department heads, and consultants offer information on facilities and service planning, trustees make the decision. They should insist on having service populations defined, use rates per person calculated and studied, and costs per person of alternative ways to provide the service presented. Efforts by trustees to frame these decisions in per person, cost-benefit terms and to make decisions to close tolerances will reduce hospital costs two ways: by removing excess facilities which cost money and increase the complexity of the cost control problem at other levels, and by providing tangible leadership and evidence of concern with the cost of hospital care.

## Occupancy Considerations

Many industries have a capacity benchmark or load factor and express their activities relative to it. The principal one in hospitals is the occupancy rate, occupied beds divided by available beds. Occupancy can be maintained at quite a high level, but it is frequently uncontrolled. Some trustees and administrators seem to regard it as evidence of divine providence rather than of management performance. The first step in its control is to divide it into reasonable components reflecting demands and specialized resources. Obstetrics, pediatrics, psychiatry, and special purpose units such as intensive and coronary care should be treated individually. The rest of the hospital, principally the adult medical-surgical units, can be treated as a single unit which can achieve occupancy of ninety percent or more in most situations.[4] This level still permits a substantial weekend shutdown and census drop. The project developed admission scheduling systems which permit ninety percent occupancies without endangering emergency patients and without unreasonable delays or cancellations for elective patients. In the study hospital occupancy increased from eighty-eight to over ninety-five percent. The number of admissions on the adult medical-surgical services also increased by more than nine percent in the first seven months. These goals can only be obtained when planning level decisions are sound. Hospitals which are overbedded are either underoccupied or overutilized. In neither case is admission scheduling a useful or appropriate venture, unless the underlying problem—too many beds—is attacked first.

Occupancy concepts can be extended to other parts of the hospital than beds. The major service departments, operating rooms, x-ray, and laboratory, can operate at "occupancies" similar to adult medical and surgical beds, and stablizing inpatient loads will help them to do so. The units with large unpredictable demands, such as obstetrics, emergency, and coronary care, cannot do as well. Even for these units, where much lower occupancies are obtainable, there are ways of establishing reasonable goals. A well run hospital will deliberately make such a determination as a guide to both the level of facilities required and the demands upon staff.

Trustees should insist on admission scheduling, on occupancy goals for all inpatient bed services, and on routine reporting of attainment of those goals. These goals should be studied in light of use rates, supply of facilities, and opportunities to gain higher levels under appropriate conditions. The contribution to cost savings from admission scheduling is intertwined with planning decisions about occupancy level. But if all community hospitals were achieving at least ninety percent occupancy in adult medical-surgical units and seventy percent in obstetrics and pediatrics (eighty-six percent overall) in 1971, the improvement would have permitted the closing of eight percent of the nation's bed supply.[5] The admission scheduling system which permits this high occupancy opens another possibility: the reduction of inpatient stay through preadmission testing. This opportunity appears to be worth about five percent of annual expenditures, according to preliminary studies, and it is discussed below.

## Medical Factors

Physicians control much of the activity of the hospital and, therefore the expenses. The indirect nature of this relationship is important. If a physician economizes by sending a patient home early or not ordering a laboratory test, that patient's bill is reduced. The cost of care to the community is not reduced, however, until some actual expenditure is eliminated. Doctors can *contribute* to hospital cost reduction, but in a poorly managed hospital they cannot *cause* cost reduction. (They can cause increased waste by creating unnecessary demand which misleads careless trustees and administrators into unnecessary expansion.) Utilization committees and other quality review committees composed mainly of doctors (peer review) are the principal devices for controlling doctors' demands, combined with a continuing education program.

The magnitude of savings available here is almost impossible to judge. It could conceivably be as great as the savings claimed for HMOs, although there is no proof that such large changes are attainable. There is evidence of substantial room for improvement, however. Lengths of stay vary by region of the country, from 5.9 days in the West to 8.0 in the East. The West has always been lowest of the four regions, but it has reduced its stay twelve percent since 1969. The East has also reduced length of stay, but only five percent.[6] A good deal appears to depend on physicians' attitudes, and it is not clear how these are formed. Certainly the formal mechanisms of peer review play a role, but so does concrete evidence of trustee concern. This area of cost control has not yet been fully explored in the demonstration project.[7]

The most interesting finding to date at the medical level has come as a result of the admission scheduling program at the high occupancy study hospital. Here most nonemergency patients are given definite dates for admission from a few days to two weeks in the future. Because the admission is reliably scheduled, much of the diagnostic work can be done early on the day of admission or the day before. New systems must be established to record the doctor's orders and provide the patient with instructions and premedications. These systems are only feasible when the admission date is reliable and they are only profitable when occupancy is high. A pilot study of the system involving 250 patients has shown a reduction in average length of stay, after adjustment for age, service, and physician, of seven-tenths of a day, or approximately six percent. Further work is underway.

The success of the preadmission testing system suggests a largely unexplored area of interaction between hospital and medical practice. It has led to investigation of the information return rates of laboratory and x-ray tests to doctors, and the results are revealing. Not only are the cycles long—twenty-five or more hours for routine reports—but they do not coincide well with the doctors' daily visits. Two or three days elapse between request for test and receipt of result. This will be an area of future investigation. Physician assistance will be an important component. For some diagnostic services, speed of reporting may become the critical measure of success, outweighing the load factor for the department or measures of cost and efficiency.

In the medical area, the trustee can be most helpful by maintaining the mechanisms which encourage reasoned and balanced communication. Planning, scheduling, and preadmission testing systems cause many readjustments in the doctors' activities. A given system may have different effects on the surgeon than on the general practitioner, in terms of personal income as well as patient care. It is clear that no group of doctors can dictate the solution for all, and also that the views of doctors must be weighed against each other as well as against costs. The project uncovered rules and procedures apparently established for the doctors' benefit which add tens of thousands of dollars a year in hospital costs. On the other hand, no one denies the necessity of doctors, their long working hours, and the need to use their time efficiently. It is foolishness to make their life unattractive, impair their income, or reduce their ability to treat patients with ill-considered, inflexible, bureaucratic procedures. Only when their viewpoint is systematically solicited and dispassionately weighed can these extremes be avoided.

## Expenditure Controls

The final cost control area is the one receiving most attention in conventional industrial engineering studies and budget oriented cost control programs. This is the design of systems to encourage the careful management of day-to-day expenditures at the department head level. Such systems involve adopting a standard for departmental performance and the frequent comparison of actual achievement against the standard. The standard is usually either the budget or some more or less scientific work measurement. A variety of approaches to performance measurement already exists. Several well-known programs of supervisory incentives[8] and hospital cost containment[9] concentrate heavily or exclusively in this area.

The study found this kind of cost reduction opportunities in the demonstration hospitals. To make the existence of the opportunities a matter of routine, rather than special study, requires a practical budgeting and reporting system to measure departmental performance. The initial requirements for such a system are presented in section III.6 and 7. The differences in available systems are relatively minor, compared to the critical importance of having some effective system. Overall the study suggests that the potential direct returns of these systems are not as promising as those attacking planning, occupancy, and medical problems. Their true importance lies in two areas, of which potential direct savings is one. Related to the tangible savings is an intangible; these systems encourage economy by hospital middle management and give evidence of trustee concern. Second, and at least equally important, the cost savings potential of facility planning, occupancy, medical utilization (and even HMOs) is not fully recoverable without such systems. A rise in occupancy does not lead to a reduction in costs if manpower and supplies increase more than the workload. Reduced numbers of tests ordered per patient do not cut the average laboratory cost per admission unless laboratory costs are reduced proportionately. Mergers and reductions in the physical facilities may avoid capital investment, but they only reduce operating costs when individual departments cut expenditures for manpower and supplies.

Department heads frequently need more than simply cost reporting systems to bring their expenditures under control. In one study hospital, eighty percent of annual expenditures were theoretically under departmental control. The other twenty percent included depreciation, top administration, insurance, interest, and other costs beyond departmental decisions. Eighty percent of the department controllable costs were in manpower, and half of these were in nursing. The nursing department wrestles daily with a complex scheduling system involving eight work locations, three shifts, and four classes of personnel. Two computer-aided scheduling algorithms were developed (section II.3 and 4) to assist with these problems. One helps with the weekly or monthly scheduling of vacations and days off. The other helps with the daily variations in workload due to changes in degree of illness, and in work force due to absenteeism. For all but the smallest hospitals, such scheduling systems are necessary to assist supervisory personnel with complicated decisions which must often be made under serious time pressure.

## The Interrelation of Cost Control Levels

The most striking finding of the demonstration is the importance of the interconnection between levels. The process of cost reduction in hospitals is similar to an arch, and the keystone of the arch is the planning decision about the supply of facilities. One of the demonstration hospitals was significantly less successful than the other. Occupancy did not go up, census variation could not be reduced, and almost no change occurred in the budgeting or expenditure patterns as a result of study efforts. This was the overbedded community where two nearly equal hospitals competed for limited revenue. Recommendations to alleviate this situation were generally acknowledged to be sound, but were not implemented by the community for reasons extraneous to the goal of economical care to all community citizens. The ultimate solution lies in building an organization which can reasonably represent the whole community, either through interlocking boards, a third board or holding company,[10] or merger. The study team is convinced that further effort at any other level is unpromising until the planning capability of this community has been improved and the excess physical resources removed.

In the other demonstration, the supply of facilities has been held equal to or less than demand by a combination of luck—a steady population growth—and a voluntary planning council which has for many years discouraged unnecessary hospital expansion. This hospital has made promising use of techniques to raise occupancy and control personnel expenditures. As a result, its per diem and per stay costs are dropping. If the bed supply were suddenly increased, rather than carefully balanced to the demand, it appears that these achievements would be lost. Occupancy would drop; census variation would rise; scheduling of personnel would become more difficult; staffing would increase to cover uncertainties in scheduling and workload; and costs per admission would rise. (Costs per patient day might remain constant if the surplus of beds encourages a lengthening in patient stay.)

Attitudes favorable to cost reduction are essential, particularly at medical staff and supervisory levels. The temptation to spend is with these people constantly. They feel less anxiety over quality of service if extra laboratory tests and x-rays are ordered and if extra employees are scheduled to protect against absenteeism. They get pressure from some patients and families to prolong hospital stays and pressure from some workers to reduce output requirements. Doctors find it is easier to avoid criticizing a wasteful colleague, and supervisors to avoid bringing up points of conflict with fellow department heads. The attitude of trustees and hospital administrators is very important in getting others to participate in cost reduction. Actions speak louder than words, and control of available facilities is the action which speaks loudest of all. (In the more successful demonstration, the trustees were actually a remote group that entered rarely into the daily life of the institution; they were exemplars by their actions.)

When facilities are available in surplus, doctors tend to assume the extra unit of use is free. "If I keep the patient overnight," said one doctor at the overbedded hospital, "it cannot increase costs. No extra nurses are hired, and even the food he eats would probably have been thrown away. Since there are plenty of beds, no other patient will be turned away. How then can you say that sending him home saves money?" There is no good answer to that question, because all possible replies lead eventually to a second question, "If you didn't want me to use the bed, why did you build it?" or "Why don't you close it?"

The supervisors do not overlook the impact of trustees' or doctors' decisions. It can appear to supervisors that neither the trustees nor the medical staff are willing to make an effort to control cost. It is not surprising, therefore, that they make little effort themselves. When the study team began its work with the high occupancy hospital, there followed a lengthy period of testing by the department heads. Ideas or suggestions about system improvement were politely ignored until it became clear that they were firmly supported by the trustees and, in some cases, the medical staff.

As viewed by the supervisor, cost containment interrelates with the levels of planning, occupancy, medical decision, and expenditures in other ways than attitudes. Slack occupancy leads to variation, and variation means occasional peak loads which are usually unpredictable to the supervisor. Staffing must be set for peaks, and the further the peaks are from the averages the more costly this becomes. At the same time, the slack tends to disperse to small unrecoverable units of resources. A ten percent drop in census implies a ten percent drop in nursing requirements. But 400 nursing employees are divided into four levels of training, three shifts, and eight work units (leaving, on the average, four people in each group). Rarely will that one-tenth saving be recoverable from any one work group.

The study team's principal conclusion is that cost reduction is a top-management-down procedure, with evidence of cost saving actions rather than rhetoric necessary at each level. Related to this conclusion is a proposition generated by this demonstration: four systems improvements (effective planning, improved scheduling, medical review and control, and supervisory review and control) are each necessary conditions for cost reduction, but none by itself is a sufficient condition. Significant cost savings rest on acknowledging and acting on all four improvements. Some value can come from any of the four, more from two, but full value only when all four are acting to reinforce and make effective the presence of the others.

The second major conclusion is that the installation of cost reduction programs is a major organizational change process requiring considerable human relations skill and change process technology. Attitudes of all major participants in the institution must be changed, including trustees and medical staff. Most groups must master new cognitive material—new measures of actual performance, new ways of analysis for decisions, and new techniques for solving old problems.

While the materials which must be learned can be held to a minimum level of technicality, learning takes a noticeable length of time. Mastery of the admission scheduling system at a study hospital, for example, took six months, not counting system design by the study team. Necessary preliminary revisions of existing systems and thorough communication of plans took three months. Despite this preparation, there was extensive reaction in the admitting, nursing, and medical staffs when the system went on-line. (These findings are discussed in section IV.4) Not until three months after start-up was the system fully turned over to departmental management. Follow-up contact by the study team continued at a less frequent rate for several months. The complexity and time involved in this process may be a function of the environment, incentives for cost reduction, and history of similar activities in the particular hospital. In any case, the installation of systems takes substantial time and continuous guidance by a responsible representative of management.

## The Role of Trustees

The trustee of the voluntary hospital holds the key to cost containment. Leadership toward the goal is what is required, rather than technical skills. (These are actually less difficult than we expected; the demonstration process has more often scaled down unnecessary sophistication than the opposite.) There is no questioning the importance of the goal, particularly for trustees associated with consumer groups, unions, and employers paying Blue Cross and insurance premiums. This component of production costs and family budgets must be brought under control.

What then can the interested trustee do? The demonstration suggests the directions trustees must support:

1. *Community-wide planning, with elimination of competition between individual institutions.* More often than not, the rivalries between the "Memorials," "Communitys," and "St. Swithinses" result in reduced occupancies, excessive investment, poor control of utilization rates, and situations where attempts at economy at one hospital are immediately offset by expenditure at another.

2. *Judicious but firm control of the community bed supply.* High occupancy and controlled use of the hospital are both related to bed supply. If excessive beds are provided, it is automatically impossible to achieve both these goals, and achieving either often becomes vastly more difficult. Governmental control of the bed supply through franchising or certification of need is frequently necessary to keep reasonable control. In those states where it exists, and in others where it is necessary, individual hospital trustees should support it.

3. *More attention to relevant direct measures of performance and less to irrelevant ones.* The study team has seen hospital trustees follow management strategies which maximize revenues, profits, local payrolls, or even prestige. If the goal is cost containment, none of these strategies is appropriate. Trustees should ask for more careful cost budgeting, consistent occupancy goals, better exception oriented reporting, and cost-benefit justification of all investment and expansion projects. They should help their hospitals develop systems which produce this information and reinforce its importance by careful and frequent monitoring of achievement.

4. *Negotiated incentive or prospective reimbursement schemes for hospitals.* There are a number of these developing in various parts of the country, and the details are not yet fully evaluated. It seems likely that flexibility and the opportunity for reasoned individual judgment will be necessary in any long-run solution to the cost containment problem, but that limits must be placed on individual hospital costs.

5. *Better communication, understanding, and coordination with the goals of the medical staff.* Many hospital actions such as preadmission testing, increased admissions, nurse staffing, and expansions have direct

economic and professional impacts on doctors which are sometimes quite subtle. Doctors' viewpoints must be heard and judiciously evaluated at the trustee level as well as in the detailed discussions which take place throughout the organization. Trustees should be particularly concerned with the supply of physicians, the balance between specialties (including family practice), the accessibility of hospital resources to individual doctors, and the accessibility of medical care to individuals in the community.

6. *Tangible and intangible support for all levels of hospital management who support cost containment goals and gain established objectives.* Hospitals are leaving an era of rapid and ungoverned expansion when management rewards went to those who could expand services and facilities and move promptly, even if uneconomically, to meet new demands. New management styles and techniques must be mastered from the administration down to the head nurse and housekeeping foreman. It is entirely appropriate for trustees to reward good performance and encourage new learning. All the available devices have a place: promotions, pay increases, reassignments to less demanding tasks, provision of data and staff assistance, and encouragement of reeducation.

The penalties to community hospitals if trustees fail in these tasks are losses in economy, flexibility, satisfaction of doctors and employees, and service and satisfaction to patients. But voluntary trustees have a long history of generous and thoughtful response to the needs of hospitals. That history is the major reason for their present important role. There is no reason to think that they cannot respond as well to the challenge of cost containment as they have to past challenges.

## NOTES

[1]This chapter is modified slightly from an article which originally appeared in *Harvard Business Review*, Vol. 51, No. 6, November-December 1973 under the title, "Practical Ways to Contain Hospital Costs."

[2]C. P. Hardwick and H. Wolfe, "Multifaceted Approach to Incentive Reimbursement: Blue Cross of Western Pennsylvania." *Medical Care*, May-June 1970, p. 182.

[3]John R. Griffith, *Quantitative Techniques for Hospital Planning and Control*. Lexington: D. C. Heath & Co., 1972, chapter 4.

[4]There are a number of exceptions where this goal is too high. They include small rural hospitals, extraordinary emergency demands, and unusually small wards.

[5]American Hospital Association, *Hospital Statistics*. Chicago: The Association, 1972, p. 13.

[6]*PAS Reporter*, Vol. 11, No. 16, October 26, 1973, p. 2.

[7]Both study hospitals had the conventional committees. Utilization rates were slightly below 900 adult medical-surgical patient days per thousand persons in both communities. In one community, growth in utilization was curtailed by the

physical facilities. The other community did not have a correspondingly higher use rate, despite its oversupply of beds, indicating a conservative attitude on the part of the medical staff toward the use of the hospital. In this aspect, they were more cost-conscious than the trustees, but they also were somewhat unusual. In many other communities use rates have risen to fill available beds and then generate demand for more.

[8]J. J. Jehring, *Increased Productivity in Hospitals*. Madison: Center for the Study of Productivity Motivation, University of Wisconsin, 1966.

[9]P. E. Ludwig, *Dollars and Sense*. Battle Creek: The W. K. Kellogg Foundation, 1971.

[10]C. N. Platou and J. A. Rice, "Multihospital Holding Companies." *Harvard Business Review*, Vol. 50, No. 3, May-June 1973.

# Section II

# Cost-Effective Planning of Hospital Facilities and Services

# II.1

# A Procedure for Rational Planning

*by William L. Dowling*

## Focus of This Section

This section describes the approaches to cost-effective planning developed by the Bureau of Hospital Administration during twenty years of service to nearly fifty Michigan hospitals. The demonstration project undertook several planning studies which permitted technical development and detailed description of the methods used. Pragmatic data gathering and decision making techniques for step-by-step planning of hospital facilities and services are presented here. Emphasis is on determining size and scope of facilities and services and evaluating opportunities for consolidating or sharing services. The discussion centers on planning at the institutional level, although hospital role is viewed as a function of the needs of the community it serves and the resources of the larger health services delivery system within which it operates. While the discussion is entirely in the context of the community hospital and its component services, applications to other health care institutions such as clinics and long-term care facilities are straightforward.

Described are methods for determining service area and population, forecasting demand for services, translating forecast demand into facility requirements, and assessing alternative ways of providing the facilities required. Architectural planning and planning at the departmental level are touched upon, although more complete discussions can be found in other sources.[1]

## Definition of Cost-Effective Planning

Planning is deciding in advance on a course of action for achieving a desired end. Hospital planning is deciding in advance how to allocate resources to provide facilities and services which meet the needs of the population served, while minimizing capital and operating costs over time. Cost-effective planning then is the process of determining the least costly arrangement of facilities and services consonant with community needs. Clearly, noncost criteria are important. The position taken here, however, is that intangible factors are best considered in the context of dollar cost implications of alternative facility arrangements.

## Implications of Cost-Effective Planning

In hospital planning, management faces the classic economic problem of conserving or efficiently using scarce resources for adding or expanding facilities and services. This can be framed either as a problem of goal maximization and fixed resources, where the planner attempts to accomplish as much as possible with the resources available, or as a problem of cost minimization and fixed goals, where the planner attempts to accomplish these goals with as few resources as possible. Although there is certainly a limit to the capital funds hospitals can raise, it is probably more meaningful to think of hospital planning as the second type of problem. The goal is to provide facilities and services which just meet community needs, with the minimum expenditure of capital and operating resources. Thus, cost-effective planning determines the minimum set of facilities and services required and the least costly way to provide them.

The application of cost-effective planning techniques can be expected to produce certain results:

Cost-effective planning should result in more careful and precise decisions about facilities and services. In many communities, this will mean more modest additions to hospital facilities and services than would otherwise occur.[2] Present or potential bed surpluses may be identified. Because the key factors affecting facility requirements are explicitly identified and measured in cost-effective planning, management can alter those factors that would otherwise lead to overelaborate plans. For example, if high admission rates or long lengths of stay are identified, actions can be taken to reduce them rather than expand the hospital plant. Also, if the capactities of different size departments or units to accommodate expected levels and patterns of use are identified, there is less reason to err on the conservative side "just to make sure." Finally, cost-effective planning provides an explicit opportunity to decide how much of a given service is desirable in a given community.

Cost-effective planning should result in more consolidations, mergers, and sharing of services among hospitals than would otherwise occur. Economies of scale, as well as an advantageous relationship between quality and size, appear to pertain for many hospital programs and services. Spitzer has reviewed both the efficiency and quality problems of small hospitals,[3] and there is growing interest in the cost and quality implications of small size, or more precisely, of low patient care workload volumes.[4]

A number of factors may make production more efficient in large hospitals or units: specialization of equipment and personnel, reduction of excess capacity of infrequently used equipment and facilities, reduction of reserve requirements for certain equipment and facilities maintained to meet fluctuations in demand, lower prices for some inputs as a result of volume buying, lower cost of borrowing money due to the lower risk associated with larger hospitals, lower costs associated with greater volumes of output as a result of knowledge and skill gained through experience and learning, and economies of horizontal or vertical integration. A number of empirical studies have found that economies of scale do in fact exist in hospitals[5].

From the hospital planner's point of view, it is important to recognize that economies of scale for the hospital as a whole are caused by economies in individual departments or units, since there are many ways for hospitals to capture departmental economies of scale, whereas the overall size of a hospital is largely dictated by the size of the population served. Certain individual services can be contracted to outside organizations large enough to achieve economies of scale; other services can be consolidated, merged, or traded among hospitals; others can be jointly operated. Cost-effective planning explicitly identifies and costs out alternative ways of providing needed services (which may include providing a given service in several hospitals, centralizing the service in one hospital, or other forms of cooperation and sharing). Thus, the cost saving opportunities available through cooperative planning are made manifest, and hospitals are discouraged from choosing more costly ways of providing facilities and services.

Cost-effective planning should result in more substantial development and use of alternatives to the hospital than would otherwise occur. Again, this shift in emphasis is caused by the explicit identification and costing out of alternative service possibilities, some of which involve substitution of out-of-hospital programs for inpatient facilities. Less costly service mixes demonstrated in this manner are difficult to ignore.

Cost-effective planning should result in lower operating costs over time. Minimizing the size of hospital facilities minimizes the areas to be staffed and maintained. There is less tendency to overuse facilities and services when the supply is correctly established. Experience indicates that hospitals are more receptive to cost saving innovations such as admission scheduling, preadmission testing, nurse scheduling, and utilization review when the supply of facilities is somewhat tight.

Cost-effective planning should result in better hospital performance under prospective reimbursement schemes. The budget review or negotiations process employed to set prospective rates makes it necessary for hospitals to cost out carefully the development and operation of new services in order to gain recognition of the costs of their plans in their prospective rates. At the same time, hospitals with good planning processes should fare better under prospective reimbursement. Thus, prospective reimbursement provides both an incentive for and a test of cost-effective planning.

### Requirements of Cost-Effective Planning

The search for the least costly arrangement of hospital facilities and services in a community requires willingness to consider all possibilities. Balanced and objective consideration must be given to allocations of resources to construction and operations, facilities and manpower, and in-hospital and out-of-hospital services. Cost-effective planning begins with the following premises. A reasonably defined community or service area must be identified. The entire population of this area rather than a single hospital's inpatient population should serve as the starting point for planning. The full spectrum of health facilities and services required to meet community needs must be considered, rather than just acute inpatient services. The facilities and services provided by nearby hospitals must be considered to avoid duplication and to avoid planning small units that are uneconomical and medically unwise.

Attention must be paid to eliminating underuse or overuse. Facilities and services should not be planned to accommodate poor utilization patterns. Attention must be paid to problems of accessibility and location, with particular reference to disadvantaged groups. The effectiveness and efficiency of existing patterns of financing and delivering health services should be evaluated and innovative methods such as health maintenance organizations should be considered.

## The Planning Process

### General Approaches to Planning Hospital Facilities and Services

All approaches to hospital planning attempt to some degree to base hospital facility and service requirements on community needs. The approach advocated here is one of explicitly estimating past demand trends and extrapolating these trends to forecast future hospital use. The forecasts so obtained may be modified by expert judgment about expected changes in the factors that affect hospital use (including deliberate efforts to decrease or increase use to more closely equal need). The approach relies mainly on *demand,* the actual decisions of doctors and patients to use hospital services, rather than *need,* an independent normative judgment of the quantities and types of services that should be used by a given community. Obviously both are important in the final decision. It is futile to provide services people will not use (services for which there is no demand), expensive to encourage use of services they do not need, and dangerous to fail to provide services they both need and want. In the approach described here, demand forecasts provide a starting point, and checks against need are built into the process.

Another approach to planning begins with estimates of need, as suggested by morbidity rates, diagnosis-specific death rates, and other indicators of health problems. We rejected these because of the cost of collecting this information and the difficulty of analyzing it to the point of specific planning decisions, and because it appears that for most U.S. communities and hospital services, the current demand or use levels are substantially higher than what would be judged as needed under a strict medical definition. In addition, health status indicators cannot be directly translated into facility and service requirements because they are determined by population characteristics and socioeconomic factors, as well as by the adequacy of available health care. They are, however, useful for identifying medically underserved subgroups in the population.

Another approach to planning employs facility-population ratios (for example, hospital beds per thousand population) as a measure of the adequacy of available facilities. Such ratios arise from empirical observations and normative judgments, often based on existing facility-population ratios in areas where health resources are felt to be sufficient. Little agreement exists, however, on what the "right" ratios are. Such ratios fail to account for factors other than population size which affect demand or need and hence facility requirements and, given the variation in hospital use from community to community, could result in planning more or fewer beds than would actually be used. In addition, the use of existing facility-population ratios tends to maintain the status quo rather than encourage change in patterns of delivering health services.

Still another approach is to specify a demand model and analyze the factors assumed to influence the use of hospital services. This approach postulates a set of economic, demographic, and social factors believed to determine the demand for health services. Multivariate analyses are used to estimate the direction (positive or negative) and degree to which each factor (independent variable) contributes to the overall use of services. Demand models can be used to estimate future use, once the effect of each independent variable on use has been estimated, by inserting predictions of future values of independent variables into the model. This approach requires that the planner predict future changes in the demand influencing factors, but these changes are frequently difficult to predict. Although conceptually sound, this approach is still in the developmental stage and is not preferred for general use in planning for existing individual hospitals. It has application in special cases, particularly where severe shortages have existed in the past and in new communities where historical data are lacking.

The cost, flexibility, and practicality of these alternative planning approaches vary. While improvements will undoubtedly be made in the need-based approaches and the multivariate demand models, they are currently difficult and expensive to apply. The method presented here, extrapolating from past trends in hospital use, gives a fairly reliable indication of future use, and is sufficiently flexible to accommodate most communities where hospitals presently exist. The approach is straightforward and understandable. Reliable data on past use are generally available at reasonable cost. Finally, this approach has proved to be as accurate or more accurate than the others[6], especially when tempered by expert judgment at certain critical points.

Two refinements should be made to the approach of extrapolating from past use to gain maximum reliability and flexibility. First, aggregate hospital use should be broken down into its component parts. Total hospital admissions and patient days should be divided into medical, surgical, obstetric, pediatric, and psychiatric admissions and days, and the total service area population broken down into age and sex groupings that represent the actual populations at risk for each component of hospital service. Only then can the use of each service be related to the relevant population, as, for instance, pediatric use to the population aged zero to fourteen and obstetric use to the female population aged fifteen to forty-four. Aggregate use of each service, such as total pediatric patient days, should be further broken down into its parts—population at risk, admission rate, and length of stay—and the future state of each of these variables projected separately.

Second, expert and normative judgment must be brought to bear in assessing factors underlying use. The possibility of over- or underuse of hospital services must be examined and plans made for correcting for these conditions, for example, building more long-term beds to encourage earlier discharge of long-stay patients, if inappropriate use is found. The possible effects of expected changes in economic and social factors known to affect use must also be judged. For example, the expectation that the Medicare Program would increase hospital use by the aged by about fifteen percent proved to be fairly accurate for many communities. In addition, the possible effects of expected advances in medical science and of changes in the organization of health services must be weighed. For example, one effect of a change from fee-for-service to prepaid group practice on hospital use is known to be a decline in inpatient days of care on the order of twenty to forty percent.

## General Presentation of the Planning Process

Systematic planning follows a series of steps leading from definition of the overall role of a hospital in meeting community needs to increasingly specific assessments of the quantities and types of facilities and services required. These steps are presented below. It should be noted, however, that good planning processes tend to be reiterative. New data or changed expectations that come up in one step force a rethinking of the decisions reached in preceding steps. To some extent, therefore, any simple list of planning steps is arbitrary and misleading. However, identification of the elements of the planning process is important because it provides a guide to all the decisions which will be made, explicitly or implicitly, as a plan becomes reality. The better these elements are understood, the better the chance that decisions will be explicit and consciously evaluated, rather than implicit or even accidental. The steps that comprise systematic planning are as follows:

1. Define a reference community and the roles of its hospitals.
   - (a) Determine the geographic area and population served by a hospital or group of hospitals.
   - (b) Assess the health needs of this population.
   - (c) Define the hospital's role in meeting these needs.
   - (d) Determine the programs and services required to fulfill this role.
2. Forecast future service volumes or workloads.
   - (a) Compute past use rates.
   - (b) Forecast future use rates.
   - (c) Forecast future population at risk.
   - (d) Compute future service volumes.
3. Transform future service volumes into facility requirements.
   - (a) Identify facility units.
   - (b) Determine the service producing capacity of facility units.
   - (c) Determine standby reserve requirements for emergencies and peak volume periods.
   - (d) Compute future facility requirements.
4. Inventory present facilities, compare present and required facilities, and determine additional facilities required to accommodate future service volumes.
5. Identify alternative ways to provide the required facilities, evaluate the total costs of each of these, and select the least costly.

Pertinent to each step are certain concepts, areas of knowledge of the health system, and quantitative techniques. The first step in the planning process will be discussed in this chapter and the balance of the steps accompanied by examples and illustrations will be developed in the chapters that follow.

## The Interplay Between Community Definition and Hospital Role

Definition of a hospital's role is the critical starting point for planning, because the role of a hospital determines the direction in which it should move and the activities, programs, and services it should provide. More specifically, a hospital's role determines the breadth, depth, and manpower requirements. It should, in general, be based on community needs, hospital resources, and the functions of other organizations serving the community.

The hospital planner needs a clear definition of the hospital's role because of the complexity of planning and the number of participants inside and outside the hospital who figure in the process. Many groups and individuals exert considerable influence in the hospital environment. Physicians, department heads, and other key personnel may desire more extensive or sophisticated facilities and programs than a balance of cost and service goals would indicate, because of their orientation to high professional standards and to their particular area of responsibility. A clear, strong sense of the hospital's role is necessary to provide balance and perspective to competing interests during bargaining and negotiation.

### Geographic Area and Population Served

The methodology for determining service area populations will be described in detail in the following chapter. It is pertinent to note here that although autonomous service areas may be found for isolated hospitals, the service areas of metropolitan hospitals commonly overlap, so that a group of hospitals jointly serves the same population. This makes cooperative planning and cooperative provision of services essential to avoid duplication and maximize the effectiveness of resources available.

### Health Needs of the Community Served

Although methods for identifying and measuring community health needs are not well developed, available information can provide general guidelines and priorities for planning facilities and services. The goal of meeting community needs provides a constant source of direction and serves as a criterion against which plans can be judged. Clearly, assessments of need require a combination of data collection and review, community and professional input, and good judgment. In the absence of specific data and analytic techniques to quantify needs, considerable judgment is required. A critical job of the planner is to develop and incorporate these "sensors" into the planning process.

Inferences can be made about needs from data on the characteristics and size of the population a hospital serves. Size obviously determines the general magnitude and scope of services needed. The age and sex distribution directly influences the distribution of adult medical and surgical, obstetric, pediatric, long-term, and rehabilitation services. Economic and social characteristics serve as indicators of health status and suggest the existence of high risk groups and possible barriers to obtaining services. Comparative use rates often indicate subgroups whose needs are not being fully met. Morbidity and mortality data and comparative ratios of health facilities and manpower to population suggest needs. Need is also represented by physical plant deficiencies in terms of current standards and obsolescence of present services. Finally, the distribution of the population suggests appropriate locations for facilities.

Obviously, the roles of individual hospitals differ; otherwise it would be possible to specify a single, universal role. The differences are subtle variations around a four-function basis, including patient care, teaching, research, and community-wide services. Evidence of the need for the fourth function, and of actual hospital activities to provide community service, has been growing. Organized emergency and outpatient services; special programs such as those for alcohol and drug abuse; programs to recruit physicians and support them in their office practice; outreach, educational, and preventive programs; home care and long-term care programs; and similar services implement a community service goal. Such activities, undertaken unilaterally or cooperatively with others, are increasingly important to community hospitals. They differ in character and organization from the more narrowly defined function of "patient care," care of patients admitted by the medical staff.

The question of role definition becomes the selection of the priority and relative emphasis of these four functions. It can only be answered in the specific setting since it depends on location, ownership, access to resources, past role of the institution, and the posture of other institutions serving or capable of serving the same community. Possibly because of its subtlety and complexity, the question of role definition is frequently poorly answered or unanswered.

A sound approach to this question involves a careful inventory of resources, the best available information on needs, an imaginative search for new and innovative solutions, and the deliberate solicitation of a wide variety of viewpoints. This solicitation should systematically include all significant consumer viewpoints, provider viewpoints, and the opinions of other institutions and agencies. Much of the data necessary to assess the opportunities for various roles in community services and patient care are developed in this planning methodology. The values that underlie alternative role definitions must be elicited from the various individuals and groups over a period of time as the data become available. The assignment of priorities among patient care functions, community service, teaching, and research must be the result of repeated reviews and study, with increasing specificity and delimitation as final decisions on facilities and services are approached.

## Programs and Services the Hospital Must Provide

The decisions which emerge about the hospital's role should be consistent with community needs. Ideally the hospital should either move to meet each unmet need or have a clear understanding that some other institution will meet it. At this stage of the process the decisions are likely to be tentative in nature, particularly when they are positive (decisions to offer certain services), and subject to further study in succeeding steps. Nevertheless, these decisions influence the areas of study. Negative decisions are especially important as they tend to "rule out" further study. Practicality usually forces the hospital to admit that it cannot be "all things to all people." What it is not and, by inference, whom it does not serve, are critical. Decisions to include facilities and services that should be excluded may overtax available resources and place the hospital in an uneconomic competitive position. Such decisions are frequently pressed for by professionals seeking expensive and highly technical clinical services, implementation of experimental technology such as on-line computer systems, and overly ambitious educational programs. On the other hand, important services may be excluded, perhaps principally because of the blinders of tradition. Examples are ambulatory and home care programs, long-term care programs, mental health programs, special purpose programs such as abortion and drug abuse, and programs for special population groups who may previously have had difficulty gaining access to the hospital's resources.

The decisions which specify and implement the hospital's role are the premises for the balance of the planning process. Yet, in the Bureau's experience they are the most likely cause of serious error. They are particularly difficult for the consumer and the trustee, for they involve complex issues and vague evidence. It is seductive to maintain tradition without assessing changes in the environment or to accept persuasive special pleadings without questioning the assumptions and validity of the arguments offered. It is easy for a trustee to assume that professionals—administrators, doctors, nurses, and even outside consultants—know what services should be provided, but frequently they do not. The only safeguards lie in the solicitation of many and diverse opinions, the review of checklists of what the hospital's role might be, and the open-minded, dispassionate consideration of the alternative roles these sources suggest.

Once these qualitative decisions are made it is necessary to make quantitative estimates of the facility size for most of the services. Frequently a decision such as the provision of inpatient obstetrical services will be made tentatively at this point, subject to quantification and economic evaluation. The techniques for quantification are taken up in the following chapter.

## NOTES

[1]D. C. Carner, *Planning for Hospital Expansion and Remodeling.* Springfield, IL: Charles C. Thomas, 1968.

R. Hadenberg, *Planning the Community Hospital.* New York: McGraw-Hill Book Co., 1967.

J. J. Souder, *Estimating Space Needs and Costs in General Hospital Construction.* Chicago: American Hospital Association, 1963

E. T. Wheeler, *Hospital Design and Construction.* New York. New York: McGraw-Hill Book Co., 1964.

E. T. Wheeler, *Hospital Modernization and Expansion.* New York: McGraw-Hill Book Co., 1971.

U. S. Public Health Service, Division of Hospital and Medical Facilities, *General Standards of Construction and Equipment for Hospital and Medical Facilities.* PHS Publication No. 930-A-7. Washington: Government Printing Office, 1967.

[2]The methods to be described identify indicators of facility and service shortages where these exist, with particular attention to the needs of the aged and the poor. The prevailing situation in the U.S., however, appears to be one of excess supply rather than shortage.

[3]W. Spitzer, "The Small General Hospital: Problems and Solutions." *Milbank Memorial Fund Quarterly,* Vol. 48, October 1970.

[4]D. Shapley, "Computers in Medicine: Hospitals Cope with Costs, Quality Review." *Science,* Vol. 48, February 28, 1975.

[5]S. E. Berki, *Hospital Economics.* Lexington, MA.: D. C. Heath and Co., 1972, p. 115.

[6]P. J. Feldstein and J. J. German, "Predicting Hospital Utilization." *Inquiry,* Vol. 2, June 1965.

# II.2

# Measuring Service Areas and Forecasting Demand

*by John R. Griffith*

## Introduction

The preceding chapter dealt with important general considerations in planning, and developed procedures for systematic decision making regarding *what* is included in a plan for a given institution, *when* it will be instituted, *how* it will be financed, organized and constructed, and *how much*, will be provided. This chapter and the one which follows deal solely with *how much*, the estimation of the appropriate size of a physical facility. They concentrate on the most expensive facility, the inpatient bed, although the methods described are frequently applicable to smaller services, such as operating rooms or other general care services such as emergency rooms or clinics. The author discusses these forecasting problems briefly on a following page.

The approach relies upon the equation:

$$
\begin{aligned}
\text{(1) Beds required} = {} & \text{Admissions/1,000 population per year} \\
& \times \text{Average length of stay} \\
& \times \text{Population (in 1,000s)} \\
& \div (\text{Occupancy} \times 365)
\end{aligned}
$$

This equation states a mathematical identity when it is applied historically. That is, given any four of the five terms, the fifth can always be calculated. It also is composed entirely of terms which are multiplied or divided, and thus is independent of order and may be recombined as desired. Some common combined forms are:

(1a) Beds required = Patient days/1,000 population per year
× Population (in 1,000s)
÷ (Occupancy × 365)

(1b) Beds required = Admissions
× Average length of stay
÷ (Occupancy × 365)

(1c) Beds required = Patient days
÷ (Occupancy × 365)

These forms are used for convenience, usually because data are available for the terms remaining but not for the others. The most general form (equation 1) can be restated in terms of facilities other than beds:

(2) Facility quantity required = Incidence of use per person per year
× Average duration of use
× Population of users
÷ Load factor

For operating rooms, for example, if:

| | |
|---|---|
| Incidence | = .5 cases per admission |
| Duration | = 1.5 hours per case |
| Population | = 20,000 admissions per year |
| Load factor | = 6 hours per day × 250 days per year |
| No. ORs required | = .5 × 1.5 × 20,000 ÷ (6 × 250) |
| | = 10 |

To solve equation 1, it is necessary to forecast each of the terms on the righthand side to an appropriate future year. It is generally preferable to avoid combining terms, and to solve the equation for each major service, although difficulties with data may make either or both of these goals impossible. The method presented here permits the use of the full set of terms or of variant 1b (that is, with admissions per thousand population and length of stay combined) in most situations.

The aim of the forecasting process is to minimize uncertainty, the unknown and unmeasurable chance of error. Uncertainty is inevitable in decisions about future events. This approach minimizes it by breaking the forecasting decision into the smallest feasible components in order to examine as carefully as possible each underlying process and to bring the best judgment to bear on its forecast. As the examples will show, there are many important component decisions buried in the overall forcasting decision. For this reason, the preparation of forecasts is a substantial test of the professional skill of the management team. The most successful managers are those who fully understand where the component decisions are hidden and by what criteria they should be made.

A variety of data is routinely collected which is relevant to health service forecasting problems, and there are several techniques for augmenting the available data. In addition, there are a considerable number of technical analyses which can be applied. On the other hand, data collection and analysis are costly in themselves, both because they consume resources and because they cause time delays which add to the total costs of a project in several different but often very expensive ways. With regard to some of the smaller components of a large project, for example, a crude estimate of the size of that component might be accepted because it would take several months to refine the estimate significantly, and the improvement in accuracy is not seen as worth the cost of the delay. In general, there is always a trade-off between the reduction of risk by further investigation of the forecasting problem and the increase in cost incurred to accomplish it. The criterion is that further investigation is desirable as long as it is likely to reduce the overall costs more than it increases them. The application of the criterion, however, is frequently a difficult managerial judgment.

The following is the general method which the Bureau of Hospital Administration has developed over a period of twenty years of assistance to Michigan communities and hospitals. Each of the major steps in this analytic process will be described in terms of the component decisions which lie within it. Illustrations will be drawn from recent applications.

1. *Identify and measure a reference community or service population.* For forecasts of the overall use of inpatient and ambulatory hospital services, this step involves counts of families and people, often within a defined geographic location. For component services, they may be populations of inpatients or other special groups of patients. In certain specialized situations, they may be populations defined other than geographically (veterans, HMO subscribers).

2. *Identify the component of the population which is at risk for the specific service in question,* such as fertile women, aged persons, children, or inpatients with a given disease or condition.

3. *Identify the admission rate (the incidence rate) and the expected length of stay.*

4. *Select a planning horizon or period for the forecast.* In general, this must exceed the resource cycle, or length of time necessary to plan and provide the resources. For beds, the resource cycle is about five years. Likely conditions past the planning horizon should also be considered, but in a less precise manner. It is the Bureau's belief that the planning horizon and quantitative forecasts should be limited to two resource cycles, to avoid overreliance on imprecise estimates.

5. *Prepare one or more projections (or tentative forecasts) of the population identified in step 2, and the rates identified in step. 3.* These tentative forecasts can, and frequently should, be prepared in a variety of ways.

Graphic and simple least squares regression analyses are always desirable where historic data exist. For population forecasts, reference to multivariate forecasts prepared by demographers serving regional or state populations is recommended. Comparisons with other communities and judgmental analyses of use rates are recommended. In rare cases, surveys of intentions and more elaborate statistical techniques are necessary for rate forecasts.

6. *Decide on one value for each of these elements which is to be accepted for the forecast.* An exploration of the amount and direction of possible errors whould be included in this decision. Specific technical procedures exist for all of these steps, except the third and the first part of the sixth and final step. While these techniques appear superficially to be straightforward and unbiased, there are numerous decision points in their application which require careful judgment. As the following discussion will show, there is a constant interplay of judgment, data, and analysis which requires surveillance by a professional health manager, preferably with prior experience. The discussion which follows covers measurement of the service population (steps 1 and 2), development of forecasts (steps 4, 5, and 6), and some unique aspects of the most important single facility requirement question, the size of the adult medical and surgical service.

## Defining and Measuring the Service Population

There are several approaches to measuring the size and geographic extent of the pupulation served by a hospital. These differ in detail, data requirements, precision, and cost. All of the good ones have the same basic approach, first identified and developed by Dr. Paul Lembcke.[1] Extensive application has been made by several hospital and health planning agencies.[2] The approach analyzes the small population areas surrounding the study hospital (towns, townships, neighborhoods, census tracts, or postal areas) in order to calculate the fraction:

$$R = \frac{\text{Admissions from area to the study hospital}}{\text{Admissions from area to any hospital}}$$

for each area. The fraction is called the relevance index. It is a measure of a hospital's market penetration or share of market in each small area. Care must be taken not to confuse this statistic with one much more easily obtained but less useful, called the commitment index:

$$C = \frac{\text{Admissions from area to study hospital}}{\text{All admissions to study hospital}}$$

There is no simple relation between the two, and forecasts based on commitment indices can be correct only by chance. The major technical approaches to measuring the relevance index are discussed in detail by Griffith in *Quantitative Techniques for Hospital Planning and Control*, chapter 4.[3] These are a number of practical systems now operating to collect relevance index and service population data on regional bases. These are usually called patient origin studies and are chiefly under the auspices of voluntary and comprehensive health planning agencies. For these regional systems, data collection using computer-coded discharge summaries such as PAS and pre-PAS is frequently used to cut cost.[4] Since the calculation involves the number of admissions to all hospitals, not just the study hospital, it is substantially cheaper to use a regional planning agency to collect and analyze the data for several hospitals at once. Improvements in the accuracy are also possible through these cooperative efforts.

The contribution of each small area to a hospital's service population is the product of its relevance index times its population. The total service population will be the sum of all these contributions. It is also possible to map service populations, showing the relevance index by the shading of each small area. A typical service area map for three hospitals (combined) in Jackson, Michigan is shown in figure II.2.1.

Limited access freeways bisect Jackson County both east and west and north and south. Hospitals lie on these roads at approximately thirty-five miles distance, with the exception of the west, where a ninety bed hospital is only seventeen miles from Jackson. The expected pattern of declining relevance index is seen, dropping off more rapidy as the distance to alternative facilities declines. The hospital draws significant relevance indices from outside its county in only one direction, to the north. (It is approximately fifteen miles east and west and twelve miles north and south from Jackson to each county boundary.) The shape of the service area is of interest because the pattern is not completely predictable. Use of Jackson hospitals from Concord and Parma Townships and the four townships in Ingham County is higher than expected, given the availability of alternative hospitals.

A number of judgments must be made in constructing and using relevance indices and service populations. One of these, the selection of which hopsitals to include in data collection, is simplified when regional planning agencies handle this task. It also is discussed in Griffith.[5] Briefly, the analysis is valid only when the data are collected for nearly all hospitalization alternatives for a given small area.

## Individual Versus Groups of Hospitals

Figure II.2.1 shows the relevance indices for all the hospitals in Jackson as a group, as though they were a single facility. This was done because a single medical staff served the two largest hospitals, and because there was no evidence of specific geographic association with either hospital. The medical staff could admit to either hospital at will and apparently controlled the occupancy of the two institutions as they saw fit. A case could be made for handling the third hospital separately because it is an osteopathic hospital. However, the hospital is small, and planning separate facilities for osteopathy is not an acceptable policy to state planning agen-

**FIGURE II.2.1**
**Density of the use of Jackson acute care hospitals by township**

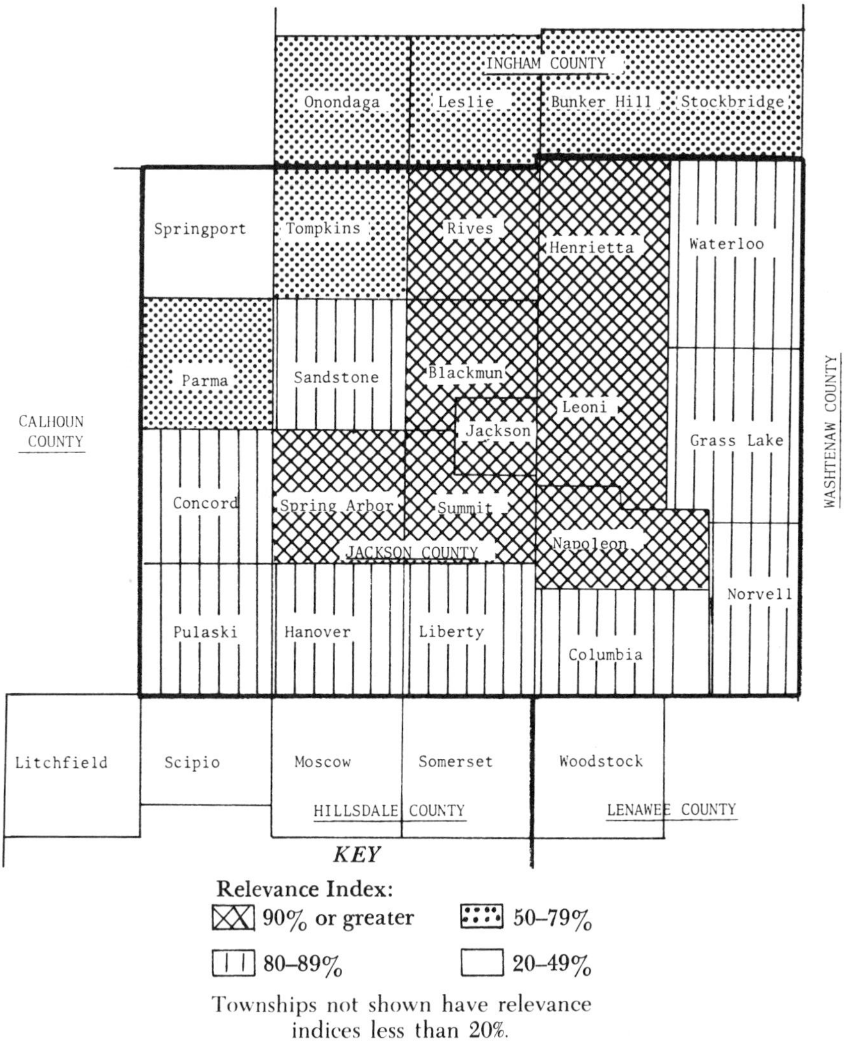

cies. The decision to combine all three is tantamount to saying that the facility supply for all three hopsitlas must be jointly rather than individually planned. This appears to be the desirable choice in situations like Jackson, where a cluster of similar hospitals is separated by some distance or by clear patterns of use from alternative care sources.

Metropolitan settings pose a different problem. It is often true that these hospitals have relevance indices of less than 0.5 for any small area, even the one in which the hospital is located. At the same time, a given small area may have similar relevance indices around 0.2 or 0.3 to several different institutions. It is possible to treat such hospitals individually, assuming that the preferences of individual citizens will continue to divide among alternative care sources as they have in the past. If each hospital in the area plans according to its historical relevance indices, the results will reflect that consumer preference in the planning decisions. Alternatively, the facilities for logical groups of hospitals may be forecast together, and allocations made among them at a later stage. These allocations might reflect individual shares of market as they could be forecast to the future and other criteria, such as opportunities to share or merge selected services or to assign certain populations to certain hospitals. This approach has strong philosophical appeal in a setting where the forecasts and decisions are made by an appropriate representative body, because it increases the understanding and flexibility of the decision process. The increased centralization places heavy demands on regional planning agencies as discussed below.

## Secondary Service Areas

Large referral hospitals tend to draw over larger and more diffuse areas than small community hospitals. It sometimes is the case that they have no area where their relevance index is more than a few percent, although more commonly there is at least a small primary service area. Rush-Presbyterian-St. Luke's Medical Center (RPSL) in Chicago draws patients from almost every neighborhood in the metropolitan region. It also has the highest relevance index of any hospital for a few nearby neighborhoods, but it does not dominate any neighborhood. (That is, it had no index over 0.5.)[6] University Hospital, Ann Arbor, however, shares a clear primary service area with the other Ann Arbor community hospital. Relevance indices for the two hospitals combined are near 0.9 for Ann Arbor and several nearby townships. However, two-thirds of the patients of University Hospital are from the rest of Michigan.[7] The RPSL case was handled by taking the population and the single relevance index for the region as a whole, since the contribution of individual neighborhoods was too small to forecast reliably. The University Hopsital case was handled by establishing and forecasting a primary service population for the two hospitals as a group, and forecasting the remaining demand for University Hospital as a secondary demand. (It is secondary in the sense of being medical referral demand from areas which also have primary service hospitals.) When secondary demand exists it is often forecast as a total patient day or admission demand (using equation 1b or 1c) since the reference population becomes so diffuse as to be difficult to investigate in more detail. The creation of separate primary and secondary demand forecasts is generally the preferred solution for large hospitals. A secondary demand may exist for many medium-sized community hospitals, as well.

## Specialized Relevance Indices

### Inpatient Services or Specialties

It is possible to construct relevance indices for individual services (such as obstetrics or pediatrics) and there is some evidence that these are not identical[8] even for the major inpatient services. The obstetrics service area might be smaller than the adult medical-surgical, particularly if the latter is large. On the other hand, the obstetrics service area would be larger if an adjacent hospital did not offer obstetrical care. Cases like Jackson, and rural counties with one general hospital, do not generally require separate service area measurement by specialty. The need for separate study is more frequent in metropolitan areas and is likely to become increasingly so as hospitals merge some specialties. The separation is a relatively simple problem to handle where large volumes of data are available through regional planning systems.[9] In isolated situations it is costly and sometimes infeasible to identify specialized service areas. (The reliability of the relevance index is a function of the sample size of admissions studied. A one-year sample of obstetrical admissions from a small area will be only about one-tenth as large as the total number of admissions. More than one year's data may be impractical to obtain.) The most reasonable solution appears to be to obtain specialty data whenever regional systems are established. Each of the major acute specialties—pediatrics, adult medicine-surgery, obstetrics, and psychiatry—should be analyzed. Data collection problems compound themselves when finer detail is attempted. Hospitals differ on the specialty classification, and individual cases are sometimes ambiguous (as, for example, the patient who is admitted on the surgical service and later transferred to the medical). The more the data are subdivided, the larger the errors these ambiguities and classification differences create.

Long-term care service areas can also be constructed if the proper facilities are included in the data collection. Numbers of cases are much more limited because of the low turnover, and the precision of the result is less. For this reason, it is frequently convenient to group facilities and select arbitrary areas such as counties. The lack of consensus on the quantity of facilities needed for these services also tends to make precise service area definition less necessary.

### Outpatient Service Areas

It is theoretically possible to extend the relevance index and service population concept to services other than inpatient. Data on the relevance index of various physicians (rather than hospitals) are sometimes helpful in analyzing doctor shortages, utilization, and ambulatory facility location. Definitional and data collection problems impede ambulatory care applications. The physicians' index is generally constructed from the admissions ordered by various physicians rather than their case loads because of the difficulty of getting case data. Ambulatory data, other than emergency room visits, are difficult both to define and to collect. Emergency visits can be analyzed in terms of relevance indices, although a separate data collection effort is necessary.

## Patient Days Versus Admissions

It is conceptually possible to prepare relevance indices based on patient days rather than admissions. The result is to weight the relevance index and the service population for differences in length of stay which occur between hospitals and between small areas.[10] The same result occurs if one-day census data are used rather than discharge or admission data. The relevance incides constructed from census data will reflect patient days, not admissions. Length of stay is known to be a function of many factors, including illness, age, source of payment, physician, and hospital efficiency. Many of these factors relate only indirectly, if at all, to geography. The factors can be identified and analyzed more directly by examining length of stay by facility rather than by geography. The service area population should be identified by geographic area, and the length of stay by facility. The use of a patient day base or one-day census is not recommended for service area determination.

## Definition of the Small Areas

Small areas can be identified by post office, zip code, neighborhood, village or township, and census tract. The first two are easily obtained from either medical or financial hospital records. The population, unfortunately, is measured by the last two. Computer programs have been written to translate between postal address or zip code and census data, but these are not uniformly available. Special programs or manual estimations are frequently required. In metropolitan areas, the data collection cost is greatly reduced if the population data are translated to a zip code basis rather than vice versa. Some loss of accuracy is incurred, but its importance, although so far unmeasured, is not believed to be great. Accuracy is also lost, and costs mount, when hospitals must identify census tracts or geographic locations other than post offices. Programs which translate urban street addresses to census tracts have been developed, but the Greater Detroit Area Hospital Council's experience with these was unpromising. Zip codes, therefore, appear to be the compromise of choice at this time. The areas are somewhat larger than would be desired, and are chosen for reasons quite different from the factors affecting hospital use or population measurement.

In rural areas, where population is less dense, the Bureau has used post offices, and has assigned populations from minor civil divisions to post offices based on judgment and rural delivery routes.[11] This is relatively inexpensive and of acceptable accuracy, and is recommended for individual community studies. Whole counties are sometimes used as "small areas," or rural portions of counties after identifying the urban areas separately.[12] These alternatives are relatively cheap, but at the cost of data which are of some value. In figure II.2.1, for example, the upper row of townships is in Ingham, not Jackson County. It is of some value to know that more than fifty percent of these citizens come to Jackson as opposed to Lansing, which is a few miles to the north. If county-wide data or rural county-wide data were used, one could say only that a much smaller percentage of the total rural Ingham County population uses Jackson hospitals.

## Small Area Admission Rates

A byproduct of the data which generate the relevance indices and the service population is the small area admission rate:

$$\frac{\text{Number of admissions from area (to all hospitals)}}{\text{Area population}}$$

At least theoretically the rate should reflect under- or overuse of hospitals and may be indicative of special problems such as poor health, disadvantaged populations, and doctor shortages. As a practical matter, however, the small area data taken individually may not be reliable. Errors between adjacent areas in assigning admissions and errors in small area population bases are apparently large. (These errors tend to offset each other when several small areas are merged as they are in calculating the total service population.) At least a review of the individual admission rate statistics to confirm or deny impressions of special needs gained from other sources is in order, however. Deliberate efforts might be contemplated to correct these problems and adjustments made to the forecasts of the population.

## Forecasting Service Populations

The service population, like the other terms of equation 1, must be forecast to the future. This problem has two components: forecasting changes in the service area, or the relevance indices; and forecasting the change in the total service area population.

### Changes in the Service Area

The service area is a market phenomenon which reflects the choice of patients and doctors among available alternatives for hospital care. As such, it is the result of a large number of factors, and only a few of these are under the control of a single hospital. The lack of control or even predictability means that great uncertainty is associated with forecasts of changes. A hospital might increase its attractiveness by improving and expanding medical service, by recruiting physicians and maintaining their loyalty, and by improving comfort and convenience to patients. In cases where the portion of the bill paid directly by patients is significant, it might also affect the service area by reducing its charges relative to other hospitals. If no other changes occurred, the result might be an increase in some or all of the relevance incides and an increase in the total service population. Other hospitals may take these actions as well, however, so the net outcome is difficult to estimate. At the same time, many of the factors affecting the service area are independent of health care activities, per se. These include geographic factors such as roads, habit patterns such as regional shopping preferences, and personal factors such as loyalty to certain hospitals or doctors. When service areas grow rapidly, as a result of suburban migration, for example, it is difficult to predict how fast patients will change from their old affiliations, or whether the newcomers' choices will be the same as the older residents'.

In the face of these uncertainties, the most conservative position to assume is that the service area will not change its shape.[13] That is, the individual relevance indices will remain constant. Only concrete and convincing plans to change the service area, such as the provision of new doctors' offices or ambulatory care, construction of new hospitals in new locations, or deliberate agreements between hospitals to change area responsibility or medical staff privilege arrangements, should be accepted for modifying the empirical service area. When these occur, modifications should be made based on judgmental revisions of the individual relevance indices and recalculation of the population.

As regional councils continue to collect data on relevance indices over a period of time, time series analysis and other statistical techniques may become useful for empirical projection of trends. Few, if any, communities are in a position to do this at present. A theoretical contribution of regional planning councils becomes clear in this context. The council might facilitate decisions such as service area revision, institutional relocation, and staff privileges on a multiple hospital basis. In some cases, it might even negotiate service area responsibilities directly, particularly to overcome problems of underserved areas.

This discussion has presumed the continued existence of hospitals for which service area populations exist, rather than the more difficult problem of the construction of new (or relocated) facilities. Limited work has been done with the forecasting of changed service areas in urban areas[14] and rural areas.[15] It appears that the safest solution is to assume that the new hospital will attract similarly to comparable existing ones, reducing relevance indices of the existing hospitals most in the small areas nearest it. The service area population of closed facilities might be distributed pro rata to remaining ones serving each small area.

## Forecasting the Service Population

Once any adjustments in the service area have been forecast, the population trends within the service area can be analyzed and forecast. Ideally, this would involve a forecast of population trends within each small area. The principal factor affecting population trends is often migration, however, and this factor is difficult to forecast at best and notoriously difficult for small areas.[16] Where such forecasts have been prepared, they should be used in conjunction with county or metropolitan forecasts incorporating the service area. (Care should be exercised with regard to utility forecasts. For telephone, electricity, water, and sewage planning purposes, it is much cheaper to err on the high side than the low, creating a built-in bias. The opposite is probably true for health care facilities and schools.)

Forecasts for the relevant population unit such as the county or the metropolitan area should be obtained from recognized demographic authorities and used as a basis for checking small area forecasts and estimating the impact on the hospital service area. Forecasts by recognized experts are generally available and are preferable to those developed by hospital or health care consultants.[17] If the service area is reasonably congruent with the county, as in figure II.2.1, there is no serious problem. Where this is not so, judgment must be made as to whether the trend of the service area will equal, exceed, or fall short of the county trend, and by how much. Growth within counties is often uneven. Local authorities should be consulted on the locations most likely to grow, particularly in the absence of small area forecasts. In these cases, the service area as a whole should generally be forecast, rather than its small areas.

If the above steps are carried out, the result will be an empirically defined service area, measured in terms of its present population. It will have been carefully reviewed for its relationship to other hospitals, its consistency with hospital goals, its application to special services, and for special problems of access which it might reveal. Finally, its size will have been forecast to future years. Attention can now be turned to forecasts of incidence rates and expected utilization per incidence.

## Forecasting Use Rates: A Simple Example

The two terms, admission rate and length of stay, require both statistical study and careful review in the light of professional judgment. Often several professional opinions are desirable. Since the forecasting process and sources of data are similar, the terms can be developed simultaneously. The process can be best understood in terms of a clearly defined and easily measured service such as obstetrical beds, permitting the reader to focus on the analytic logic rather than data collection, definitional problems, and other confusing elements. The following example is a real one, forecasting obstetrical demand for Jackson, Michigan, the service area shown in figure II.2.1.

The population at risk is the fertile female population living in the service area. This can be conveniently defined as women between the ages of fifteen and forty-five. The hospitals will plan to serve all these women at the time of their delivery, and there are no serious problems of diagnosis of the condition. Finally, the process is unusually carefully counted and forecast because of its economic and social implications.

### Projection Based on Total Use, Rather than Use Rate

One approach might be to ignore specific knowledge of trends in the population and in the fertility rate and simply to project the past total number of obstetrical patient days into the future using least squares regression techniques.[18] This approach would use equation 1c. Figure II.2.2 shows the historic data. The patient days of care have been plotted for the past ten years, and a least squares linear regression line has been estimated for these data.[19]

Inspection of the trend reveals immediately that such an approach might be dangerous. Patient days have been falling in an irregular manner but, on the average, 283 days per year. Sooner or later, a simple forecast of 283 fewer days each year will be wrong. It implies no obstetric patient days at all in three decades. This forecast can be improved by considering the three component factors: the number of fertile women (the population), their admission rate (the fertility rate), and the obstetrical length of stay (the expected days per delivery). The cost of investigating each component will not be great, relative to the cost of unnecessary beds or insufficient beds.

**FIGURE II.2.2**
Postpartum patient days by year

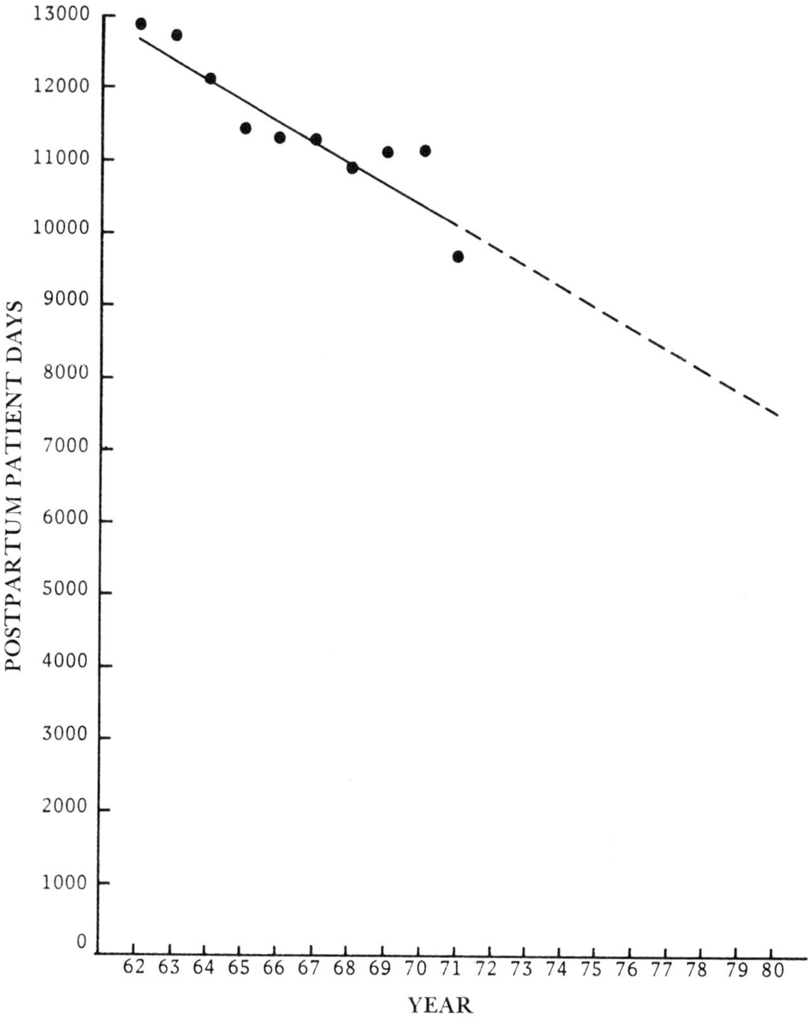


REGRESSION:
Days = 13,000 − 283 (year − 1961)
$R^2 = .84$
Significance < .01

## Projections of Use Rates

### Population Projection and Forecast

Figure II.2.3 shows the population at risk. These data are available from actual census counts in the decennial years and frequently are projected for the future by state or regional planning agencies. The projection shown was prepared by the State of Michigan Executive Office. It accommodates aging of the known population of young girls, mortality, and migration, and therefore differs from the linear extrapolation of the decennial census data. Adjustments made for differences between the county and the service area were minimal. Most of the growth is expected in the townships around Jackson City. There are certain risks, or unmeasurable errors, principally that the area migration rate will change. A sudden change in an area industry, for example, might attract many new young families. Sudden large changes can be deliberately ignored. They are unlikely, and if they occur the hopsitals can change their plans. Those with greater likelihood can be included by adjusting the statistical projection upward or downward using good judgment. In the case of Jackson, the Bureau staff, after discussions with local leadership, decided to accept the projection unchanged.

In accepting the population projection for 1975 shown in figure II.2.3, the planner has made a clear-cut decision which brings to bear both statistical and analytic capabilities and detailed knowledge of the environment. Such a decision can be called a forecast, which will deliberately distinguish it from projections and statistical analyses by the element of judgment. The decision to accept a forecast is always part of the planning process, even though the projections and analysis may be done by others.

### Projection and Forecast of the Incidence Rate

The next item to investigate is the incidence rate. For obstetrics it is desirable to use births rather than admissions because comparable data already exist on the rate of births per thousand women age fifteen to forty-five (the fertility rate). The number of births is shown in figure II.2.4, and the fertility rate is shown in figure II.2.5.

Two projections of the fertility rate are shown in figure II.2.5. The first, shown by the solid line, is the result of simple linear regression. The second, shown by the dotted line, is the result of expert judgment. A third, nonlinear regression, was tried in the forecasting process and rejected as inferior to linear regression on technical grounds. For these data, eighty-nine percent of the variation in fertility rate is explained by the line: Fertility Rate = 7,616 − 3,823 (Year), shown in figure II.2.4. The statistical significance of the line exceeds ninety-nine percent.[20]

The statistical analysis is technically very satisfying. It indicates that the decline in patient days shown in figure II.2.2 is related heavily to the change in fertility patterns of the Jackson population. This change has been steady over the past decade and can easily be projected into the

**FIGURE II.2.3**

Estimated female population aged 15–44

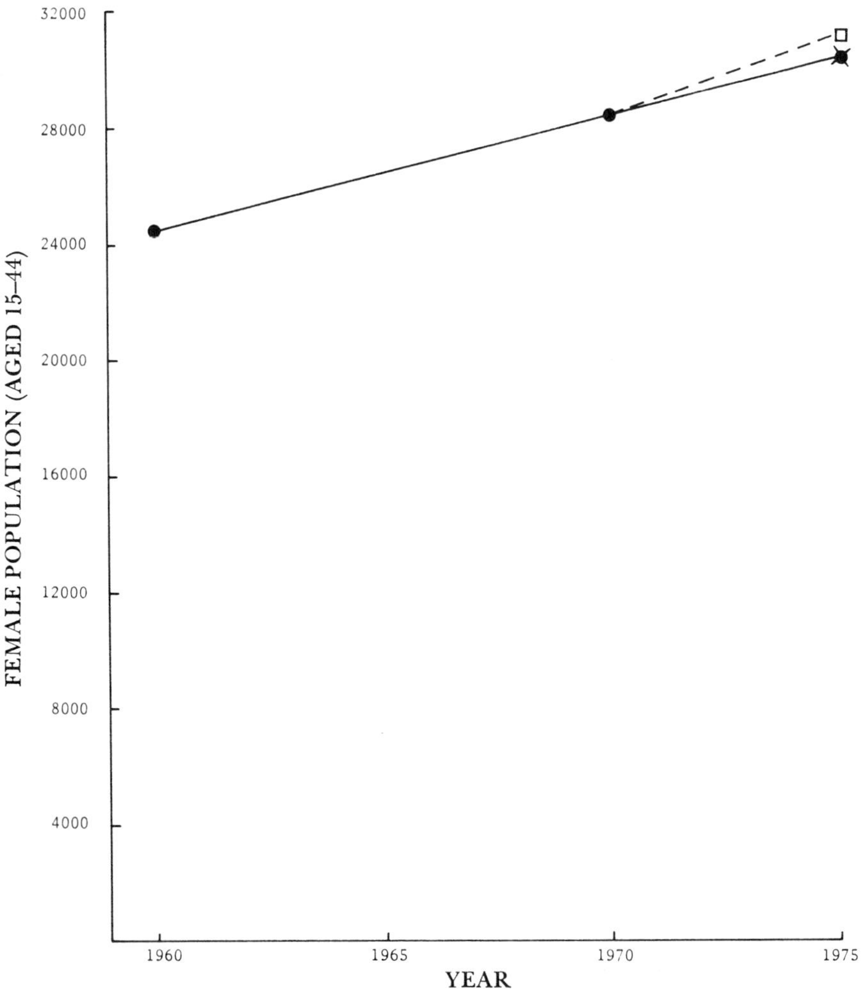


—— Linear Extrapolation
– – – Projection to 1975 based on the aging of cohorts and adjusted for emigration and mortality (31,470 in 1975)

**FIGURE II.2.4**
Trends in births 1960–1972

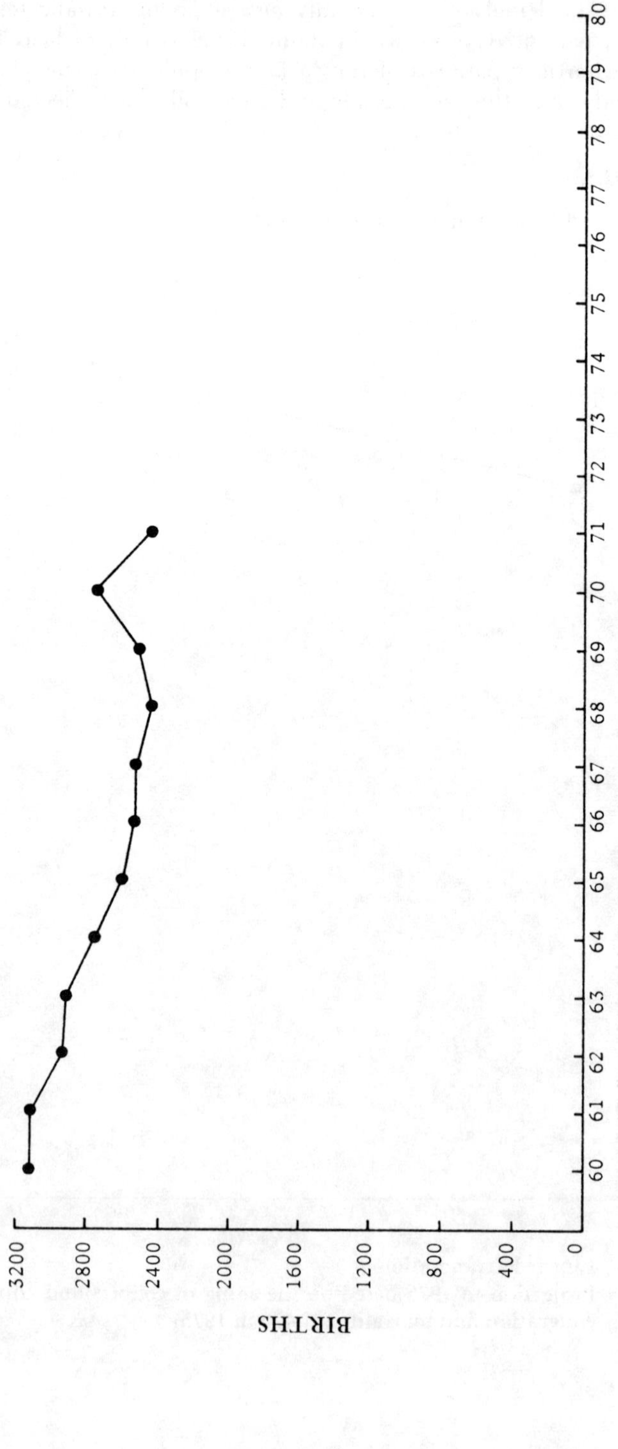


Data on births obtained from State Department of Health, Center for Health Statistics

future. Substituting the values of the years 1975 and 1980 into the regression equation yields projected rates of 65.6 and 46.5 respectively.

If the decline in fertility rates continues in the next decade as it has in the present one, those projections can be accepted as forecasts. However, good judgment indicates considerable caution with regard to such a decision. A check of historical fertility rates for U.S. women shows that the rate has fluctuated over relatively long cycles and in this century has been no lower than seventy (in the 1930s and in 1972) and no higher than 120 (around 1950). A review of national rates indicates that Jackson is following the national trend but lagging behind it by a few years. Further, there have been studies of the so-called zero population growth fertility rate. These studies indicate that rate is also about seventy births per thousand

**FIGURE II.2.5**

Births per 1,000 females aged 15–44

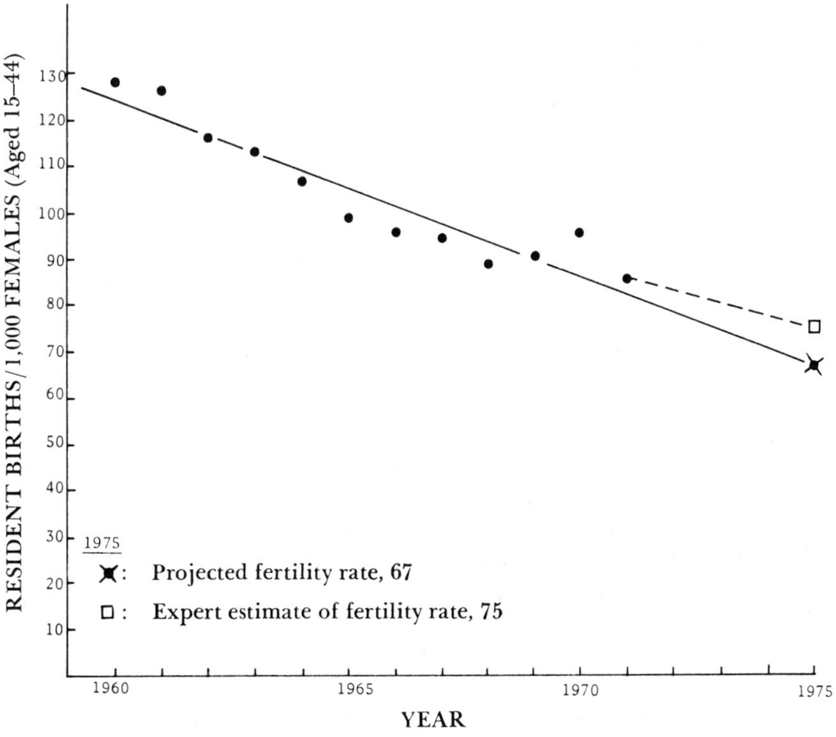


LINEAR REGRESSION:

Fertility Rate = 7,616 — 3.82 (year)

$R^2$ = .89 Significance = .005

women. If the statistical analysis projections are accepted as forecasts, the planner is assuming a demographic situation in which the Jackson population will eventually decline and in which fertility will be less than has been recorded in the country in this century. This set of assumptions seems radical. An alternative, conservative assumption would be to assume that the fertility rate may continue downward for a while but will, within the decade, rebound at least to the 1971 level of 85.5.

Still another alternative would be to seek advice from demographers who are accustomed to forecasting this rate and who can take into account additional information such as surveys of birth intentions of young women near the start of their family formation years. Such surveys could be conducted in Jackson, but they are expensive, time-consuming, and would require staff not normally available. Also, the chance that they would make an important change in the forecast is limited. The most likely result of a survey of the Jackson population would be that its young women have child bearing intentions not unlike those of similar young women in other situations. Finding a skilled demographer is not nearly so difficult.[21] The demographers providing the population forecast generally know of, or will supply themselves, expert judgment on fertility rates. After review of the data and conversations about local conditions, the consultant estimated that the rate would level off at seventy-five births per thousand females and suggested this as the forecast. In his deliberations, he considered such factors as the average family size in Jackson, abortion reform legislation, and court actions under consideration but not resolved at the time of the forecast. His forecast is lower than the most recent level (85.5) but considerably more credible than the radical regression projection. It appears to be the projection of choice to adopt as the forecast. In doing so the planner is trading risks. The most conservative projection (85.5) would require about fourteen percent more beds than the demographer's estimate. What is implied in the decision is that the risk the demographer's projection is too low is not worth the cost of providing obstetrical beds to meet it. At the same time, the risk that his projection is too high is not worth the cost of further investigations to improve knowledge. The planner could have conducted a household survey at a cost on the order of $25,000 to $50,000 and at a delay of several months. He has implicitly said that he does not believe such a survey would add enough to his knowledge to convince him to lower construction requirements by an equivalent amount to be worth the cost and delay.

## Projecting and Forecasting the Length of Stay

The third demand component, length of stay, is relatively simple to analyze by examining days of care per birth, using a method identical to that used for the incidence rate. (This number is slightly different from the length of stay, which is days of care per admission, because the number of births is not the same as the number of admissions. The difference is a combination of false labors, stillbirths, and multiple births and is likely to remain proportionally constant. Thus, the two numbers can be expected to follow the same trends.) Using this measure allows a straightforward calculation of the final forecast.

Figure II.2.6 shows the statistical analysis. Length of stay has been declining, but the association with time is marginally significant, and the rate of change is slight. Judgment is clearly desirable before adopting the projection of 4.1 days per birth in 1980. In this case, the judgment of the local obstetricians is probably the best. When asked, they suggested that the 1971 level (3.9) was acceptable. The forecast adopted agreed with that position.

## Summary Forecast

Three of the terms of equation 1 have been analyzed and forecast. The forecast of postpartum days in 1975 and 1980 is their product:

| | (Fertility Rate) | × | (Population) | × | (Days/Birth) | = | Pt. Days | (Births) |
|---|---|---|---|---|---|---|---|---|
| 1975: | 75/1,000 | × | 31,500 | × | 3.9 | = | 9,200 | (2,400) |
| 1980: | 75/1,000 | × | 34,500 | × | 3.9 | = | 10,100 | (2,600) |

The last step of the forecasting method is an estimate of risk, or the known error attached to the forecast. The planner has only limited knowledge of this. Large errors are clearly possible in components where considerable variation existed between judgment and statistical projection. The estimates were conservative, however, in the direction of avoiding too few beds. It is unlikely that the fertility rate will be greater than seventy-five, and it is clearly possible to operate at 3.9 days per birth. While attaching a numerical value to the risk is speculative, it seems likely that the likely direction of the error is downward. That is, the true values, when they become known, are likely to be less than the forecasts. Provision might be made for such a reality by building the facility with a view toward conversion of part of it to other uses, although such refinement may be impractical.

In this section, a simple example was used to trace the analysis of demand phenomena, so that a forecaster might improve his understanding and reduce the risk of error. The process can be briefly restated:

- The component statistics are analyzed in preference to aggregates wherever data collection problems permit. Thus obstetric demand was divided into fertility rates, fertile population, and length of stay.
- Each component is reviewed in the light of historical trends, comparative data, and expert opinion to the extent possible.

• Several alternative projections of each component are prepared and one of these is selected normatively as being the most likely to represent the future situation. (The selected estimate or projection can be conveniently identified as the forecast.)

**FIGURE II.2.6**
Postpartum days per birth

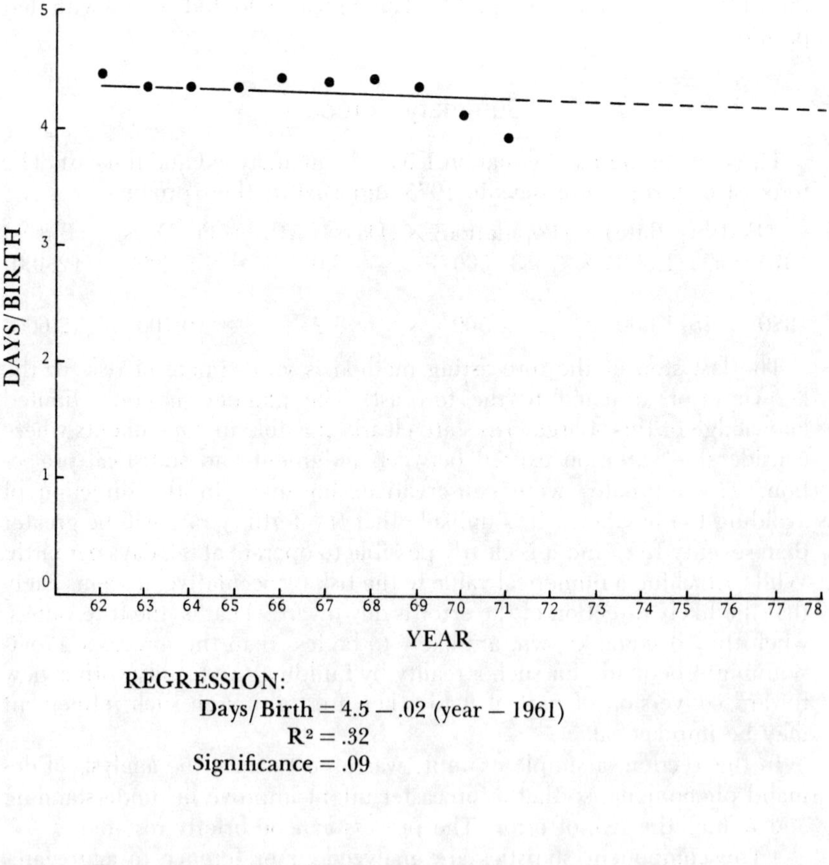


REGRESSION:
Days/Birth = 4.5 − .02 (year − 1961)
$R^2 = .32$
Significance = .09

The use of this technique in the example substantially changed the final forecast. If the initial regression line, shown in figure II.2.2, had been used, the forecast would have been 7,600 patient days in 1980. If the last year of available data on patient days had been used, the forecast would be 9,600 for both years, missing the likely increase after 1975. In neither case would there be any knowledge of the underlying dynamics, nor reasonable consultation with experts to consider statistics that were familiar to them, but none of these experts could have commented intelligently on figure II.2.2. As a byproduct, the forecast generated part of the data necessary to establish the size of the rest of the obstetrics service.

Despite the apparent complexity of these techniques to novices, experienced persons working in well organized states can prepare these forecasts in a few man days, although these days will be scattered over a few-week period. It is unlikely that the direct cost of forecasting would ever exceed a few thousand dollars. If the planning decision is made to meet an expected need of 10,100 patient days in 1980, rather than 9,600 patient days, an additional two beds will be provided, reducing the chance of an unsatisfactory result. Finally, the likely long-run conclusion appears to be that a change in the size of obstetrical services may be necessary again in the 80s, and this probability can be considered in the planning process. These improvements in knowledge and confidence are clearly worth their cost.

In the following section, this basic technique will be explored still further, in application to the largest single component of inpatient facility costs, the adult medical-surgical bed supply.

## Forecasting Admission Rate and Length of Stay: The General Case

Obstetrics beds were selected for the simple example because both the need for hospitalization and the population at risk are readily apparent for this hospital service. This is not the case for all areas of hospital care. In fact, for most areas substantial variations in demand exist in different settings, and unnecessary or undesirable use has been shown to exist in substantial amounts. The supply of beds itself, among other factors, has been cited as a cause of unnecessary use.[22] The range of current practice in total hospital use is strikingly broad, from less than 600 patient days per thousand persons in some of the prepaid group practices, which stress prevention and ambulatory care, to over 1,600 days per thousand in some communities with conventional health insurance, fee-for-service medical practice, and large supplies of hospital beds.[23] The large part of the total use, and most of the variation between communities, lies in the adult medical-surgical component. The argument of causality is difficult to establish, because it is never clear whether the demand for care led to the construction of beds or the availability of beds encouraged demand. What is considerably clearer is that there is little or no evidence that populations with higher use rates are healthier as a result, and that there is no possibility of using beds which are not built.[24] Since inpatient care is the largest single component of cost, the bed size decision is one of the most important decisions affecting community expenditure for hospital facilities. Not only does it determine capital expenditure, it affects the operating costs for several years into the future.

There is growing sentiment that the solution to these problems lies in curtailing or reducing the acute bed supply in a deliberate planning decision closely coordinated with the expansion of alternative sources of treatment and carefully considered in the light of special factors in the local situation. The special factors are those legitimately increasing need, particularly aged or poor populations,[25] and doctor shortages. These however must be drastically different from the usual U.S. community to justify a shift in the rate. Modest fluctuations in the percent of aged or poor, or in the physician supply, are unlikely to result in large changes in bed need. The alternative sources which are necessary include ambulatory services, adequate long-term care facilities, and home health services. Rogatz has provided not only a review of this argument, but a specific procedure for implementing it.[26] Others have joined him in advocating a reduction of the bed supply.[27]

Given this concern, it is probably more desirable to make a judicious normative decision about the adult medical-surgical use rate than to rely on extrapolations of past trends, although these should certainly be examined.[28] The questions which must be answered in each planning situation are:

Is this a community in which the use rate should be reduced?

If so, by how much, and over what time period?

The Bureau's general posture toward the first question has been positive in all cases where the rate exceeded the state average and no persuasive ameliorating factor can be found. The forecast rate has been approximately the current state average. In situations where the current rate is average, the Bureau has allowed no increase. Below average rates present an interesting problem which is discussed below. The Michigan rate, 1,200 patient days per thousand, is essentially the same as the national average. In states where the average state rate is above average, a more restrictive policy may be in order. It should be noted that the Bureau policy will not reduce the existing bed supply except in the more overbedded areas, and only there when population growth is not expected to absorb the excess.

Even this policy, however, is sometimes received with alarm. It is viewed by some as increasing the risk of turning away patients in need. There is plenty of evidence in the diversity of present practices, however, that this need not occur. When populations in the millions are satisfactorily treated at much lower rates than the Michigan average, it is hard to believe that any normal community cannot do at least that well. (The entire state of California, with 20,500,000 persons in diverse living conditions, had 1,089 patient days per thousand of care in 1972.[29]) The development of professional standards review organizations (PSROs) is likely to assist with the problem by seeing that it is the unneeded and not needed care that is eliminated, even if existing mechanisms are inadequate.[30] In fact, if PSROs are as successful as some hope, the Bureau's policy may be too lenient. Reductions in the use rate may be in order for all communities above the best conventionally organized communities, which appear to require from 700 to 900 patient days per thousand population. Deliberate system efforts to reduce the length of stay, such as preadmission testing and the use of ambulatory surgery, also will help meet the reduced rates in a satisfactory manner. It is the belief of Rogatz and other authorities that the development of these alternatives is enhanced by curtailing the availablity of acute general beds.

Below are some of the problems to be considered in reducing the use rate.

## Impact of Length of Stay

While the patient day use rate is the statistic most closely related to the bed size decision, it is the product of the admission rate and the length of stay. In most situations the Bureau has studied, these two statistics tend to parallel each other. When one is above average, so is the other. However, the length of stay statistic is much better undersood, as a result of years of study. National and regional comparative statistics, such as the Length of Stay Package of PAS, exist which take into account the major causes of variation: patient age, sex, disease, complication, and whether the treatment was surgical or medical.[31] The development of professional service review organizations is likely to increase the sophistication in this area and the availability of data. Standardized, adjusted comparisons such as the Length of Stay Package are a desirable starting point for comparing any single institution to others. If length of stay adjusted for the major causes of variation remains significantly above or below regional means, an adjustment of the forecast use rate should be considered. This can be a simple factor:

$$\frac{\text{Adusted expected length of stay}}{\text{Actual length of stay}}$$

where the numerator is supplied by the length of stay data analysis, and represents an age-, sex-, and disease-adjusted estimate for the patient load of the hospital in question. If possible, it is much safer to supplement the statistics with a medical review indicating which diseases show the significant variation, why, and how (and whether) the situation can be corrected. Below average stays, for example, might represent superior care which should be continued. Medical factors, such as the existence of highly selected populations which occur in referral teaching hospitals, might make changes undesirable. Also, length of stay is affected by the efficiency of the hospital (in providing requested services without delay) as well as the judgment of the doctor. If stay is to be reduced, services must be delivered more efficiently, or poor quality of care will result. (See section III.2 and 5 for service improvements which reduce length of stay.)

Another problem exists, particularly with regard to shorter than average lengths of stay. It is possible to maintain a very short length of stay by admitting "simple" cases. Thus an area might have an average patient day use rate, below average length of stay, and an above average admission use rate. This would occur if excessive numbers of short stay elective operations were admitted, for example. Using the disease-adjusted length of stay alone might not identify the problem, because the care of each patient was not excessive within the data base of the length of stay analysis. Studies of the rates of admission per thousand population by disease would be necessary to prove the existence of the problem, but these are not commonly available. The analyst would be forced to rely on gross admission rates. The forecasts of the admission rate and the length of stay should be adjusted to more usual patterns of hospital use. Arithmetically, this the same as adjusting the patient day use rate directly to regional expectations. Some analysts believe that the exact opposite of the above situation exists when access to care is difficult. Then admission rates are low, and length of stay high, because care is deferred until illness is more severe. If such a situation is suspected in an area where patient day use is below average, an upward adjustment of the forecast may be in order.

## Impact of Population Age

The rates cited above are calculated as the ratio:

$$\frac{\text{Adult medical-surgical patient days}}{\text{Total community population}}$$

where the numerator is the sum of all patient days at the study hospital from the small areas included in the community population. A theoretically better method, with which the Bureau has been experimenting, is the use rate for the adult population:

$$\frac{\text{Adult medical-surgical patient days}}{\text{Adult community population}}$$

The final refinement is the use of age-specific use rates for several groups; such as:

$$\frac{\text{Medical-surgical patient days for 15-29 year-olds}}{\text{Community population 15-29 year-olds}}$$

Age-specific rates would presumably be highly comparable across several communities, and forecasts based on them would accommodate differences in the age distribution of various communities. Age-specific use rates require both estimates and forecasts of the age groups of the population, however. Such data are difficult to obtain, particularly in forecasts. It also should be noted that the use of age-specific rates makes no contribution to the analysis unless the study community is markedly different in its age structure or will change drastically in the future. Washtenaw County, Michigan, for example, has over twenty-five percent of its population between eighteen and thirty because of the universities located there. Its use rate, as might be expected, is low. The forecast, however, should remain correspondingly low unless the fraction of young people is expected to change.

Forecasts of the age distribution are often difficult to make reliably. Further, only large changes in the distribution are likely to matter. Consider the aged population, for example. It typically uses about three times the amount of care as the younger population and comprises about ten percent of the total. A hypothetical community of 100,000 might have total use of 100,000 patient days per year, divided as follows:

| | | | |
|---|---|---|---|
| 10,000 | aged use | 25,000 days or | 2,500 days/1,000 |
| 90,000 | other adults use | 75,000 days or | 833 days/1,000 |
| 100,000 | total adults use | 100,000 days or | 1,000 days/1,000 |

A change to a twelve percent aged population (which is a large—twenty percent—change) would contribute only a three percent change in the overall use rate:

| | | | | | |
|---|---|---|---|---|---|
| 12,000 | aged | × | 2,500 days/1,000 | = | 30,000 days |
| 88,000 | non-aged | × | 833 days/1,000 | = | 73,300 days |
| 100,000 | total adult | | | = | 103,300 days |

or 1,033 days/1000 population.

At the present time, with use rates ranging as widely as they do, and forecasts of the population contributing the largest errors in the final outcome, such embellishments are unjustifiable.

## Evidence of Unmet Need

Review of the admission and patient day use rates of the small population areas, calculated in the service area determination, together with study of the economic, cultural, and geographic characteristics of these communities may reveal pockets of very low use in situations suggesting poor access to care. The combination of low or average admission rates, high patient day rates, and low income is the syndrome of chronic unmet primary care needs.[32] Unusual patterns of travel outside the service area (that is, unexpectedly low relevance indices) may also reflect unmet needs, at least unmet within the appropriate community. Adjustments may be made in the overall rate by estimating the desired rates for these populations and averaging them into the total community. Such areas must constitute a large fraction of the total service area and must be widely different from the average patient day rates, or the adjustment will be trivial, as noted in the case of the aged. It is also wise to combine such an adjustment with a specific planning strategy, such as the provision of a neighborhood health clinic, to meet the underlying problem.

Areas which are very rural may require an above average use rate, because hospitalization is necessary to eliminate doctors' travel time. Self care and long-term care facilities may be more appropriate than acute beds, however. Severe physician shortages may require a similar treatment, although it is better to treat the problem directly, investing in other incentives than hospital beds to attract doctors.

## Lower Than Average Use Rates

In a community with a below average patient day rate, examination of the community situation may reveal unmet need which would justify increasing the rate. Often this will not be the case. In fact, the community may be high income, well doctored, and with excellent health insurance coverage. An analogous situation applies to states below the U.S. average use rate. What is to be done in such a situation? In the absence of evidence of unmet need, there is only one justification for increasing the use rate, and that is in the notion of equity or entitlement to funds. A low use community may argue that additional hospital beds will improve the general attractiveness of the town, and help recruit new industry, more doctors, and other good things. Further, there is the idea that most costs are shared. A community with a below average rate pays relatively more health care premiums or taxes for the care they receive. This may in fact be true, but it is a weak case for several reasons:

- There is no evidence that the U.S. average is necessary for health.
- Raising below average rates has a negative impact on the cost, and encourages other communities to do likewise.
- Hospitals are not the only community resource for recruitment, even for doctors. Parks, schools, libraries, transportation, police and fire protection, homes for the aged, and a host of other items are also attractive. As for doctors, it may be cheaper to pay them in cash than to build them unnecessary hospital beds. It is certainly preferable (and cheaper) to build them offices and supporting services.

For society as a whole, it seems that increases in the use rate should be accepted only on the most rigorous grounds, even for those communities which are now below average.

## Cost Implication of the Use Rate

The total inpatient admission rate multiplied by the overall average length of stay and the average per diem cost of care directly expresses the cost per person of hospital care. This figure relates closely to the expected insurance premiun. The results of the forecasting decisions can thus be compared directly to the community's expected insurance premium which will have to be supplied for a given level of facilities. This rate (called the "pure premium")—can be multiplied by the community average family size and adjusted for claim processing and other costs to indicate the relative impact of various levels of facilities upon employees, unions, and tax revenues which supply the financial support for hospital care. The adult medical-surgical service (AM-S) in most hospitals accounts for about seventy-five percent of total beds. Thus it should attract a major share of the planning resources and attention.

Even though the AM-S patient day or admission rate may show a steady upward trend, the best decision may be to curtail its further growth. Figure II.2.7 shows such a situation for a single hospital in a Michigan community of 60,000. The dotted line shows the regression projection of patient days per thousand population, which would reach 1,350 in 1880 if beds were provided and admission trends continued as they were in 1965-71. The Bureau's recommendation was to maintain facilities only for 1,000 days per thousand. This rate was below the adult medical-surgical average for the state at that time, but was higher than many apparently healthy and similar communities. It was, of course, much higher than rates under HMOs or prepaid group practice organizations. The impact on the community per capita costs is the elimination of a thirty-five percent increase in pure premium, plus inflation and whatever other hidden costs are associated with unnecessary use. The dollar amounts are impressive:

| | |
|---|---|
| At 1,000 days per 1,000 pop. × \$65.80/day | = \$65.80 per person-year |
| At 1,350 days × \$65.80/day | = 88.83 |
| *Savings per person per year* | = 23.03 |
| *Savings per family per year* | |
| \$23.03 × 2.7 persons per family | = 62.18 |
| *Annual savings to the community* | |
| \$23.03/person × 60,000 persons | = \$1,381,800 per year |
| *A hypothetical employer of 500 persons would save:* | |
| \$62.18 × 500 | = \$31,100 per year |

Inflation would increase these costs, of course. And if the extra hospital days represent extra days lost from work, these must be considered as well. The figures for this community are relatively low because hospital operating costs were low. The same change for a nearby industrial city where costs averaged $105 per day would be $99 per family. Clearly, the use rate decision is an important one.

**FIGURE II.2.7**
Adult medical and surgical utilization 1965–1980

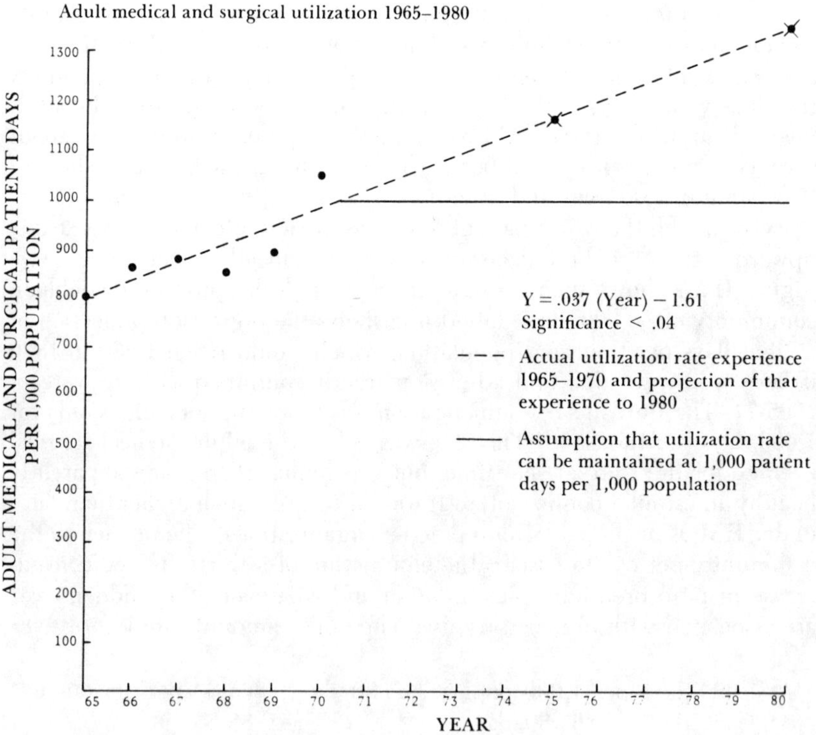


Source: "Health Facility and Program Needs
The Memorial Hospital, Owosso, Michigan"
The Bureau of Hospital Administration
School of Public Health
The University of Michigan, 1971

## Other Forecasting Requirements

For some services, notably pediatrics, and in some locations, notably resorts, there are marked seasonal variations in demand. These must be analyzed and eliminated if possible, by changing the policies of the institution. Only if they cannot be eliminated should they be incorporated in the future forecasts of the eventual facility size. Urgent medical demand (that is, medical emergencies which cannot wait) and similar situations should be projected and included in the forecast. Otherwise, it will pay the community to defer service for a few weeks to nonurgent patients in order to avoid construction simply to meet peak demand. Techniques for preparing the forecast are described in Griffith[33] and many standard time series analysis textbooks. They will not be reviewed here.

Another necessary step is to forecast service outputs for the major diagnostic and therapeutic departments such as operating rooms, laboratory, and x-ray. Demands for the service of these departments can be viewed as derived demands generated by the number and types of in- and outpatients a hospital treats. Stated another way, the patient population rather than the service area population is the population at risk for these services. Data can be collected to indicate the average quantities of different diagnostic and therapeutic services received by in- and outpatients, expressed as use rates per admission or per visit. If possible, service use rates should be calculated separately for each major hospital service. Substantial variation exists from service to service in diagnostic and therapeutic service use, and determinations of service-specific use rates will permit planners to correct for changes in patient mix over time. For example, a hospital that expects pediatric and obstetric admissions to decline and medical-surgical admissions to increase can expect the demands for operating room, laboratory, and x-ray services to increase even if its overall patient load remains the same. Ideally, service use rates should be calculated by diagnostic category, but data are not available to achieve this degree of specificity in most hospitals. Data on service use rates could be presented as shown in figure II.2.8.

Average service use rates of this type can be derived by dividing departmental output by admissions or visits. Aggregate per admission rates are calculated by HAS for participating hospitals, and comparisons are provided by hospital size and region. In most hospitals, however, special studies might be required to develop service use rates by major service. Several sources report such rates as rules of thumb for planning purposes, but the great variation that exists from hospital to hospital makes reliance on these questionable.

Diagnostic and therapeutic service use rates for past years can be extrapolated into the future by the usual projection methods.[34] HAS data indicate substantial upward trends in the quantities of services provided per admission in hospitals of all sizes. For example, between 1969 and 1972 laboratory tests per admission increased 21.9 percent and x-ray procedures per admission 13.1 percent.[35] Projections should be reviewed by experts and modified where indicated by expert judgment. They should also be modified if it is anticipated that hospital policies or programs that might change service rates will be implemented. Factors that should be considered include:

- The addition of new services
- The addition of specialists to the medical staff
- New hospital policies (for instance, that all patients have a chest x-ray or certain laboratory tests as a part of their admission work-up)
- The addition of new services by nearby hospitals.

Implicit in the above discussion is the assumption that the measures of service output used actually reflect department workloads (or stated more precisely for facilities planning purposes, accurately reflect the demands placed on departmental facilities). However, most departments provide a greater variety of services, some of which place heavy demands on facilities and some of which do not. The mix of services provided by departments like surgery, laboratory, and x-ray may vary from month to month and may shift permanently over time. Hence, facility requirements may not be accurately reflected by aggregate output measures like OR visits, laboratory tests, and x-ray procedures. This represents an important problem in planning that data are often not available to solve.

## Accuracy of Forecasts

The overall accuracy of forecasts is difficult to assess because of their self-fulfilling characteristic. If a specific bed supply is constructed, the

**FIGURE II.2.8**
Diagnostic categories for service use rates

| | *Operating Room Visits/Admission or Visit* | *Lab Tests/ Admission or Visit* | *X-ray Exams/ Admission or Visit* | *Etc.* |
|---|---|---|---|---|
| *Inpatients* Medical | | | | |
| Surgical | | | | |
| Pediatric | | | | |
| Obstetric | | | | |
| Psychiatric | | | | |
| Other | | | | |
| *Outpatients* Clinic | | | | |
| Emergency | | | | |
| Referred | | | | |
| | | | | |

outcome is partially determined. Use cannot exceed the available capacity. If this capacity is insufficient, measures of "error" will then be indirect: physician and patient dissatisfaction, excessive delays, overcrowding, and so forth. If too many beds are built, it is likely that the use rate will rise or occupancy will be diminished. The error will appear as a departure from the forecast in these measures and in the population forecast.

When an error occurs in the forecasts, it is most likely to be in the population forecast, rather than the size of the service community or various components of the use rate. Unfortunately, population forecasting for small areas remains inexact, and it is likely to be most difficult and controversial in those places where hospital facilities planning is most important. Allowance can always be made for error in the forecasts, but it is wise to note that it is usually easier to expand a facility than to contract it, and the cost of building it, once spent, is forever gone. Thus forecasts which avoid excessive growth are conservative, in most situations, in the sense of minimizing public expenditure while satisfying health care needs. This is particularly true if the opposite approach is taken in selecting the use rate. If use rate reductions are taken cautiously, population increases should be handled in the same manner.

## NOTES

[1]E. Poland and P. A. Lembcke, "Delineation of Hospital Service Districts: Methodology and Statistical Appendices." (Multilith) Kansas City: Community Studies, Inc., 1962.

[2]See work by P. DeVise of the Chicago Hospital Council and papers by R. L. Morrill and E. Earickson in *Inquiry,* Vol. 5, No. 4, December 1968 and in *Health Services Research,* Vol. 3, No. 3, Fall 1968.

[3]John R. Griffith, *Quantitative Techniques for Hospital Planning and Control.* Lexington, Mass.: D.C. Heath and Co., 1972, chapter 4.

[4]Services of the Commission on Professional and Hospital Activities, 1968 Green Road, Ann Arbor, Michigan 48105.

[5]Griffith, *Quantitative Techniques,* p. 68.

[6]A. Richard Thonander, "Ascertaining a Hospital Service Area and Service Population from Discharge Survey Data." Master's thesis, The University of Michigan, 1972.

[7]Bureau of Hospital Administration, "Analysis of Demand for Services, University Hospital." Ann Arbor: The Bureau, The University of Michigan, 1968.

[8]Daniel L. Drosness and Jerome W. Lubin, "Planning Can be Based on Patient Travel." *Modern Hospital,* Vol. 106, No. 4, April 1966, pp. 92-94.

[9]Greater Detroit Area Hospital Council, "Patient Origin and Hospital Utilization Study." Detroit: The Council.

[10]One way to visualize these distortions is to consider a community hospital with a five-day stay (for all patients) and a teaching hospital with a ten-day stay which each admit fifty percent of a small area's hospitalization. Then the relevance index based on admissions or discharges will be 0.5, but an index based on patient days or a one-day census will be $5 \div (5+10)$ or 0.33 for the community hospital, and

0.67 for the teaching hospital. A similar kind of distortion would exist if the lengths of stay of two small areas were different at the same hospital, but this problem seems to be less common.

[11]Griffith, *Quantitative Techniques,* p. 71.

[12]Health Planning Council of Michigan, "Origin of Acute Care Patients." Lansing, Michigan: The Council, 1967-1969.

[13]An interesting variant of this problem is the impact of suburban migration upon downtown institutions. In effect, the downtown hospital is saying its service area will grow as it continues to serve migrants in new suburbs. The facts apparently do not support this assumpution. The migrants prefer suburban hospitals. The service area of the downtown hospital remains constant, and the population in that area declines or changes character.

[14]Morrill and Earickson, *Inquiry,* Vol. 5, No. 4.

[15]J. Meade, "A Mathematical Model for Deriving Hospital Service Areas." *International Journal of Health Services,* Vol. 4, No. 2, 1974, pp. 353-364.

[16]In some minor civil divisions in the Detroit area, even the preliminary 1970 census counts were in error by ten percent. The forecasts obviously depend on many chance elements, including economic growth.

[17]Griffith, *Quantitative Techniques* has further discussion of criteria for judging population forecasts, pp. 85-86.

[18]*Ibid.*, chapter 2.

[19]The least squares regression technique is commonly used to analyze time series data. It identifies the line passing closest to the points, and can be used to estimate either straight or curved lines. Further discussion of the technique appears in most statistics textbooks and in Griffith, *Quantitative Techniques*, chapter 2. The use of the coefficient of correlation, $R^2$, is discussed in footnote 20.

[20]Technically, the percentage of variation explained by the line is called the "coefficient of determination," and the probability that the line exists in fact rather than as an accident of the sample is called the "significance" and is tested by the F statistic. For these data, the F statistic is 81.5 at one and ten degrees of freedom. A check of the nonlinear regression showed no apparent improvement in the F statistic and was rejected on those grounds. The standard error of estimate, a measure of the uncertainty of placement of the line, was 5.06 in the linear case.

[21]For Jackson this was Dr. David Goldberg, Professor of Sociology and Director of the Population Studies Center, The University of Michigan.

[22]S. E. Berki, *Hospital Economics*. Lexington, MA: D. C. Heath and Co., 1972. Pages 145ff. provide discussion of these issues with reference to primary sources.

[23]Bureau of Hospital Administration, "Health Facility and Program Needs for Bay City, Michigan." Ann Arbor: The Bureau, The University of Michigan, 1968.

[24]Cf. V. R. Fuchs, *Who Shall Live*. New York: Basic Books, 1975, pp. 96-97 especially.

[25]G. Sparer and L. Okada, "Differential Patterns of Poverty and Health Care Utilization in Eight Urban Areas," American Association for Public Opinion Research, Pasadena, California, 1971.

See also T. W. Bice, "Medical Care for the Disadvantaged," final report of Contract HSM 110-69-203, National Center for Health Services Research and Development, DHEW, 1971.

[26]Peter Rogatz, "Excessive Hospitalization Can be Cut Back." *Hospitals*, August 1, 1974, pp. 51ff.

[27]Reduction of hospital beds received attention from the Nixon administration from the veto of Hill-Burton legislation in 1970 (*Hospitals*, Vol. 44, No. 14, July 1, 1970, p. 20) through a Social Policy Statement to Congress in February 1973 (*Hospitals*, Vol. 47, No. 9, May 1, 1973, p. 39). Mothballing oversupply of beds was suggested by Dr. Peter Rogatz, Senior Vice President of Blue Cross of Greater New York in a keynote session of the American Health Congress August 20, 1973 in Chicago (news, *Hospital Progress*, Vol. 54, No. 10, October 1973, p. 19). The concept has been adopted by the Health and Hospital Corporation of New York City in response to reimbursement penalties for low occupancy rates imposed by state regulations applying to Medicaid and Blue Cross (Max H. Seigel, "City's Hospitals Drop 1,700 Beds," *New York Times*, June 2, 1974, Sec. 1, part 2, page 53).

[28]R. M. Grimes, et al., "Use of Decision Theory in Regional Planning." *Health Services Research*, Vol. 9, No. 1, Spring 1974. Uses extrapolations combined with Bayesian analysis of error implications. Such an approach might be combined in future work with the one developed here.

[29]R. A. Chernow, "Use Rates for Community Hospitals." Ann Arbor: The Bureau of Hospital Administration, The University of Michigan, January 1974. (unpublished) Data are from AHA *Guide Issue* and include military population and federal hospitals.

[30]Public Law 92-603, Section 1123, and publications of The Office of the Secretary, DHEW on PSRO.

[31]The Length of Stay Package of the Commission on Professional and Hospital Activities, Ann Arbor, and publications of CPHA. Also see Griffith, *Quantitative Techniques*, chapter 12.

[32]Sparer and Okada, *Differential Patterns*.

[33]Griffith, *Quantitative Techniques*, chapter 3.

[34]*Ibid.*, especially chapter 5.

[35]J. Phillips, "A New Perspective in Cost Inflation." *Hospitals*, Vol. 47, No. 41, October 1973.

# II.3

# Converting Demand Forecasts Into Facility Requirements

*by William L. Dowling*

## Steps in Converting Demand to Facility Requirements

The previous chapter described methods for forecasting the quantities of hospital services that will be demanded by a defined population in future years. Such forecasts, from the point of view of the hospital or hospitals serving this population, represent estimates of the service outputs they must be capable of providing. The next step in the planning process, discussed in this chapter, is to convert expected service outputs into facility requirements. For example, if 2,600 deliveries are expected in some future year, how many labor room beds, delivery rooms, postpartum nursing unit beds, and nursery bassinets will be required to provide this quantity of service? The goal of cost-effective planning is to determine the minimum facility set that will accommodate expected demands for services. Once facility requirements are determined, alternative ways of providing them can be identified and evaluated.

The required number of facility units (beds, operating rooms, x-ray units) depends on the quantity of service outputs to be provided, the pattern of demand for service, the service producing capacity of a unit, and the desired level of protection against peak periods.

Once the estimate of demand has been developed, arrival or demand patterns must be considered. These patterns may be cyclic or stationary. Demand may be of an emergency nature, where arrivals are unpredictable and delays in service not permissible, or schedulable, as is the case for elective surgery. The service producing capacity of a facility unit (its output during a defined period given hospital policies regarding hours and methods of operation) will be affected by cyclic and emergency demand patterns. Extra capacity protects against demand peaks. The estimation of these reserves is discussed below.

The following general formulas can be applied to convert forecasts of services into facility requirements:

- Expected annual service output ÷ Days per year services provided = Average daily workload.
- Average daily workload ÷ Daily service capacity per facility unit = Average number of facility units utilized.
- Average facility units utilized ÷ Reserve facility units required = Total facility units required.
- Average facility units utilized ÷ Total facility units required = Load factor.

To illustrate, consider the planning of beds for the obstetric service. Using the methods described in the previous chapter, a hospital forecasts 2,600 deliveries for the planning year and extrapolates an average length of stay on the postpartum nursing unit of four days. The expected annual service output for which facilities will be required is 10,400 patient days of care. The postpartum unit is, of course, in operation 365 days per year, so the average daily census or average number of facility units utilized will be 28.5 (10,400 ÷ 365). However, because of the need to accommodate peak workloads which cannot be anticipated or delayed, an additional reserve, determined by techniques described below, of about 10.5 beds will be required. The total bed requirement is thirty-nine (28.5 + 10.5), and the average occupancy level (load factor) will be seventy-three percent (28.5 ÷ 39).

The approach to facility units not used around the clock, such as operating rooms, is similar. Suppose a hospital forecasts 5,000 operations per year and maintains a surgical suite use policy of seven and a half hours per day, five days per week (260 days per year). The average daily workload will be 19.2 operations (5,000 ÷ 260). If operating times average one hour with an additional half-hour to clean up and set up between operations, the daily service capacity of a single operating room is five (7.5 hours ÷ 1.5 hours per procedure), and the average number of operating rooms required is 3.8 (19.2 ÷ 5). If all emergency surgery occurs at night, if the operating suite is not otherwise in use, or if elective surgery can be cancelled when necessary to accommodate emergencies, it may be decided that no reserve operating rooms are required. In this case, four operating rooms are required, and the load factor will be ninety-five percent. Adjustments would be necessary to provide additional reserve capacity if emergencies were handled differently.

The above examples emphasize the process of converting expected service output into facility requirements in five separate steps:

1. Identify the facility units associated with the service.
2. Determine the service producing capacity of a single facility unit.
3. Determine the number of facility units required to accommodate the average demand for service.
4. Determine the number of additional facility units necessary to accommodate emergency demands or peak loads (the reserve or standby requirement).
5. Calculate the total number of facility units required and the load factor using the results of steps 3 and 4.

These steps are sometimes combined through the application of formulas or rules of thumb for converting service output into facilities. They should be handled as distinct steps, however. Cost-effective planning may be subverted by shortcutting this process. This chapter emphasizes identifying factors such as hospital policies and patterns of operation which bear on each step, because many of them can be controlled or influenced by management. Unquestioning acceptance of existing policies may lead to planning more facilities than are actually required. Hence, policies and procedures affecting facility requirements should be made explicit and their implications examined.

## Identifying Facility Units

For most hospital services, facility units are fairly obvious. For departments providing several services, the facility unit corresponding to each must be identified. Equipment, manpower, and space requirements can frequently be related to facility units so that once facility requirements are determined, other resource requirements can be planned.

## Determining the Service Producing Capacity of Facility Units

Service capacity is the number of units of service that can be accommodated or produced by a single facility unit during some defined period of time. The time period should reflect the normal availability of the facility, usually a month or a year. Because hospital policies and patterns of operation influence service capacity, it usually falls far short of technical capacity—the facility's maximum output or physical capability. For inpatient bed facilities, service capacity and technical capacity tend to be quite close. But for most facilities like operating rooms and x-ray equipment, technical capacity is two or three times greater than service capacity as equipment is deliberately left idle much of the time.

The actual service producing capacity of a facility unit depends on four factors: average duration of service (service time); average wait time between arrivals for service (down time); amount of time the facility is available or in operation; and policies and methods of operation (the operating discipline).

The average service time for beds is the average length of stay, differentiated by hospital service. The average duration of clinical activities such as surgical procedures, x-ray procedures, and emergency and outpatient visits, can be determined from data on current operations. Several sources report average actual service times or standard service times which can be used for planning,[1] but for expansions or replacement of existing facilities in-house studies are preferred, at least for verification. Service times are affected by the breadth and sophistication of services provided as well as by the age and characteristics of patients served, and these factors can vary greatly from hospital to hospital. In addition, in-house studies provide an opportunity to assess and improve patterns of operation. Average service times are generally sufficient to plan for nonemergency demand. When arrival patterns and service times fluctuate widely and unpredictably, as for emergency type services, a frequency distribution of service times often must be obtained.

In studying service times, special attention should be paid to preparation time and clean-up time before and after services are provided. "Requirements" for these activities tend to mount when excess capacity is available. If the down time experienced in a particular facility or unit is caused by a low level of demand, the alternatives of discontinuing the service or expanding the hospital's market should be considered in cooperation with nearby hospitals. Patient scheduling and personnel staffing should also be reviewed. Poor scheduling practices can greatly reduce the efficiency of facility use. Patient arrivals to a department for service either from outside the hospital or from the nursing units should be formally scheduled where possible (although allowance for emergency arrivals may be necessary). Investments in appointment systems or patient transportation personnel may be more than offset by reductions in facility requirements. Effort should also be made to even out demand levels by rescheduling elective work from peak hours. Waiting lists, waiting rooms, and surgical prep rooms may be planned to assure that patients are available to be served as soon as a facility unit is free. Poor scheduling practices can generate *both* idle facilities and excessive delays.

Down times may be due to staffing shortages or inefficient use of personnel. For example, if x-ray technicians are required to do work which might better be done by clerks (such as log in patients, find their previous films, and fill in charge slips), between procedures, the technicians are prevented from making full use of the x-ray equipment. Investments in ancillary personnel to free technical personnel to perform the most essential tasks would be wise. In addition, where facilities must be adapted or changed over to accommodate different types of procedures, as is common with operating rooms and x-ray rooms, an attempt should be made to schedule all patients requiring a particular procedure during the same period.

Obviously, the amount of time per day or per week facilities are staffed and available for use affects the service output. In general, this is measured by staffed hours. Beds and facilities for emergency demands are available around the clock, but many hospitals limit the hours of elective services to one or two shifts and to five or five and one-half day weeks. The cost of additional staffing to permit fuller use of such facilities and hence to reduce facility requirements should be evaluated. Another cost to be considered is that of keeping patients in the hospital an extra day when services are not available on weekends. This practice adds to both facility and bed requirements.

In industrial engineering, the term "operating discipline" refers to the set of all policies, procedures, staffing, scheduling, and work methods that affect productivity. Methods of improving departmental productivity through revision of operating discipline are the subject of section III. (See especially section III.5, on x-ray department operations.) No further discussion of this is offered here, except to reiterate that current patterns of operation should be questioned in planning.

Administrators might well monitor departmental performance in terms of both the load factor and the ratio of service capacity to technical capacity. This is rarely done, except for the inpatient occupancy statistic. Such statistics might be quite revealing. In a recent study of a 300 bed hospital, the Bureau of Hospital Administration found that the laboratory was staffed at thirty-four percent of technical capacity (3,000 of the 8,760 hours in a year), x-ray thirty-seven percent, and the operating rooms forty-two percent.[2] Another study, conducted in a hospital planning a sixty percent bed expansion where the radiologist was requesting a 100 percent increase in the number of x-ray rooms, the load factor was found to be only 30.1 percent. That is, the facilities were only in use 30.1 percent of the available staffed hours. Further, it was found that, by increasing the load factor to eighty percent of the available capacity (still only twenty-four percent of the technical capacity) no additional rooms would be required in the expanded hospital.[3] A third study indicated load factors of nine percent for the delivery rooms, thirty-one percent for labor rooms and fifty-seven percent for postpartum recovery rooms in a major teaching hospital.[4]

The load factor and the ratio of service capacity to technical capacity have some valuable planning properties which will be explored further in the following chapter. Specifically, whenever the service capacity can be increased as a proportion of the technical capacity, additional output is possible without additional capital investment. (This follows from the definitions. The service capacity is simply the utilized portion of the technical capacity for a given set of facilities.) This means that the marginal cost of additional service capacity will be lower than the cost of equivalent technical capacity expansion whenever the overtime and shift differential payments and other costs of extended operation are less than the equivalent annual cost of new facilities.[5] Many of the "other" costs are intangible, but the comparison should be made whenever expansion is being considered. (One would not wish to perform elective x-rays at 3:00 A.M., but the intangible cost of doing them at 6:00 P.M. might be quite acceptable, in preference to a capital expansion.)

Whenever the load factor can be increased, the marginal cost of meeting the additional demand is theoretically zero. (It may in practice be higher because of concessions to the operating personnel or minor adjustments in staffing and equipment.) This means that load factor improvements are almost automatically the first choice in cost-effective planning. Frequently they involve systematic reorganization of demand, through mergers and shared services. Investigation of such possibilities will always be high on the agenda of rational planners as long as actual load factors remain substantially below maximum feasible levels.

## Determining Reserve and Total Facility Requirements

The average daily output of a particular service a hospital expects to provide along with the daily capacity of one facility unit determine the average number of facility units that will be required. Additional standby facility units may be required where arrivals or demands for service fluctuate around the average output. Arrival or demand patterns experienced by hospital facilities or units can be characterized along two scales:

| | Schedulable (Deterministic) | Emergency (Stochastic) |
|---|---|---|
| Stationary | | |
| Cyclic | | |

### Stationary, Schedulable Demand

A stationary demand pattern is one in which the average quantity of service sought (or provided) is essentially the same from day to day and from season to season, or one which can be arranged this way by having a waiting list of reasonable length. Stationary and deterministic demands are consistent *and* predictable (not subject to chance or random variation). An outpatient department handling about the same number of patient visits each day, with an appointment system to schedule patients, and few walk-in patients would be an example. Planning facility requirements for such services is a simple matter. Dividing the expected daily service output by the daily service capacity per facility unit determines the number of units required. No allowances need be made for emergency demand or cyclic variation. Unfortunately, few hospital facilities experience stable and deterministic demand patterns (OPDs included).

## Cyclic Variation

A cyclic demand pattern is one in which the quantity of services sought rises and falls in a recurring systematic manner, usually by day of the week or season. Cyclic and deterministic demands rise and fall in a recurring pattern *and* are free of chance variation; that is, the average demand level rises and falls systematically, but the demand on any given day is predictable. The demand for surgical procedures might follow this pattern. Most operations can be scheduled so that the number to be performed each day is known. However, the demand may be consistently higher on certain days (typically Mondays and Tuesdays) and during certain seasons (typically the winter months). Planning facilities which must accommodate a cyclic and deterministic demand pattern is also quite simple. Daily service output divided by daily service capacity per facility unit is used, but the numerator is the expected daily output for days during high volume days or seasons. This can be estimated by an examination of monthly and daily outputs for previous years and weeks.[6]

A cautionary point has been made about cyclic demand situations. Because facility requirements for peak periods may greatly exceed those that would be required were demand more stable, the administrator should make every effort to level out cyclic demand patterns. This might be accomplished by a number of means:

- Identifying certain elective procedures (such as T&As) and explicitly scheduling them for low volume months
- Encouraging physicians to stagger their vacation times
- Identifying new services that might be performed during low volume months
- Employing waiting lists to reduce seasonal variations
- Operating departments on weekends during peak periods
- Interchanging the use of different facilities for which high and low demands occur at the same periods

## Stochastic Variation

Planning facilities to accommodate arrivals or demands for service that are random or stochastic (and that cannot be delayed or held in a waiting line) is more difficult. In such situations, the planner must determine the number of standby or reserve facility units required (in addition to the facility units required to accommodate the average expected service output) to meet unpredictable demand peaks. More information is needed by the planner. Both the expected (average) demand and the probability of demands above the expected are pertinent. In addition, the desired level of protection against not having enough facilities to meet arrivals or demands for service must be decided. Clearly, facilities planned to accommodate the average service output would be insufficient, since demand would exceed capacity half or more than half the time. For example, an analysis of the census of the postpartum nursing unit of one of the study hospitals, which provided a total of 5,100 days of patient care during a recent year, showed the pattern in figure II.3.1.

The average daily census on this unit was fourteen (5,100 ÷ 365 = 13.97), but the individual days ranged (unpredictably) from a low of three patients which occurred one day during the year to a high of twenty-five which also occurred once. Obviously, mothers could not be asked to wait, so scheduling could not be used. Inspection of the frequency distribution indicates that a twenty-four bed unit would have been overcrowded one day during the year; a twenty-three bed unit, two days; a twenty-two bed unit, four days; a twenty-one bed unit, ten days; and so on. What, then, is the proper size for the unit? Twenty-five beds would always be sufficient, but if this number of beds were provided, twelve or more would be empty half the time (the median occupancy is slightly over twelve patients), and the average occupancy level of the unit would be only fifty-six percent (14 ÷ 25).

Clearly, there is a trade-off between the cost of the OB unit based on its size (or its efficiency expressed in terms of percent of technical capacity actually used on the average—its average occupancy level) and the frequency of not having enough beds. Thus, in cases where demand is stochastic, and cannot be scheduled, the correct size of a unit depends on management judgment about the proper balance or trade-off between these two factors. More will be said below about the protection levels commonly used in planning facilities of this type.

Four general approaches can be used to determine total (and hence, by inference, reserve) facility requirements in situations where arrivals or demands for services are stochastic:[7]

- The use of normative occupancy levels
- The use of empirical data such as the frequency distribution in figure II.3.1 or data on the experience of comparable hospitals

**FIGURE II.3.1**

Frequency distribution of obstetric census* Memorial Hospital 1971

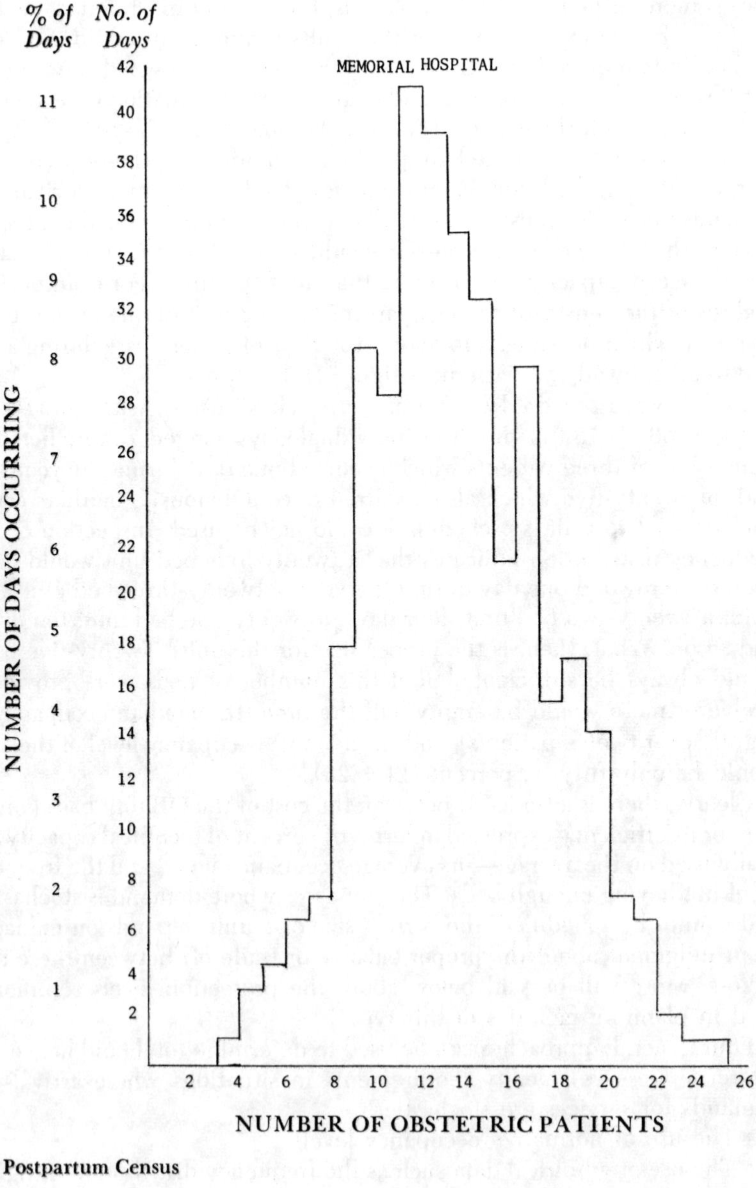


* Postpartum Census

- The use of mathematical models based upon theoretical distributions
- The use of simulation techniques

The first two approaches are the simplest and most frequently used. A hospital's past experience, the experience of other hospitals, or normative standards are referred to in deciding on an acceptable occupancy rate or, more generally, a rate expressing average actual facility use to capacity facility use. Eighty or eighty-five percent occupancy is commonly used in planning adult medical and surgical bed requirements. Ninety percent is achievable, and is recommended by the Bureau of Hospital Administration in most circumstances. It is practical when combined with a scheduling system such as that described in section III.2.

Empirical figures tend to vary with hospital size. For example, HAS reports the average occupancy levels for nursing units in participating hospitals as shown in table II.3.1.

Areawide planning agencies frequently establish occupancy norms to be used in planning. The Greater Detroit Area Hospital Council incorporates in its formula for determining bed need an overall occupancy rate of eighty-eight percent, based on a ninety-one percent occupancy rate for medical-surgical units and a seventy-five percent occupancy rate for obstetric and pediatric units. Third-party reimbursement organizations also may establish norms. The New York Blue Cross plan adjusts payment rates downward for hospitals which do not achieve sixty percent occupancy in OB units, seventy percent occupancy in pediatric units, and eighty percent occupancy in adult medical-surgical units.

It should be noted that empirical and normative occupancy levels usually reflect both cyclic and stochastic demand patterns. That is, these two factors are not accounted for separately. Also, the use of these occupancy levels to determine the total bed need does not enable the planner to make probabilistic statements (to state how many days per year given numbers of facility units will be insufficient) and hence does not make explicit the trade-off between costs and degree of protection.

The empirical approach can be expanded to incorporate distributions of arrivals, census, or other measures of demand patterns. Data on past demand levels can be collected and presented in the form of a graph (histogram) showing the frequency (in days, hours, shifts) with which different demand levels occurred as in figure II.3.1 or in the form of a table.

It can be seen from the table II.3.2 that the census of this unit was twenty patients or more 6.3 percent of the time (twenty-three days out of 365), twenty-one or more 4.4 percent of the time, twenty-two or more 2.7 percent of the time, and so forth. A twenty-one bed unit should be planned if the desired level of protection against not having enough beds or against overcrowding is ninety-five percent. This would mean there would be crowding no more than five percent of the time or eighteen days per year.

Note that the use of an empirical frequency distribution for determining facility requirements is based on the assumption that future arrival or demand patterns will be similar to those experienced in the past. When this assumption cannot reasonably be made, this approach should not be used. If demand forecasts indicate that the average demand level will change slightly, bed needs can be estimated by shifting the entire frequency distribution up or down to determine standby requirements based on the desired degree of protection. However, the larger the shift in the forecast average the greater the error in using the old empirical distribution.

The third approach is to apply a formula based on the assumption (which can be tested) that the arrival or demand pattern for a particular service approximates that described by a known theoretical distribution. It is frequently assumed that the process generating arrivals or daily census levels for OB, CCU, ICU, and ER units can be closely described by the Poisson distribution. If so, once the average daily census (or more generally, the average daily service output) has been forecast, total facility requirements can be determined either from tabulated values of the Poisson distribution[8] or from the formula:

$$\text{Bed need} = \text{Average daily census} + Z\sqrt{\text{Average daily census}}$$

Z in this formula is the value from the cumulative normal distribution tables. Since the probability of $Z > 2$ is .025, a value of $ADC + 2\sqrt{ADC}$

**TABLE II.3.1**
Average percentage occupancy levels for nursing units in HAS hospitals

| *Hospital Bed Size* | *CCU/ICU Units* | *OB Units* | *Med-Surg Units* |
|---|---|---|---|
| Under 50 | 25.0% | 25.3% | 64.3% |
| 50–74 | 38.3 | 30.8 | 74.6 |
| 75–99 | 46.7 | 37.1 | 74.1 |
| 100–149 | 56.7 | 45.0 | 80.0 |
| 150–199 | 63.3 | 50.0 | 83.4 |
| 200–299 | 68.5 | 56.7 | 84.6 |
| 300–399 | 73.3 | 59.8 | 85.7 |
| Over 400 | 74.1 | 66.2 | 87.9 |

Source: HAS six-month national comparison for month ending June 30, 1973, American Hospital Association, Chicago, Illinois.

would protect against 97.5 percent of the expected variation in demand, if two assumptions are correct. The first assumption is that demand varies according to the Poisson distribution, and the second is that the normal distribution approximates the Poisson. The first assumption is conservative; that is, it yields higher capacity and lower occupancy than is truly necessary. The second assumption is mathematically verifiable for any Poisson with a mean greater than fifty, and is frequently satisfactory for Poissons greater than twenty-five. Below that value (ADC < 25), the use of the normal distribution increasingly *understates* the true capacity needs and should be avoided.

**TABLE II.3.2**
Frequency distribution of hospital census

| *Census* | *Days Occurring* | *% Days Occurring* | *Cumulative % of Days* |
|---|---|---|---|
| 0 | 0 | 0 | 0 |
| 1 | 0 | 0 | 0 |
| 2 | 0 | 0 | 0 |
| 3 | 1 | 0.27 | 0.27 |
| 4 | 3 | 0.82 | 1.09 |
| 5 | 4 | 1.10 | 2.10 |
| 6 | 6 | 1.64 | 3.83 |
| 7 | 7 | 1.92 | 5.75 |
| 8 | 18 | 4.93 | 10.68 |
| 9 | 31 | 8.49 | 19.17 |
| 10 | 28 | 7.67 | 26.84 |
| 11 | 41 | 11.23 | 38.07 |
| 12 | 39 | 10.68 | 48.65 |
| 13 | 35 | 9.59 | 58.34 |
| 14 | 32 | 8.77 | 67.11 |
| 15 | 21 | 5.75 | 72.86 |
| 16 | 30 | 8.22 | 81.08 |
| 17 | 15 | 4.11 | 85.19 |
| 18 | 17 | 4.66 | 89.85 |
| 19 | 14 | 3.84 | 93.69 |
| 20 | 7 | 1.92 | 95.61 |
| 21 | 6 | 1.64 | 97.25 |
| 22 | 6 | 1.64 | 98.89 |
| 23 | 2 | 0.55 | 99.44 |
| 24 | 1 | 0.27 | 99.71 |
| 25 | 1 | 0.27 | 99.98 |
| | 365 | 100% | |

For many years it was common practice to use the Poisson assumption approach for planning *all* hospital beds.[9] However, the use of scheduling systems for adult medical-surgical patients and other methods of controlling the census (such as a simple waiting list) make higher occupancies possible. (See the discussion in section III.2.) The Poisson approach is useful for low cost estimates of facility requirements for highly stochastic services and is not otherwise recommended. The most common appropriate applications are to small intensive care and coronary care units. Larger stochastic services, such as OB, might be simulated. Other services can be normatively or empirically estimated.

The fourth approach to solving the stochastic demand situation is Monte Carlo simulation. In applying simulation techniques, the stochastic process of interest is modeled, and the digital computer used to try a variety of alternatives which might be too difficult or expensive to try in real life. For example, the operation of a service producing unit could be modeled, and different configurations of facilities tested against actual or expected arrival patterns and service times to determine the adequacy of each configuration to meet alternative demands for service. The output of the simulation would be estimates of the amount of time facilities would be in use and the probability of demand exceeding their capacity, for each configuration tested. Simulation requires large quantities of data, describing not only the average parameters for demand arrival and service time but frequency distributions as well. It yields a corresponding richness of results, however, and is recommended for any major facility planning problem with substantial stochastic variation. The ease and flexibility of the technique have increased in recent years, and the cost has fallen. Data collection is the major cost element for most practical problems. Applications to obstetrics units and emergency units are now straightforward.[10]

Following is a discussion of the obstetrical simulation application for two hospitals which together served most of the demand described and forecast in the preceding section. These hospitals were contemplating merger. The discussion illustrates the form of data requirements and the use of simulation in determining the total facility requirements under two important alternatives for the provision of care.

Analysis of the arrival patterns of OB patients to "Memorial" and "Church" Hospitals during four selected months of 1971 showed that, although arrivals fluctuated widely, they did not follow the Poisson distribution closely enough for the formula presented above to give a reliable estimate of bed needs. Therefore, simulation techniques were employed to determine 1975 OB facility requirements.

This approach required data on the actual distributions of: arrival times of mothers in labor; arrival times of births; and service times in labor, delivery, recovery, postpartum care, and nursery care. It was used to calculate the number of facilities required for: labor rooms; delivery rooms; recovery rooms; postpartum beds; and nursery bassinets. The input data could be carefully tailored to the local situation. For example, a high percentage of mothers were found to arrive between midnight and 10:00 A.M. This particular finding is inconsistent with the Poisson assumption but can be accommodated in simulation. High percentages of induced deliveries or complicated deliveries could also have been handled without difficulty once the data were collected. In the study described here, recovery room facility use was estimated by the chief of obstetrics, because this service did not exist in the two hospitals but was strongly recommended for the future.

The output of the simulation is information on the facilities required to accommodate the expected service volume. In this study, the objective was to determine the number of labor room beds, delivery rooms, recovery room beds, and postpartum nursing unit beds that would be required to accommodate 2,200 deliveries per year in a single location. This information is given in figure II.3.2, which is the actual computer printout from the simulation. As shown in the upper left corner of the table, the results are to be compared to the present array of facilities in the two hospitals, which total twelve labor room beds, five delivery rooms, and fifty postpartum nursing unit beds. Ten recovery room beds were added to evaluate this improvement. The column headed "Entries" shows that the OB service was required in the simulation to accommodate 2,205 arrivals over the period of a year. The column headed "Maximum Contents" indicates the largest number of each facility which would have been occupied in a year. For example, no more than eight labor room beds would ever have been filled at one time. The greatest number of delivery rooms that would have been simultaneously in use is four, postpartum nursing beds forty-seven, and recovery room beds five. These figures indicate the number of each type of facility that would be required to accommodate 2,200 deliveries without being short as often as once a year or once in 2,000 deliveries. However, the cost of providing and staffing such facilities is substantial, and, therefore, in hospital planning a trade-off is made whereby this cost is reduced somewhat by providing fewer beds than would be required to be certain of having enough beds 100 percent of the time. Typically, delivery facilities are planned to be adequate 99.5 or 99.9 percent of the time, and the patient who delivers when facilities are fully occupied is accommodated using a labor room. Sometimes a labor room is specifically designed for this purpose.

The section of the table dealing with labor rooms indicates that only eleven times during the year would six labor room beds be filled when another patient arrived needing a bed. (From the first page of figure II.3.2. under "Labor" an "Upper Limit" of six is exceeded nine plus two, or eleven times in "Observed Frequency.") Only two times would seven

**FIGURE II.3.2**
Consolidated OB service simulated output

PAGE 1

| STAGE | CAPACITY | AVERAGE CONTENTS | AVERAGE UTILIZATION | ENTRIES | AVERAGE TIME/TRAN | CURRENT CONTENTS | MAXIMUM CONTENTS |
|---|---|---|---|---|---|---|---|
| LABOR | 12 | 1.403 | .116 | 2205 | 67.435 | 3 | 8 |
| DELIV | 5 | .178 | .035 | 2202 | 8.588 | | 4 |
| POSTP | 50 | 23.658 | .473 | 2218 | 1130.101 | 21 | 47 |
| RECOV | 10 | .422 | .042 | 2202 | 20.329 | 3 | 5 |

TABLE LABOR

| ENTRIES IN TABLE | MEAN ARGUMENT | STANDARD DEVIATION | SUM OF ARGUMENTS | |
|---|---|---|---|---|
| 2203 | 1.507 | 1.250 | 3321.000 | NONWEIGHTED |

| UPPER LIMIT | OBSERVED FREQUENCY | PER CENT OF TOTAL | CUMULATIVE PERCENTAGE | CUMULATIVE REMAINDER | MULTIPLE OF MEAN | DEVIATION FROM MEAN |
|---|---|---|---|---|---|---|
| 0 | 504 | 22.87 | 22.8 | 77.1 | -.000 | -1.205 |
| 1 | 726 | 32.95 | 55.8 | 44.1 | .663 | -.405 |
| 2 | 546 | 24.78 | 80.6 | 19.3 | 1.326 | .394 |
| 3 | 266 | 12.07 | 92.6 | 7.3 | 1.990 | 1.194 |
| 4 | 113 | 5.12 | 97.8 | 2.1 | 2.653 | 1.994 |
| 5 | 37 | 1.67 | 99.5 | .4 | 3.316 | 2.794 |
| 6 | 9 | .40 | 99.9 | .0 | 3.980 | 3.594 |
| 7 | 2 | .09 | 100.0 | .0 | 4.643 | 4.394 |

REMAINING FREQUENCIES ARE ALL ZERO

TABLE DELIV

| ENTRIES IN TABLE | MEAN ARGUMENT | STANDARD DEVIATION | SUM OF ARGUMENTS | |
|---|---|---|---|---|
| 2202 | .188 | .429 | 414.000 | NONWEIGHTED |

| UPPER LIMIT | OBSERVED FREQUENCY | PER CENT OF TOTAL | CUMULATIVE PERCENTAGE | CUMULATIVE REMAINDER | MULTIPLE OF MEAN | DEVIATION FROM MEAN |
|---|---|---|---|---|---|---|
| 0 | 1822 | 82.74 | 82.7 | 17.2 | -.000 | -.437 |
| 1 | 347 | 15.75 | 98.5 | 1.4 | 5.318 | 1.890 |
| 2 | 32 | 1.45 | 99.9 | .0 | 10.637 | 4.219 |
| 3 | 1 | .04 | 100.0 | .0 | 15.956 | 6.547 |

REMAINING FREQUENCIES ARE ALL ZERO

CONSOLIDATED OB SERVICE

SIMULATION OUTPUT

PAGE 2

TABLE RECOV

| ENTRIES IN TABLE | MEAN ARGUMENT | STANDARD DEVIATION | SUM OF ARGUMENTS | |
|---|---|---|---|---|
| 2202 | .513 | .730 | 1130.000 | NONWEIGHTED |

| UPPER LIMIT | OBSERVED FREQUENCY | PER CENT OF TOTAL | CUMULATIVE PERCENTAGE | CUMULATIVE REMAINDER | MULTIPLE OF MEAN | DEVIATION FROM MEAN |
|---|---|---|---|---|---|---|
| 0 | 1339 | 60.80 | 60.8 | 39.1 | -.000 | -.702 |
| 1 | 639 | 29.01 | 89.8 | 10.1 | 1.948 | .666 |
| 2 | 184 | 8.35 | 98.1 | 1.8 | 3.897 | 2.034 |
| 3 | 37 | 1.68 | 99.8 | .1 | 5.846 | 3.402 |
| 4 | 3 | .13 | 100.0 | .0 | 7.794 | 4.770 |

REMAINING FREQUENCIES ARE ALL ZERO

TABLE POSTP

| ENTRIES IN TABLE | MEAN ARGUMENT | STANDARD DEVIATION | SUM OF ARGUMENTS | |
|---|---|---|---|---|
| 2199 | 23.854 | 5.648 | 52457.000 | NONWEIGHTED |

| UPPER LIMIT | OBSERVED FREQUENCY | PER CENT OF TOTAL | CUMULATIVE PERCENTAGE | CUMULATIVE REMAINDER | MULTIPLE OF MEAN | DEVIATION FROM MEAN |
|---|---|---|---|---|---|---|
| 0 | 0 | .00 | .0 | 100.0 | -.000 | -4.223 |
| 1 | 0 | .00 | .0 | 100.0 | .041 | -4.046 |
| 2 | 0 | .00 | .0 | 100.0 | .083 | -3.869 |
| 3 | 0 | .00 | .0 | 100.0 | .125 | -3.692 |
| 4 | 0 | .00 | .0 | 100.0 | .167 | -3.515 |
| 5 | 0 | .00 | .0 | 100.0 | .209 | -3.338 |
| 6 | 0 | .00 | .0 | 100.0 | .251 | -3.161 |
| 7 | 0 | .00 | .0 | 100.0 | .293 | -2.983 |
| 8 | 0 | .00 | .0 | 100.0 | .335 | -2.806 |
| 9 | 0 | .00 | .0 | 100.0 | .377 | -2.629 |

CONSOLIDATED OB SERVICE

SIMULATION OUTPUT

PAGE 3

| | | | | | | |
|---|---|---|---|---|---|---|
| 10 | 0 | .00 | .0 | 100.0 | .419 | -2.452 |
| 11 | 5 | .22 | .2 | 99.7 | .461 | -2.275 |
| 12 | 12 | .54 | .7 | 99.2 | .503 | -2.098 |
| 13 | 19 | .86 | 1.6 | 98.3 | .544 | -1.921 |
| 14 | 32 | 1.45 | 3.0 | 96.9 | .586 | -1.744 |
| 15 | 56 | 2.54 | 5.6 | 94.3 | .628 | -1.567 |
| 16 | 64 | 2.91 | 8.5 | 91.4 | .670 | -1.390 |
| 17 | 92 | 4.18 | 12.7 | 87.2 | .712 | -1.213 |
| 18 | 108 | 4.91 | 17.6 | 82.3 | .754 | -1.036 |
| 19 | 136 | 6.18 | 23.8 | 76.1 | .796 | -.859 |
| 20 | 142 | 6.45 | 30.2 | 69.7 | .838 | -.682 |
| 21 | 145 | 6.59 | 36.8 | 63.1 | .880 | -.505 |
| 22 | 146 | 6.63 | 43.5 | 56.4 | .922 | -.328 |
| 23 | 150 | 6.82 | 50.3 | 49.6 | .964 | -.151 |
| 24 | 139 | 6.32 | 56.6 | 43.3 | 1.006 | .025 |
| 25 | 128 | 5.82 | 62.4 | 37.5 | 1.048 | .202 |
| 26 | 131 | 5.95 | 68.4 | 31.5 | 1.089 | .379 |
| 27 | 130 | 5.91 | 74.3 | 25.6 | 1.131 | .556 |
| 28 | 113 | 5.13 | 79.4 | 20.5 | 1.173 | .733 |
| 29 | 100 | 4.54 | 84.0 | 15.9 | 1.215 | .910 |
| 30 | 83 | 3.77 | 87.8 | 12.1 | 1.257 | 1.087 |
| 31 | 74 | 3.36 | 91.1 | 8.8 | 1.299 | 1.264 |
| 32 | 49 | 2.22 | 93.4 | 6.5 | 1.341 | 1.442 |
| 33 | 37 | 1.68 | 95.0 | 4.9 | 1.383 | 1.619 |
| 34 | 27 | 1.22 | 96.3 | 3.6 | 1.425 | 1.796 |
| 35 | 22 | 1.00 | 97.3 | 2.6 | 1.467 | 1.973 |
| 36 | 19 | .86 | 98.1 | 1.8 | 1.509 | 2.150 |
| 37 | 8 | .36 | 98.5 | 1.4 | 1.551 | 2.327 |
| 38 | 6 | .27 | 98.8 | 1.1 | 1.592 | 2.504 |
| 39 | 5 | .22 | 99.0 | .9 | 1.634 | 2.681 |
| 40 | 6 | .27 | 99.3 | .6 | 1.676 | 2.858 |
| 41 | 4 | .18 | 99.4 | .5 | 1.718 | 3.035 |
| 42 | 4 | .18 | 99.6 | .3 | 1.760 | 3.212 |
| 43 | 3 | .13 | 99.8 | .1 | 1.802 | 3.389 |
| 44 | 2 | .09 | 99.9 | .0 | 1.844 | 3.566 |
| 45 | 1 | .04 | 99.9 | .0 | 1.886 | 3.743 |
| 46 | 1 | .04 | 100.0 | .0 | 1.928 | 3.920 |

REMAINING FREQUENCIES ARE ALL ZERO

beds be filled when an eighth patient arrived needing a bed.[11] Although a hospital might not wish to face this pressure nine times a year, it should be willing to provide temporary accommodations twice a year to save the cost of providing and staffing an eighth labor room bed. The need for delivery rooms, recovery room beds, and postpartum nursing unit beds can be analyzed in the same manner using the appropriate sections of the table. If the delivery rooms are planned so that they are adequate to meet the demand for service 99.9 percent of the time and the other units 99.5 percent of the time, it is concluded that a single OB service would require six labor room beds, three delivery rooms, four recovery room beds, and forty-two postpartum nursing unit beds to accommodate the expected 2,200 admissions in 1975.

Postpartum beds are sometimes handled less conservatively. An "overflow" is easy to spot twelve or twenty-four hours in advance, and it is usually a simple and safe matter to find a few healthy mothers who can be discharged a day early. If such a possibility were acceptable eighteen days a year—once every three weeks—the postpartum bed complement could be reduced to thirty-three. Doctors, nurses, and trustees might agree that this was too much restriction, but that a rate of once every six weeks was acceptable. Such a level is the equivalent of overflow one time in forty, or 2.5 percent of the time, and would require thirty-six beds. Obviously the final decision is subjective, depending on the cost of an overflow in terms of quality, convenience, and patient satisfaction. The simulation permits a reliable, factual exploration of the alternatives.

If the final decision were to be as indicated:

| *Facility* | *Required Size* | *Protection Level* | *Present Size* | *Reduction* |
|---|---|---|---|---|
| Labor | 6 | 99.5% | 12 | 6 |
| Delivery | 3 | 99.9 | 5 | 2 |
| Recovery | 4 | 99.8 | 0 | (4) |
| Postpartum | 36 | 97.5 | 50 | 14 |

a substantial facility reduction is possible. It should be noted that this does not automatically make the action desirable. The question of costs remains to be studied, and this is discussed in the following chapter. Hypothetically, however, the single unit solution is preferred.

## Summary

This chapter traced the steps of translating demand forecasts to facility requirements. Emphasis has been placed on the importance of separating the steps and dealing specifically with each one rather than relying on rules of thumb and conglomerate decisions. The five steps are:

1. Identify the facility units associated with the service.
2. Determine the service producing capacity of a single facility unit.
3. Determine the number of facility units required to accommodate the average demand for service.
4. Determine the number of additional facility units that must be available to accommodate emergency demands or peak loads based on the desired level of protection sought (the reserve or standby requirement).
5. Calculate the total number of facility units required and the load factor from the results of steps 3 and 4.

The sources of information for each step have been discussed and the procedures for calculating each component identified. It is notable that the service capacity is frequently much less than the technical capacity, and that load factors in actual practice are below maximums known to be practical. Increases in either of these elements are generally cheaper than new construction and may be cheaper than continued operation of multiple facilities.

The difference between the expected load factor and one of 100 percent is largely a matter of reserve or standby capacity. Several approaches to the estimation of standby capacity requirements have been presented—normative, empirical, mathematical, and simulation—and their relative merits discussed. It should be noted that most of these approaches yield relatively lower reserve requirements and higher load factors for larger facilities. The approaches listed here tend as a result to favor reductions in the numbers of facility units and the aggregation of service in fewer geographic locations. The results are not automatically desirable, however. Considerable further analysis is necessary to evaluate their implications in specific situations. The methods for that analysis are described in the following chapter.

## NOTES

[1]Karl Bartscht, et al., *Hospital Staffing Methodology: Radiology, Manual MM5.* Ann Arbor: Community Systems Foundation, 1968.

L. Shuman, et al., *Manual for Implementing Radiology Micro-Listing.* Pittsburgh: University of Pittsburgh, 1972.

The Chicago Hospital Council, *Clinical Laboratory Study Manual.* Chicago: The Council, 1968.

Committee on Laboratory Management and Planning, *A Workload Recording Method for Clinical Laboratories.* Tampa: College of American Pathologists.

[2]W. L. Dowling, "Linear Programming Approach to the Analysis of Hospital Production." Doctoral dissertation, The University of Michigan, 1971.

[3]R. Conrad, et al., "Utilization Study Saved Hospital from Needless Expansions of Radiology." *Hospital Financial Management,* September 1973.

[4]Larry K. MacDonald and Louis F. Reuter, IV, "A Patient-Specific Approach to Hospital Cost Accounting." *Health Services Research,* Vol. 8, No. 2, Summer 1973, p. 111.

[5]Capital costs can be equated to annual expenses by using an accounting depreciation schedule, or preferably by finding the equivalent discounted value of the investment. Techniques for doing this are described in Griffith, *Quantitative Techniques*, chapter 9 (see note 6), and in most finance books.

[6]John R. Griffith, *Quantitative Techniques for Hospital Planning and Control*. Lexington, MA: D. C. Heath & Co., 1972, chapter 3.

[7]In cases where the range of actual arrivals or demands around the expected mean is small, where there are few emergency patients, and/or where services for nonemergency or scheduled patients can easily be delayed to accommodate emergency patients, facility requirements can be planned as though the arrival patterns were deterministic. This greatly simplifies the planning problem. However, for many hospital services (CCUs, ICUs, ERs, OB units, being the most common examples), the random component of demand is so large and the need to service arrivals immediately so important that the stochastic nature of the demand process must be considered in planning.

[8]Herbert Arkin and Raymond R. Colton, *Tables for Statisticians*. New York: Barnes and Noble, Inc., 1963.

[9]See, for example, W. Shonick, "Understanding the Nature of Random Fluctuations of the Hospital Daily Census," *Medical Care*, Vol. X, No. 2, March-April 1972, pp. 118-142, which gives an excellent summary of this approach and its weaknesses, together with some alternatives to the Poisson assumption. In the Michigan State Plan for Hospital and Medical Facilities, ca. 1960, in the early years of Hill-Burton, the formula $ADC + Z\sqrt{ADC}$ was used with Z values as great as 4. When applied to a 100 daily census, 140 beds were required. The last ten would be necessary about once every eighty years!

[10]This method has been well described by John D. Thompson and Robert B. Fetter in various publications through the 1960s. See also Griffith, *Quantitative Techniques*, chapter 7, and O. Ray Hurst, Charles G. Richie, et al., "Simulation Tells What Really Will Be Needed," *Modern Hospital*, Vol. 122, No. 1, January 1974.

[11]Although this format is typical of simulation output, the labels are frequently arbitrary and the format varies. The authors have not attempted to explain this example because each specific example must be explained by its programmer or analyst.

# II.4

# Evaluating Shared Service Opportunities

*by John R. Griffith*

## Introduction

If the steps outlined in the preceding chapters of this section were followed in a specific community, the result would be forecasts of the demands for different kinds of hospital and health care services, decisions about the amounts of these demands to be met, analyses of the facility size required to meet the demand for each service, and statements of the expected load factors. This, however, falls well short of the total information necessary to decide on a specific array of facilities. The remaining questions are where and by which institutions the services will be provided. In a new, not previously existing community, one might solve this problem by the construction of a single health care facility or multiple facilities designed in a coordinated, integrated manner. Such an opportunity is rare. Thus the questions at hand are: Where will expansions and contractions of specific services occur within the array of presently operating facilities and services? When will additional locations for facilities be added to the existing array? Another way to state the question is, "Which of the existing services should be centralized and which decentralized and to what degree?"

It is immediately obvious that this problem is extremely complex and that one of the first requirements for its solution is a sound and reliable procedure to guide the analyst quickly towards a rational solution. The method presented below is directed to the selection of feasible alternatives, the identification of all issues relating to each feasible alternative, and their thorough evaluation. Insofar as possible, this evaluation will be unbiased, quantitative, and cast in economic terms.

Once the likely alternatives have been selected and analyzed, there are still substantial problems remaining, including both the final decisions for the array of services and the problems of implementation of the agreed-upon array. The method proposed does not eliminate either the debate necessary to reach the solution or the problem of implementation.[1] Rather, it is specifically designed to improve the equality of debate by measuring and describing as much of the situation as possible in uniform, factual terms.

It should be noted that the problem exists quite independent of the management structure of the community. If one organization owned all the hospitals serving the community, it would still be faced with the problem of optimizing the use of this array of facilities. The problem might be easier to solve because of the existence of the unified management, but the quantitative and technical requirements of the problem would remain the same. In the work which follows, the existence of a decision body representing the community interest and a reasonable process for the collection and expression of diverse views is assumed. This discussion addresses the technical content of evaluating the centralized versus decentralized service question; it assumes that there is a body, such as a well-organized comprehensive health planning agency or well-selected board of trustees, to which the findings can be presented for debate and discussion. In this we assume that the professionals providing care, the consumers, and the so-called community establishment all have an opportunity to comment and to understand the options presented. At certain points in the procedure, alternatives are explicitly referred to such bodies for evaluation in light of important but difficult to quantify community views. For many important elements of the decision, this will be the cheapest and most democratic way of obtaining the necessary information.

## Conceptual Framework

There is general agreement that substantial economies of scale can operate in enterprises such as hospitals. Thus there is an inherent economic pressure for aggregating hospital services into larger rather than smaller units. On the other hand, there are some frequently noted difficulties with larger service institutions. These include, particularly, the loss of human relationships important to patients' emotional well-being, the loss of efficiency in complex interactions of large teams of people, and the loss of local control of decisions.[2] There is an obvious tendency for larger hospitals to use whatever savings they have generated in ever more elaborate services for their community. While these might be desirable, they are not automatically so.

The arguments favoring economies of scale can be summarized according to three areas of interest—the operating cost, the capital cost, and the technical quality. In the operating cost area, it is noted that larger units have fewer staffing situations where one person of a given skill level is required regardless of demand; that they tend to have higher occupancy or load factors and thus higher utilization of personnel and lower standby allowances for personnel; that they achieve better purchasing advantages because of their size and better negotiating advantages with third parties; and that they offer the opportunity for more training and job specialization of personnel and specialization of equipment with the result that the personnel and equipment are more efficient. These, essentially, are the arguments of mass production translated to the health care field. The same extensions can be made with the capital costs. There will be higher load factors, less standby capital, and less investment in single facilities which may be necessary occasionally and which must therefore be provided regardless of demand.

Some of these arguments obviously are aimed both at reduction of cost and improvement of quality. It is argued that more job specialization yields a higher quality of performance in such areas as x-ray, laboratory, and surgical team procedures; that improved training programs increase the quality of performance; and that specialization in the overhead departments, purchasing, personnel, accounting, and general management, also increases the general quality of the operation at a given level of cost. It is argued, for example, that larger hospitals are able to pay for the services of trained personnel in the overhead areas whereas smaller hospitals cannot. Prescriptions such as a minimum of 2,000 births per year for an individual obstetrics service[3] are based as much on quality considerations as cost. There is a growing tendency to note these restrictions in the highly specialized clinical services such as kidney and heart transplants.[4]

The arguments against centralization are harder to illuminate and substantiate. They boil down to the comment that all this might be true theoretically, but it doesn't really happen, or doesn't happen with the uniformity that the theoretical arguments would imply. In fact, it does not. The data compiled by HAS (table II.4.1) indicate that while some service units in large hospitals are noticeably more efficient than in smaller ones, there are several large units (including the frequently cited labor and delivery rooms) which, in fact, are much more expensive.[5]

At the same time, say the opponents of centralization, technical quality isn't everything. The presence of exactly the right equipment or the best trained personnel does not make up for the lack of continuity in medical care, the distances traveled to reach the centralized facility, the loss of motivation that comes with the treatment of large masses of relatively unidentifiable people and the other unfortunate characteristics of a mass production society. These arguments are harder to substantiate. Table II.4.2 shows the perceived disadvantages of centralization as noted by people who managed the centralization of one or more hospitals' services. It is worthy of note that some respondents saw increased problems in communication costs, community support, morale, medical staff integration, and travel, and that increased management was perceived to be necessary.

The same respondents were more uniform in accepting the advantages of merger, although this may reflect their bias from involvement in the in-

**TABLE II.4.1**
Comparison of departmental labor productivity 50–75 and 300–399 bed hospitals

| | *50–75 beds* | *300–399 beds* | *Percent Increase in Productivity* |
|---|---|---|---|
| Laundry (pounds per manhour) | 24.4 | 39.6 | 62.0 |
| Dietary (meals per MH) | 2.6 | 3.3 | 26.4 |
| Central Supply (line items per MH) | 3.5 | 4.3 | 25.2 |
| Pharmacy (line items per MH) | 9.6 | 11.5 | 19.2 |
| Social Service (MH per case) | 6.6 | 5.8 | 12.9 |
| Nursing Service (MH per patient day) | 6.7 | 5.9 | 11.5 |
| Medical Records (MH per discharge) | 2.3 | 2.2 | 6.9 |
| Housekeeping (MH per 1,000 sq. ft.) | 45.5 | 44.2 | 3.0 |
| Laboratory (tests per MH) | 3.9 | 4.0 | 2.3 |
| | | | *Percent Decrease in Productivity* |
| Physical Therapy (treatments per MH) | 1.4 | 1.3 | 9.4 |
| Operating Rooms (MH per visit) | 9.1 | 10.4 | 14.4 |
| Radiology (MH per procedure) | 1.0 | 1.3 | 25.2 |
| Blood Bank (MH per unit drawn) | 1.4 | 2.7 | 97.1 |
| OPD (MH per visit) | .7 | 1.5 | 108.5 |
| ER (MH per visit) | .7 | 1.6 | 120.8 |
| Delivery and Labor Rooms (MH per delivery) | 5.6 | 17.5 | 210.3 |

Source: Hospital Administrative Services, The American Hospital Association, September–November 1971.

itial decision. Table II.4.3 shows agreement with many of the economies of scale arguments. Some of the perceived advantages are potential disadvantages as well. The possibility of providing "many more specialized services" and of obtaining "more independence in the planning function" can be cited as steps away from community control. That is, once a large enterprise has been established, it takes on a life of its own and tends to pursue its own goals rather than those of the community at large.

On balance, the trend seems to favor the growth of further centralization. Holper, in his administrative review of shared and consolidated services for the American Hospital Association in 1973, noted the trend as continuing and extending to more clinical services.[6] Given the general trend towards more centralization, but the existence of strong negative

**TABLE II.4.2**
Possible disadvantages of mergers

| *Description of Disadvantage* | *Percentage of Respondents Agreeing to the Idea That These Represent Real Problems After Merger* |
|---|---|
| 1. Affiliation agreement could have solved the existing problems with greater care | 6% |
| 2. Employee layoffs occurred | 7% |
| 3. Higher cost result due to the need for expanded managerial staff | 16% |
| 4. More traveling by hospital personnel and patients to come to the hospital | 30% |
| 5. Problems of low morale among one or all of the employee groups | 33% |
| 6. Problems of integrating the medical staffs due to long-standing ties within each of the premerged hospitals | 42% |
| 7. Communication costs rose within the organization (e.g., telephone, intercom) | 55% |
| 8. Problems in trying to rally the former auxiliaries and other community supporters | 59% |

Source: Weil, Peter Allan, "An Investigation of Preconditions and Effects of Mergers Among Hospitals in the United States as Perceived by Hospital Administrators." Master's thesis, Graduate College of the University of Iowa, June 1969, pages 192–193.

arguments, the wise community will select carefully and develop over a period of time a strategy for integration of services as the opportunities for maximal gain occur.

The remainder of this chapter will present and discuss a technical procedure in some depth with comments drawn from the experience of the Bureau of Hospital Administration in applying the procedure to several Michigan communities. Following that, there will be a specific presentation of two cases of interest, the Jackson County obstetrics case and the Bay City hospital merger analysis, and a summary discussion.

**TABLE II.4.3**
Postmerger advantages

| *Description of Advantage* | *Percentage of Respondents Agreeing to the Existence of the Advantage after Merger* |
|---|---|
| 1. Administrative economy through organizational consolidation (e.g., planning, managing) | 94% |
| 2. Economics through physical consolidation—combining departments like clinical services | 91% |
| 3. Many more specialized services can be provided | 91% |
| 4. Improved educational program | 89% |
| 5. More capital available for expansion and/or modernization | 82% |
| 6. Improved position with respect to recruitment of house staff | 82% |
| 7. Physicians may devote more time to patient care by saving travel time | 72% |
| 8. Stronger bargaining position in relating to third party payers | 63% |
| 9. Easing of manpower shortages | 58% |
| 10. More independence in planning function (less restricting governmental intervention or greater cooperation from areawide planning agency) | 40% |

Source: Weil, Peter Allan, "Preconditions and Effects of Mergers Among Hospitals," pp. 191–192.

## A Method For Evaluating Alternatives For The Provision Of Service

The business cycle of health care is that services are translated by the providers into costs which form the basis of revenues which are in turn a major component of the insurance premium which when paid by the customer provides for the services. One of the technical questions in the design of a method to evaluate alternatives for providers is the selection of the point of measurement. The authors strongly favor the selection of costs which would be incurred as a result of pursuing the alternative. Costs may be either tangible, that is, evaluated in dollar terms, or intangible. Cost reductions or benefits may be counted when connected with a specific alternative, but not income changes. This approach attempts to minimize double counting, speculative and unattainable savings, overemphasis on tangible costs, and the artificialities introduced by various methods of reimbursement of hospitals. In the application of the method, an effort will be made to subdivide the various costs of an alternative into elements. If all cost elements could be measured in dollar terms, then the total cost of each alternative could be calculated and the least costly selected. Where some elements remain intangible, they can be described in comparable terms and evaluated subjectively. In such cases this approach will yield a direct dollar comparison between the tangible costs of each of the alternatives. The value attributable to the intangible items can then be discussed in comparison to the difference between the tangible dollar values.

The method can be stated in four steps, of which two are essentially data gathering and analysis steps and two are decision making steps:

1. Review the feasibility and approximate costs of the alternative. Identify the cost elements which are likely to dominate the final cost. Identify special conditions which impact on feasibility such as interrelation with other projects which may be necessary to release space or other particularly difficult resources. Identify the nature of major opportunity costs which are involved in the adoption of the alternative.
2. Decide on the set of alternatives which are feasible and which include the most attractive alternatives for further investigation and development.
3. Conduct a detailed review and evaluation of the cost elements for each of the selected alternatives.
4. Present the results of the detailed analysis to the decision bodies and establish final evaluation and decisions.

It should be noted that the likely outcomes of the process are not single decisions but rather multiple sets of decisions which inevitably become intertwined and which are maintained over a period of years as part of the long-range plan. The typical decisions from a set of alternatives might be to abandon some; to defer others to incorporate with future activities, particularly the development of other proposals which change the opportunity costs and related services costs; to defer an alternative for a specific future event such as the obsolesence of a building; and finally, to implement one or more of the alternatives under study. A community which has been conscientious in its planning is likely, therefore, to have before it several propositions in differing stages of evaluation and adoption. Rather than a simple program for immediate action, it will develop a strategy of several different conditional alternatives which it plans to implement over the next five to ten years.

## Review of Feasibility and Conditions

Given the large number of possible arrangements which can potentially be used to meet a given demand in most communities, the first step has to be some reasonable search for the elimination of infeasible arrangements and the identification of the more desirable. This is, however, a dangerous step because it is so easy to claim infeasibility in defense of a special interest. Here as elsewhere in the data collection, the best protection is a neutral party collecting the data. Frequently, an arrangement can be made feasible by attaching it to certain other activities which may have values of their own. The combinations which make an alternative feasible must be incorporated into the analysis. It is better to state the situation or condition which would make an alternative feasible and to evaluate both the desirability of that condition and of the combination than it is to dismiss the alternative as infeasible.

Step one should contain a statement of all theoretical possibilities, the conditions necessary for the feasibility of each, a review of the feasibility of the conditions themselves, and a recommended rank order of the alternatives from the most feasible down to the obviously infeasible. This method is reasonably safe against both oversight and bias. The review of all theoretical possibilities can be audited by another analyst or member of the policy making committee. The emphasis on conditions for feasibility presents each possibility in its most favorable light and tends to eliminate the possibility of bias in ruling out given alternatives.

A second and closely related purpose of the initial review is the identification of dominant or unique cost elements. It is frequently the case that most alternatives are relatively similar in many cost elements. For example, the cost of operating a delivery suite will be essentially the same over a number of different locations and even over a fairly wide range of patient activity. On the other hand, a hospital which does not now have an adequate suite will face those operating costs plus a capital investment which will increase its total cost for the provision of obstetrical services by a large amount. These major component differences in the alternatives may be used in rank ordering the feasibility. Obviously, if two hospitals face costs which are different by large magnitudes, one does not need to investigate with great precision to rank order the alternatives in favor of the lesser cost ones. The information may also be used to guide further investigation. When the operating costs between two desirable alternatives may not differ very much but the capital costs may differ substantially, the force of the investigation in step three will go primarily toward evaluation of the capital cost. The major or dominant cost elements in the final decision are frequently related to the conditions of feasibility. In fact, the large or unique investments and expenses are likely to be the costs of the conditions themselves.

## The Initial Decision

The actual process of selecting alternatives for further investigation is not the subject of this discussion, but it should be noted that this process is a decision and one which has important policy considerations. Certain projects will be dropped as infeasible or unpromising, others will be accepted for further investigation, and with these decisions may come implicit commitments to a variety of conditions which had been attached to the initial alternatives. Decisions at this level should be subject to the same sort of policy making review as the final decisions. That is, they should be reviewed by the top policy making body of the organization.

## Detailed Evaluation of Cost Components

This step requires the identification and measurement of as many as possible of the additional direct expenditures which will be incurred in the implementation of the given alternative. The costs, however, have been subdivided into a number of elements to encourage comprehensive review and unbiased evaluation. These elements range from explicit, relatively easily measured accounting costs to implicit and difficult-to-measure opportunity costs and intangibles. While theoretical or research oriented measures of a given cost element may exist, such as the technical quality of care, it may be more practical and preferable in planning situations to treat that cost as an intangible. The elements are capital costs, operating costs, costs of changes in related operations, opportunity costs, and several kinds of intangible costs. These are discussed in detail below.

### Capital Costs

These are all the costs of construction, renovation, and additional equipment. They should be broadened to include one-time costs such as temporary facilities, training programs, and similar items which are part of the start-up for a given alternative. For major proposals, it is desirable to have these costs estimated by architects and purchasing agents, and to estimate the applicable interest rate either in loan costs or loss of investment revenue. Construction codes and licensure requirements with detailed specifications frequently require a careful analysis of the capital costs, particularly in renovation and replacement. The cost of capital should not include any evaluation of capital already in place, that is, buildings, equipment, and land already owned. These capital costs are "sunk," and potentially serious distortions result from incorporating them into the comparison of alternatives. A method of dealing with the value of these facilities in place will be discussed under opportunity costs below.

Capital costs by definition are single time expenditures which are useful for many years in the future. Most of the other costs to be discussed in the evaluation are recurring in nature. It is necessary to translate these two costs to a common base by some method. Present value methods for doing this, involving assumptions about the likely interest rate, are presented in *Quantitative Techniques for Hospital Planning and Control* and finance texts.[7] These methods equate annual expenditure expectations to single-time capital expenditures at given interest rates and expected life. The conventional straight line accounting depreciation, which divides the capital expenditure by its expected life, implies an interest rate of zero percent. This is probably the most unreasonable interest assumption which can be made, and, therefore, present value methods are to be preferred.[8] The analyst has a choice between translating the capital to annual rates or vice versa. It appears that the decisions are most easily presented to and handled by lay and mixed lay and professional groups if the capital costs are translated to annual rates.

The treatment of depreciation, or capital recovery, is clear under this procedure. If the capital cost is expressed in terms of the debt service charge which results from borrowing the capital (either from internal endowments or from external sources) at a specified interest rate, other estimates of capital cost such as straight line accounting depreciation must be excluded from the cost calculation. The debt service charge includes an annual payment for capital which repays the entire initial investment over the life of the project. At the end of the project the original capital facilities and equipment are worn out or obsolete and the indebtedness is repaid. The institution may then evaluate the continuation of the project by reapplication of the same method. More funds may be borrowed to continue the activity, if justified. If the analysis is conducted this way, not only the consumption of capital (estimated by accounting depreciation) but also the opportunity cost of capital (the interest paid) is included in the total cost estimate.[9]

### Operating Costs

The operating cost of a proposal is an estimate of the annual cost of all of the manpower, supplies, leased equipment, and contract services involved in the ongoing operation of a service. It explicitly excludes overhead and other costs which would be incurred even if the service was not offered, but it may be adjusted for additional costs incurred in other departments.

Operating cost data can be obtained from accounting data and special studies of the existing situations, from similar situations elsewhere, and from standards developed by engineers and others. Combinations of approaches are frequently necessary. Data from present situations must be adjusted for future conditions, reflecting changes in size, location, revised capital equipment, and other factors. For alternatives which are radically different from the data sources, simulation models may be required. The best estimates of trained professionals familiar with situations resembling the proposed alternative can also be used. In Jackson, for example, there was no combined large obstetric service. To estimate operating cost, the directors of nurses of the two hospitals were asked independently what staffing they would require for the centralized service of the combined size. This method could have been improved by finding still a third institution in the southeast Michigan area which operated at the proposed size, reviewing its actual staffing and expenditure patterns, and obtaining estimates from its managers.

With so many alternative ways to estimate cost, one of the problems becomes the selection of the correct alternative. It is possible to become very precise with the investment of large quantities of time in data collection, analysis, and construction of hypothetical future situations. On the other hand, the specificity of the forecasts of the future situation is likely not to be precise. The actual operating conditions are not known. New technical innovations may influence future operating costs. Finally, it is not likely that major decisions will hinge on narrow distinctions between the operating costs of two alternatives. An alternative is rarely selected over another because of a small operating cost advantage. It is much more likely to be selected for reasons such as the other requires a capital investment and it does not, or the other has a substantial opportunity cost attached to it. The need for precision in the operating cost estimate is thus rarely as great as the available technical methods for estimating. It is important to avoid unnecessary precision because of the cost and time involved in preparing these estimates.

### Impact Upon Other Departments

It is rare that centralization of a given service will affect only that service. There are usually related changes which must be made in other services or departments. These are divided into two groups. One is the so-called overhead departments, such as administration and plant services. The second group is the other medical services. Costs in either group can be positive or negative. (The removal of a service may justify a reduction in expenditures in another service or department.) The general rule in estimating the costs of these adjustments on other departments or services is to avoid tangible estimates unless explicit plans are developed. Extensions of average unit costs (e.g.,10,000 square feet of new space to be cleaned, at $2.00 per square foot) should be avoided or at least carefully reviewed. Specific budgets (two additional janitors, one floor machine, $1,000 per year for supplies) are less likely to be biased. Particularly when responsibilities are reduced, the average cost savings may never be realized. A good procedure calls for a systematic review of the overhead departments with the question, "What additions or reductions in resources will be required in this department after the centralization or decentralization of the service?"

The impact of centralization or decentralization on other medical services is approached similarly to the overhead question. Special studies of the volume of service rendered by certain ancillary services are frequently necessary. The quantities of services involved usually must be studied by a special data collection endeavor. In the Jackson obstetrics merger study, estimates of laboratory and x-ray usage by obstetrical patients were obtained. It was found that these were only a modest portion of the total and the impact could be ignored. There are two considerations involved in this decision. The first is the absolute size of the demand on related services, and second is the changes in resources of the related services which are necessary to meet this demand. When a department is operating below its desired load factor, an increase in demand can often be handled at a low or even negligible price increase. When a department is at capacity, a modest increase may trigger a costly expansion. If the cost of this expansion is of value only for the proposed alternative, it may be extremely burdensome. The only method to estimate these costs is a set of ad hoc reviews of the impact: first a qualitative assessment, second a quantitative forecast of volume, and third an assessment of actual resource requirement changes and their costs. All such costs, positive or negative, must be entered into the statement of the costs of the alternative.

Closely related to this question is the question of certain necessary residual services. The centralization of laboratories is frequently contemplated using transport systems to remote institutions. Such a centralization is quite feasible given that certain kinds of emergency laboratory services are provided in the decentralized sites. The costs of providing these decentralized services must, of course, be included in the costs of the alternative. In all such estimations, attention must be paid to feasibility. Thus, the centralization of x-ray services is frequently viewed as infeasible because it would involve the transportation of patients from remote sites.

## OPPORTUNITY COSTS

An opportunity cost is a cost incurred when a unique physical resource is consumed for one purpose and thus made unavailable for another. For example, suppose that the service in question is a centralized laundry. A piece of ground on which a new centralized laundry can be constructed is owned by one of the nonprofit institutions, and no other use for the land has been proposed. The purchase price of the land was not included in pricing the capital costs of the laundry. There it was noted that all resources already purchased were "sunk," and their additional cost was zero. However, it is known that the land could be sold, and its sale price is $100,000. (Considerable effort is necessary, obviously, to make sure that the sale price is a realistic one. The best proof is a firm offer at $100,000.) Then, the opportunity cost of using the land for the laundry is the $100,000 revenue foregone by that decision. If there is no market for the piece of land, or no alternative use, the opportunity cost is zero.

This distinction may, at first glance, appear unnecessarily complex. However, the value of an asset or resource is frequently different at different periods of time and for different owners. In certain situations an opportunity cost substantially higher than any market price would be incurred. Suppose, for example, that the land proposed for the laundry was also useful for an ambulatory care program which was strongly desired by the community. Then, if the land were used for a laundry, an alternative site would have to be found for the ambulatory care program. The alternative site might be substantially more expensive to own or to operate because of its inferior location. If that increased expense could be quantified, it would be the opportunity cost of that placement of the laundry. If it could not be quantified, which would often be the case when dealing with such elements as location, it would have to be treated as an intangible. In all these cases,—sale of asset, quantifiable alternative use, and intangible alternative use—the opportunity cost is quite different from the purchase price or the book value of the asset.

The measurement of opportunity costs is troublesome at best. It is wise to proceed conservatively, taking only firm offers or explicit decisions as a basis for opportunity costs. Where these are lacking because the alternative opportunities have not been fully developed, or because the market has not been tested, it is best to treat opportunity costs as intangible costs of the appropriate alternative.

Despite the measurement difficulties, opportunity costs can frequently be very large and can trigger action at a specific point in time or can cause deferment or abandonment of an alternative. Thus the case for prompt centralization of a service might depend upon the existence of alternative uses for the space freed in one or more of the decentralized units. Without this savings there might be no sound cost justification for the centralization. Large sums are involved because at today's land and construction prices, even a modest service such as obstetrics can free valuable space to be devoted to other activities.

Like capital costs, opportunity costs are usually one-time expenses which must be translated to annual rates over the project life. The same form of translation, the equivalent annual expense to the present value, can be used.

## The Evaluation of Intangibles

Intangibles are by definition all those elements of value which enter into a decision and which are difficult to state in economic terms. They include a number of aspects which can be quantified under some circumstances, at least to the extent of the number of people affected, or the extent of the impact. It will be impractical, however, to state this impact in dollar values. In some cases, no quantification of any kind will be possible. Any of the preceding elements can be intangible although they should be, and usually will be, tangible.

Intangibles should be stated as clearly and precisely as possible, including estimates of the number of people affected and precise definition of the impact. A statement such as "access is difficult for the ten thousand people living west of the river" is much preferable to a vague one which says access is not as good. In a given situation, the intangibles can be either positive or negative. Both will frequently occur. The eventual aim will be for each member of the policy making body to evaluate in his own mind the total value of all the intangibles taken together. As much specificity as possible will help each policy maker and improve the debate.

The important areas of intangible considerations reflected in the prior work of the Bureau are as follows:

1. **Quality**—This includes all aspects of the centralization question which impact on the quality of medical care and frequently includes considerations on both sides. The technical aspects of quality are likely to be favored by centralization whereas the attitudinal aspects of quality are believed to be favored by decentralized operations. While the impact upon quality may sometimes be specified in terms of the improved outcomes or better performance on such issues as utilization control, even this step is frequently impractical. The translation of estimates of these kinds to dollar values so that they can be treated in the equation is fraught with expense and difficult assumptions.

2. **Uncertainty**—Whenever a capital investment is made, there is some uncertainty that it will not yield the anticipated results. This is a combination of the uncertainties and risks involved in all the component forecasts. It is impossible to quantify uncertainty although various projects can be compared as to uncertainty because most decision makers will have a subjective sense of the uncertainty involved.

**3. Liquidity**—Closely related to the question of uncertainty is the intangible of the desirability of retaining a cash position or a liquid position. The value of such a position is reflected by its earnings from investment in liquid assets such as stocks, bonds, notes, and bank accounts. Nonliquid investments are those which cannot easily be sold. Health care facilities are often very permanent, and not liquid at all. A policy making body may defer a nonliquid investment on the grounds that it does not earn as much overall return as retaining the money in the bank, when it is adjusted for uncertainty and other intangibles. Such a decision is a decision for liquidity. An important justification for liquidity lies in the possibility that there are other alternatives which still have not been expressed or understood. Thus, one might pass up a centralization alternative showing only modest yield and limited opportunity cost savings on the proposition that a proposal making better use of the resources freed by centralization could be developed if further time were spent in exploration. A high liquidity preference is thus reflected in a slow rate of adoption of proposals. It is often associated with a high sensitivity to the uncertainties of change.

**4. Control**—Another intangible element which is very difficult to assess in any but a purely judgmental framework is the question of who controls the resources under the alternative in question. It may be better to retain decentralization if it facilitates domination by the special interest group to which one is personally attached. Thus, if one favors the further development of osteopathy, one favors the existence of osteopathic hospitals rather than centralized management of hospitals, because it permits better control by the interests with whom one agrees. There are many complex ramifications of this intangible. A centralized situation may actually favor domination by a special interest group, or on the other hand it might facilitate the development of a broad range of community representation. Religious-owned institutions, special medical groups, proprietary hospitals, and similar situations introduce the intangible of control in an important manner into all centralization and merger decisions.

**5. Access**—Closely tied to the control question is the question of access to hospitals and related institutions. It refers both to the access for various consumer groups in the population and also to access by various medical groups. Thus, the access of osteopaths and general practitioners to institutions is an important intangible. Control of a facility or resource is a way to insure access, but sometimes access can be insured by less drastic measures. It may be infeasible to gain centralization unless the access question is handled equitably. Lingering doubts about the success of this arrangement would be reflected in the access intangible.

**6. Amenities**—There are, in most communities, a number of problems having to do with architecture, location, traditions of service, and convenience which influence people's judgments. Hopefully, these are of little importance in a major centralization question, although they may not be. In considering the centralization of a service at a city-owned or governmental institution which has had the reputation of a charity institution, there may be substantial negative reaction because the facilities are not as convenient, because of ethnic or economic integration, or because the service is perceived as "charity."

**7. Equity**—There is a feeling that a nonprofit institution such as a hospital has certain ownership rights and prerogatives. This is frequently expressed in mergers and centralization arguments as a quid pro quo statement. Thus, if Hospital A is to have the centralized obstetrical service, Hospital B will have the centralized cardiology service. The question of equity in health care facilities is difficult to handle because it has no apparent legal basis. It is explicit in the law of nonprofit corporations that there will be no equity which accrues to any individual or group of individuals. Thus, when a board of directors or a group of concerned citizens steps forward and says something about "our hospital," it is not legally their hospital, and they have no legal foundation for this proprietary expression. Implicitly and politically, the situation may not be so simple. There are long histories in some communities of contribution of time, money, and other items of value to a specific institution, and at the very least these contributions may be lost if the charitable proprietorship concept is lost. In Table II.4.3 above, the loss of support of volunteers was noted by some of the institutions responding. How much weight is to be put on these allegiances and beliefs is a matter for local community decision. Like the control issue, it is necessarily a policy decision and one which cannot be made by a staff.

## The Final Review

Each of the alternatives agreed upon in step two should be presented to the board with detailed summary of the various tangible and intangible costs connected with it. These should be presented in terms of the cost element showing the annual dollar values, the lump-sum dollar values involved in the capital and opportunity costs, and the statements describing the intangibles. A project can be summarized as having two costs, an annual dollar cost and an unmeasured intangibles cost. For two hypothetical proposals, these costs can be stated as follows:

**Costs of proposal A** $= \mathbf{X_A + I_A}$ (1a)

Where $X_A$ = Dollar costs at annual rates

$I_A$ = Intangibles

**Costs of proposal B** $= \mathbf{X_B + I_B}$ (1b)

If one were to say that one was indifferent between proposal A and proposal B then it would be mathematically true that:

$$X_A + I_A = X_B + I_B \qquad (2)$$

This, however, is the same as saying that:

$$I_A - I_B = X_B - X_A \qquad (3)$$

or that the net difference in the intangibles is exactly equal to the difference in the tangible costs. Thus, a statement of equal preference between two alternatives implicitly prices the total set of intangibles in dollar terms. The dollar values assigned to these intangibles may be compared against other proposals and other alternatives which would yield the same kinds of intangible results to improve the consistency of policy decisions.

Intangibles are implicitly priced even if one proposal is selected over another. Consider that a decision is made in favor of proposal A even though its tangible costs may be higher than those of proposal B. This is stating that the total cost of proposal A is less than the total cost of proposal B or:

$$X_A + I_A < X_B + I_B \qquad (4)$$

This, mathematically, is the same as saying that the difference in dollar cost is less than the difference in intangible cost:

$$X_A - X_B < I_B - I_A \qquad (5)$$

Again, the intangibles have been implicitly priced, although this time the price is less complete and states only that the net cost of the intangibles of B over A would exceed the tangible cost difference.

The complexity of the approach outlined here is such that only major, expensive consolidations are likely to be carried through in this formal manner. Thus, the dollar values expressed under $X_A$ and $X_B$ are likely to be quite large. The difference will also be large in situations where action is seriously considered. Small dollar values are easily outweighed by the intangibles, particularly those of uncertainty, and tend not to get very serious consideration. The differences in the tangible costs become large principally when the capital costs, impact on other departments, and opportunity costs enter into the alternatives in very different ways. When one alternative incurs a large capital expenditure and the other does not, when one takes advantage of certain opportunities and impacts upon related departments and the other does not, and in similar situations, the tangible cost differences become quite large. It becomes increasingly difficult for defenders of intangibles to justify their arguments that the intangible costs exceed the tangible costs. On the other hand, it becomes easier to make adjustments in the cost differences to try to overcome some of the deficiencies the opponents attribute to intangibles. Thus, if control is a critical intangible, a larger board of directors or a different board structure can be contemplated. If access is a difficulty then additional investment in improving access can be made. The large dollar savings available will be tempting for expenditures and compromises of this sort.

Often an alternative will turn out to have little immediate merit because it incurs heavy capital costs for modest results, but it can be shown that under other circumstances such as when competing alternatives face capital expenditures or when certain opportunities for cost savings can be attached to the proposal, its value becomes much greater. Situations of this kind lead to the deferring of alternatives contingent upon certain developments. These may occur either naturally, such as the aging and depreciation of existing plant, or by further development of interrelated alternatives to capture opportunity cost savings.

The next section presents two applications of the method as carried out by the Bureau of Hospital Administration for local community planning groups in 1973.

## Two Case Studies

### The Jackson Obstetrics Merger[10]

Setting: Jackson County, Michigan. The obstetrics service area, the forecast of 2,200 births, and the estimated merged facility requirements of:

| | |
|---|---|
| Labor beds | 7 |
| Delivery rooms | 3 |
| Recovery beds | 4 |
| Postpartum beds | 42 |

have been discussed in the preceding chapters. The county is served by three hospitals. Two have essentially the same medical staff and collaborated on this study through a joint committee. The third is osteopathic and is forecast to have about 200 births per year. (Since the actual identification of these hospitals is irrelevant to the illustration, they will be designated as Memorial, Church, and Osteopathic.) Memorial was the largest hospital. It had traditionally operated the county's only school of nursing, and emergency care for all three hospitals was centralized there two years before this study. The religious nature of Church Hospital was an important intangible. So was the historic split between traditional medicine and osteopathy. Finally, it should be noted that all six M.D. obstetricians initiated the study by requesting immediate merger.

#### Alternatives

The various merger combinations considered were:

(1) Status quo: three units continue operation
(2) Merge at Memorial
(3) Merge at Church
(4) Merge at Osteopathic
(5) Merge at Memorial and Osteopathic
(6) Merge at Church and Osteopathic
(7) Merge at Memorial and Church
(8) Alternatives involving obstetrics mergers and other mergers (e.g., obstetrics at Memorial, pediatrics at Church)

## Initial Review of Alternatives

It immediately became clear that inclusion of Osteopathic Hospital would attract substantial opposition. Only the M.D. obstetricians favored it. The Bureau pointed out that there were considerable costs in unnecessary expense and reduced technical quality of care in continuing a unit with only 200 births per year. That was conceded by the committee, but not felt to be sufficient to change any position. Thus alternatives (2), (3), (4), and (7) were dropped as politically infeasible.

Alternative (8) received considerable attention because of Memorial's dominant "equity" position. The "equity" intangible was particularly strongly felt, because the "control" intangible—the religious issue over sterilizations—had already been noted and many people were certain that alternative (5) was likely to be the final outcome. That would mean that both emergency and obstetrics were centralized at Memorial. The only available service to offer Church Hospital for equity reasons was pediatrics. The pediatricians immediately complained, noting both the quality impact and their personal difficulties from having pediatric care split into two locations for newborn and non-newborn. It was noted that even the pediatric merger would require much additional effort and delay the completion of the study. Any other equity exchange was so far from consideration that it was not even clear where to begin. (Administrators and doctors were asked to suggest opportunities; none did.) Alternative (8) was therefore deferred with the agreement that it would be reconsidered before any decision was implemented.

This action left three alternatives:

(1) Status quo

(2) Merge at Memorial (and Osteopathic)

(3) Merge at Church (and Osteopathic)

(Since Osteopathic Hospital had been dropped from consideration, it could be ignored in all three alternatives.) Initial investigations revealed that capital investment would be necessary for either (2) or (3) but not for (1), and that either (2) or (3) was feasible with investment in renovation. No significant contingencies or opportunity costs were noted. The space freed by merger at either Memorial or Church would apparently remain idle, except as necessary to replace medical-surgical beds lost in obstetrics expansion at the other institution.

## Summary of Costs

**Capital Costs**—An architect was hired to prepare cost estimates for alternatives (2) and (3). He reported in summary:

> Program should require about 21,000 square feet. This is about the area available at [Church] Hospital on one floor. [Memorial] Hospital has about 1,000 square feet of surplus area and is planning an addition which may

affect maternity services on this floor or the desired isolation of maternity services.

The enlarged Obstetrical Department as planned and programmed necessitates a reduction of beds on the floor of 11 beds at [Church] and 23 beds at [Memorial]. Conversely, the removal of the department could add about 30 general service beds to [Church] and about 25 to [Memorial] Hospital.

Cost estimates indicate that the move could be made for about $750,000 at [Church] and $850,000 at [Memorial].

Both hospitals have a required internal stair problem that affects existing specifications for the whole structure and a permanent correction should be negotiated with the State Fire Marshal.

Considering cost, use of space, adjacency of services, we recommend that the consolidation be made at [Church] Hospital.[11]

The important element of this report was the unexpectedly high capital costs at both hospitals. This was caused by steady upgrading of the new construction elements of the fire, safety, and licensure codes. Although Church Hospital had a relatively new building, the code requirements for individual room toilets, improved air conditioning, and stair tower access had changed since initial construction. Any renovation would have to include bringing the entire unit, not just the expansion, to new construction standards. On the other hand, the present unit could be operated for a period of time without revision, because the code provisions are not automatically retroactive. The hospitals would be forced to upgrade the facilities, but much of this would probably be at least a decade away. It appeared that $100,000 to $300,000 would soon be necessary without a renovation. The cost of merger alone would be about $600,000 with the difference at each hospital attributed to upgrading. Assuming a twenty-year life and six percent interest, this is equivalent to $52,300 per year.[12]

The architect's report included several quality and amenity specifics favoring the Church Hospital alternative:

- It did not commit excess space to obstetrics.
- It permitted the nursery to be located in a cul-de-sac rather than on a traffic corridor.
- The father's waiting room was better located.

The different availability of medical-surgical or other beds cited by the architect was of no value. It was agreed that these beds were surplus.

**Operating Costs**—It was noted that medical fees, supplies, and other nonsalary costs were likely to be almost the same under either merged situation as under the status quo. These items could be dropped from consideration, leaving staffing salaries as the determining operating cost. The status quo alternative was evaluated based on actual staffing and salaries. The data showed that the average staffing per patient was higher at Church. The merged alternatives were evaluated by asking each director of nursing to propose a staffing pattern for the merged service at his or her hospital. The volume forecasts and schematics of the suite were supplied to aid them in these decisions. The estimates were made independently, and for different units. The results of these investigations are shown in Table II.4.4.[13]

**TABLE II.4.4**

Current and consolidated OB units nurse staffing costs

| *Current Units*** | *FTE Personnel/Day* | *$/Day** | *$/Year** | *Cost Savings* |
|---|---|---|---|---|
| Memorial | 28.4 | $ 828.00 | $302,000 | |
| Church | 29.0 | 860.00 | 314,000 | |
| Total | 54.7 | $1,688.00 | $616,000 | |
| *Consolidated Unit**** | | | | |
| Memorial | 48 | $1,398.00 | $510,000 | $106,000 |
| Church | 45 | $1,371.00 | $500,000 | $116,000 |

* 1972 salary and including fringe benefit levels.
** Based on present staffing levels for a typical day.
*** Based on desired staffing levels for consolidated unit.

The variations in both FTEs per day and cost per FTE can be taken either as changes which would reflect the differing locations or as measures of error or lack of precision in the results. Because there was no ready explanation, the Bureau chose to take them as error measures. The cost of the merged unit was assumed to be independent of location and cheaper than the status quo by about $110,000 per year at 1972 prices.

**Costs Incurred in Related Departments**—The centralization would result in changes in patient day volume of about ten percent. Neither administration felt that any tangible changes would result in overhead departments. (Partly this reflected the assumption that medical-surgical patients would occupy some or all of the vacated beds, because the expansion of obstetrics would reduce the medical-surgical complement at the other hospital)

Impact on other service departments was estimated by a study of accounts receivable for obstetrics patients. Data were collected in this study for the revenue implications, which must be treated as a "liquidity" intangible in this method. The information is shown in table II.4.5.[14]

Each department head was consulted about the capital, manpower, and supplies costs necessary to accommodate changes of these magnitudes. No department head felt the changes would affect operating expenditures

**TABLE II.4.5**
Percentage of workload attributable to OB service

| | *Memorial* | *Church* |
|---|---|---|
| Discharges*—delivered | 10.0% | 14.9% |
| —total | 12.7% | 15.9% |
| Patient days—total | 6.5% | 9.6% |
| Central supply | 4.8% | 6.2% |
| Laboratory | 6.4% | 8.3% |
| Pharmacy | 7.0% | 8.8% |
| Radiology | 1.5% | 1.8% |

* Not including newborn

enough to be predictable. (Again, the answer is contingent upon other adjustments.)

**Opportunity Costs**—The same survey of administration and department heads was used to identify potential uses of the available space or special problems likely to arise from merger. (The capital costs of expansion of related departments might have been treated as opportunity costs if any had been noted. This would have been particularly true if contingent cost reductions and service improvements would have accompanied the expansion.) None was noted, either favorable or unfavorable.

**Intangibles**—A special survey of the obstetricians, general practitioners with sizable obstetric practices, and some pediatricians was conducted using a formal protocol and a forty-five minute interview with each. Considerable data resulted, indicating the physicians' emphasis on the quality, control, and equity intangibles. From the report:

> To summarize the findings of the interviews, all of the physicians interviewed feel that the advantages of a consolidated OB service outweigh the disadvantages. Most feel that a larger, more active, higher volume, OB service would result in higher quality medical and nursing care. . . . In addition, most of the physicians mentioned the favorable impact on quality of specialized services, such as anesthesia coverage, fetal cardiac monitoring, or recovery services, which are not available in either hospital but which could be supported by a larger OB service. Although all of the physicians interviewed feel that a consolidated unit would be desirable, they differ in their opinions about how to move toward this objective in the face of two critical issues: (1) the issue of sterilization policies, and (2) the issue of the continued viability of or balance of services between the two hospitals. The overwhelming majority of the physicians feel that a woman should have a right to request sterilization, and that physicians should be free to respond to such a request. Since [Church] Hospital cannot permit elective sterilizations and

> since the number of sterilizations performed following delivery has been increasing and is expected to continue to increase, the overwhelming majority of the physicians interviewed feel that the consolidation should take place at [Memorial] Hospital. However, different views about the importance of the issue of balance between the two hospitals give rise to differences of opinion about the pace at which a consolidated unit should be implemented.
>
> A few physicians who attach great importance to maintaining a balance of services between the two hospitals, would like to see the balance issue more or less formally resolved before anything is done about the obstetrics service. The majority of physicians wish to see action taken promptly to consolidate OB services, with discussions of the balance issue initiated simultaneously.[15]

The doctors were also asked about the patients' preference. They placed no great importance on this, primarily because they were able to ask patients to change their initial selection at the last minute when it suited the doctor.

Separate surveys of nurses, trustees, and patients were contemplated but rejected because of the cost in time and money. The liquidity issue regarding revenue was checked and found to be unimportant. The critical intangibles can be summarized as follows:

**Quality**—Technical quality strongly favored by merger, at either site. The physical plant proposed at Church was preferred by both architect and physicians.

**Uncertainty**—A major capital investment, about $600,000 is to be made. Its effectiveness will depend upon the correctness of the forecasts. It would be disastrous if the total births rose to a level exceeding the capacity of the new suite. This possibility was viewed as remote, however.

**Liquidity**—Funds for the merger were available, without serious difficulty. Revenue implications were not troublesome.

**Control**—The religious issue became one of the critical intangibles for evaluation.

**Access**—No difference was detectable among the three alternatives.

**Amenities**—Modestly favored Church according to the architect, Memorial according to the doctors. But the doctors did not know the extent of renovations required at Church.

**Equity**—Favored Church because of the immediate history.

### OUTCOME

Technically, the outcome is not part of the methodology, but the purpose of the methodology is to facilitate rational decisions. The report delivered by the Bureau showed capital expenditures equivalent to $53,000 per year more than offset by $110,000 per year savings through centralization. The capital cost was approximately $600,000 yielding a pay-back period of

$$\frac{\$600,000}{\$110,000} = 5.45 \text{ years}$$

and an internal rate of return of seventeen percent over twenty years. Inflation, which was not considered in the operating costs, would tend to increase the rate of return. The expected capital costs were higher at Memorial, the operating costs at Church. The intangibles strongly favored centralization, as noted above.

The relatively (and unexpectedly) small return generated considerable pressure for delay. This came particularly from the supporters of "equity" because it was clear that the religious issue was not going to be overcome by the modest physical plant advantages of centralization at Church. Extensive investigations were undertaken to find ways to permit sterlizations on the Church Hospital site. No acceptable method could be found. After about a year, the religious group sponsoring Church Hospital announced that it was for sale. Obstetrics services at Church were reduced to six beds. Memorial Hospital made temporary renovations in its obstetrical services, gaining fourteen postpartum beds and providing two delivery rooms, one delivery-labor room, and the postpartum recovery area. By 1974, eighty percent of the births were at Memorial. The cost of this revision was only $80,000, and the underlying licensure problems were not corrected. Temporary licensure was extended on an annual basis with the agreement that the issue would be reopened and a fully acceptable single facility would be built as soon as the ownership of Church was settled.

## Discussion

The technical application of the method by the Bureau required four specific studies over and above those needed for forecasting facility size. They were:

- Architect's analysis of feasibility, intangibles, and capital cost for each accepted alternative
- Operating cost estimation for each alternative
- Study of implications for revenue and for other departments, including review with department heads of contingencies, opportunity costs, and intangibles
- Interviews with medical staffs on quality and other intangibles

Many additional steps could be taken to improve the precision of these data. Each would have increased the cost and time required for the survey, and in the Bureau's opinion, would not have substantially changed the result. We believe every *major* consideration was identified and accurately described. If time and funds had been available, more studies of contingent plans and opportunity costs, direct studies of patient reaction and personnel reaction, and more precise operating cost estimates could have been prepared. (For example, obstetrical nursing consultants could have been asked to prepare staffing plans.) The order of importance is as listed.

The use of the architect consultant was the most costly survey item, but also the most rewarding in terms of new information. His comments on code compliance and intangibles were valuable, and his cost estimates for both hospitals were rude shocks. This is the kind of information that is critical to get early in the planning process, because it requires much rethinking and adjustment.

It is worth noting that almost no subgroup had all the facts straight, and each study, therefore, had to be interpreted by someone knowledgeable about the whole. The architect, for example, noted extra beds as an advantage, but did not know that these beds were unnecessary. The doctors did not know that patient toilets would be added at Church to comply with the new construction code.

Finally, the most serious weakness remains, in the Bureau's opinion, the exclusion of the Osteopathic alternatives. It is impossible to estimate the cost of this decision, but it is whatever is now spent on obstetric care at Osteopathic Hospital, less the modest adjustments necessary to accommodate those 200 births in a merged location, plus the technical quality implications. There are many who feel that it is impossible to give adequate care at this level of activity. Whatever this cost is, it is being paid each year as a hidden price of the historical bitterness between the two groups of doctors.

## The Bay City Hospital Merger

In 1967, Bay City had four hospitals serving slightly more than 100,000 persons. The overall use rate was greater than 1,500 patient days per thousand population, and was one of the highest in Michigan. A study by the Bureau of Hospital Administration recommended that two of the hospitals be closed, forcing a drastically reduced use rate.[16] By 1973, the community had named a subregional planning committee which agreed to this general concept, and requested more help in implementing it. There were then three hospitals:

- Bay Osteopathic (BOH) 101 beds
- Bay Medical Center (BMC) (with two divisions to be merged into one with new construction) 432 beds
- Samaritan (SAM) 70 beds

A number of difficult decisions were involved, but this example will be limited to the acute hospital location, and will emphasize only the major issues of that decision. The overall future use rate was set at 1,225 patient days per thousand population. As a result 532 beds were required for all services for 1975, growing only to 550 by 1985.[17] This was fifty-three less than available in 1973. Modest changes in this complement caused by centralization of specific services are discussed in the report, but will be ignored here.

It should be noted that immediate reconstruction of the BMC was inevitable. The only question was the size. BOH had capability for low cost expansion of 100 beds, and land enough to accommodate the entire 550 beds. BMC owned land for its replacement at 450 beds and could also accommodate 550 beds, though less conveniently. SAM faced an immediate capital expenditure to retain its license and had no feasible expansion capability.

## Alternatives

The bed distributions under the various merger alternatives would be:

| | | |
|---|---|---|
| (1) | BMC | 550 |
| (2) | BOH | 550 |
| (3) | BMC | 449 |
| | BOH | 101 |
| (4) | BMC | 349 |
| | BOH | 201 |
| (5) | BMC | 379 |
| | BOH | 101 |
| | SAM | 70 |
| (6) | BMC | 279 |
| | BOH | 201 |
| | SAM | 70 |
| (7) | BMC | 480 |
| | SAM | 70 |
| (8) | BOH | 480 |
| | SAM | 70 |

There are intermediate alternatives, such as BMC 379, BOH 171. These will be ignored. In general, they can be treated as "fine tuning" from one of these general positions.

## Initial Review

All of the alternatives were physically feasible. Questions were immediately raised about equity—the continuation of SAM, which had a particularly devoted board and clientele; control—over the elimination of the separate osteopathic hospital which was implicit in alternatives (1), (2), (7), and (8); and access—explicit for osteopathic doctors in the same alternatives. Also alternatives (4) and (6) drastically changed the relative numbers of beds available to each M.D. and D.O.

It was decided that alternatives (1) through (4) were essentially identical to (5) through (8) except that the latter set expected that SAM would continue to exist as an acute facility. To reduce the data collection effort involved, it was assumed that the construction costs of all BMC sizes were pro rata fractions of the existing architect's estimate for 550 beds. This assumption could be revised later if it appeared critical. It was agreed that the total centralizations (1), (2), (7), and (8) were less likely to be acceptable. As a result these were given less thorough analytic treatment. The central alternatives became (a) to continue SAM or not and (b) if decentralized, to expand BOH or not.

## Cost Estimation

**Capital Costs**—Each of the possibilities in table II.4.6 was priced by architects hired by the hospital involved. Because of a "bargain" price for the BOH expansion, alternative (3) is the cheapest, and alternatives (1) and (4) substantially the same. (See table II.4.6).[18] At 6.75 percent interest and forty-year life, the new construction and BOH expansions cost $72,000 per year per million invested. The SAM renovation however, must be considered at eight percent interest, because no better rate was available to it, and also on some shorter life. The building which is being renovated is already ten years old, suggesting a thirty-year residual life. On the other hand, to have licensure difficulties within a decade of construction is not reassuring. It indicates either poor planning or a rapidly changing environment which may foreclose the useful life of the facility well short of the expected forty years. The annual cost is thus a forecasting decision. At varying life, the 1.2 million capital will have annual costs of:

$107,000 per year for 30 years
$122,000 per year for 20 years
$179,000 per year for 10 years

The Bureau's opinion was that ten years was a conservative estimate. This relates both to the noticeable design difficulties of the renovation and a conviction that small hospitals in cities have limited futures.

**Operating Cost**—Samaritan claimed substantial economies of operation. Its costs were about $65.00 per patient day, while BMC and BOH were over $90.00. For the seventy beds at ninety percent occupancy, this amounts to a difference of $575,000 per year. There was some feeling that this saving was more a matter of case mix than efficiency, however. The same patients would be below average cost regardless of where they were treated. This might have been analyzed through a diagnosis-specific survey of changes and length of stay, but was not, because it was felt relatively unimportant in view of other cost elements. The operating costs of the other two hospitals were not significantly different, and no significant cost savings could be forecast as a result of the various reconstruction proposals.

**Cost of Related Services**—This element is not relevant unless departmental or partial adjustments are brought into the discussion.

**TABLE II.4.6**
Facilities alternatives for Bay City hospitals to meet 1985 bed need of 550 beds

| *Hospital* | *Beds Proposed* | *Present Beds* | *Beds to be Constructed (+) or Closed (−)* | *1974 Capital Investment* | *Type of Construction* |
|---|---|---|---|---|---|
| *Alternative 1* | | | | | |
| Bay Osteopathic | 101 | 101 | 0 | 0 | — |
| Samaritan | 70 | 70 | 0 | $1,160,000 | Renovation |
| Bay Medical Center | 379 | 0 | +379 | $22,140,000 | New Construction |
| | | | | $23,300,000 | |
| *Alternative 2* | | | | | |
| Bay Osteopathic | 101 | 101 | 0 | 0 | — |
| Samaritan | 0 | 70 | −70 | * | (Liquidation) |
| Bay Medical Center | 449 | 0 | +449 | $25,318,000 | New Construction |
| | | | | $25,318,000 | |
| *Alternative 3* | | | | | |
| Bay Osteopathic | 201 | 101 | +100 | $2,500,000 | Addition |
| Samaritan | 70 | 70 | 0 | $1,160,000 | Renovation |
| Bay Medical Center | 279 | 0 | +279 | $17,497,000 | New Construction |
| | | | | $21,157,000 | |
| *Alternative 4* | | | | | |
| Bay Osteopathic | 201 | 101 | +100 | $2,500,000 | Addition |
| Samaritan | 0 | 70 | −70 | * | (Liquidation) |
| Bay Medical Center | 349 | 0 | +349 | $20,768,000 | New Construction |
| | | | | $23,268,000 | |

* No liquidation value for the sale of Samaritan Hospital is assumed, since the facility's value will likely vary depending on the proposed use. Any use which would eliminate other investments (such as long-term care facility) would be valued as a deduction from the total investment of alternatives 2 and 4. The same consideration holds for any net assets realized from the sale or alternative use of the present General and Mercy Divisions of Bay Medical Center (since we have not taken their liquidation value into account, either).

**Opportunity Costs**—The critical opportunity cost turns out to be the continued use of Samaritan as an acute facility. If it could profitably be diverted to long-term care or mental health care, the cost of construction avoided for the service selected can be claimed as the opportunity cost of alternatives (1) and (3). Thus, if the facility could be used without renovation, for long-term care, and would eliminate seventy long-term beds of necessary construction in that area at $20,000 per bed, the cost of using it for acute care is:

| | *Capital Cost* | *At Annual Rates* |
|---|---|---|
| Renovation: | $1,200,000 | $179,000 (10-year life 8%) |
| Opportunity: | 1,400,000 | 71,000 (40-year life 6.75%) |
| | $2,600,000 | $250,000 |

(The word *necessary* is critical in the preceding sentence. If the long-term care beds are not necessary, the opportunity cost of foregoing them is zero.) In fact, both long-term and mental health possibilities existed. They were treated as intangibles because of the shortage of time.

Opportunity costs would also be involved if construction began to crowd the land available at either BMC or BOH. Under the deferred alternative of centralization of all care at the BMH site, this might have been a consideration. It probably would have been handled as an intangible because of difficulties in establishing a dollar value. The all-BMH alternative soon disappeared from consideration however. It was several million dollars more expensive than centralization at BOH because it involved replacement of BOH's existing beds.

## INTANGIBLES

**Quality**—It was noted that technical quality was enhanced by having one large center, which could support a wider array of specialized equipment and technical skills. Thus alternative (3) carried negative quality implications, and to some extent alternative (4).

**Access**—Studies of the admission practices of physicians were revealing. First, some DOs used BMC routinely, and did not admit to BOH. Second, when the estimate was made as favorably as possible for BOH, assuming that any doctor who used BOH relied upon it solely for privileges, there were already more beds per using doctor at BOH than BMC[19] (see table II.4.7). If additional beds were constructed at BOH without changes in control and privileges, this situation would be ridiculously exaggerated. BOH users would have nearly fourteen beds apiece. BMC beds per doctor, meanwhile, would drop, because the reduction in the total was being taken from this hospital. These data produced a substantial reaction from the non-BOH doctors. Their view was shared by many community leaders, because BOH expansion meant that the available use rate for patients of BOH doctors was going up, while that for other patients was being forced down. The result was that neither of the two alternatives (4) and (6) was acceptable without revisions in controls which created a total reorganization of BOH and which were tantamount to a merger of BOH and BMC.

A second access question was of a different kind entirely. The Saginaw River divides Bay City and the surrounding service area almost in half. BMC and SAM are on one side; BOH is on the other. A proposal to centralize all care at BOH thus raises an access question. There are four bridges, but all are draw bridges. Openings are infrequent, and can last as long as fifteen minutes. This would be annoying but not critical except in an emergency. Information collected from bridge authorities verified that all four bridges were never open at once, that pleasure boat openings could be delayed, and that freighter openings took longer but carried a longer warning time. On the basis of these data, it was agreed that radio equipped ambulances could always be detoured around open bridges in a satisfactory manner.

With this conclusion, the total centralization solution was reduced to a single alternative. If adopted, it would be at the BOH site because it avoided replacement of 101 useful beds, and avoided opportunity costs related to potential land shortages at BMC.

**Uncertainty**—Because expansion possibilities over 550 beds abounded, there was little uncertainty in the construction program. If use rate or population forecasts proved too low, additional beds could be constructed.

The price of the additional 100 beds at BOH, $25,000 per bed, was extraordinarily low for Michigan in 1972, but it was a firm offer for a period of time. Even so, a prudent person would question it. Contingencies arise; contractors go bankrupt; and firm prices evaporate.

Substantial uncertainty was involved in the selection of the life of Samaritan after renovation. While the Bureau's advice to take a short life

**TABLE II.4.7**
Ratio of beds per active practitioner by type of practitioner 1972

| *Hospital(s) and Type(s) of Practitioner* | *Number of Active Practitioners* | *Number of Beds* | *Ratio of Beds Per Practitioner* |
|---|---|---|---|
| Bay Osteopathic (D.O.)* | 15 | 101 | 6.73 |
| All Other Hospitals (M.D., D.O., and D.D.S.)** | 89 | 502 | 5.64 |

* The DOs using Bay Osteopathic may have also had admissions to the other Bay City hospitals.

** The MDs, DOs, and DDSs included for "All Other Hospitals" had *no* admissions to Bay Osteopathic.

appears conservative, it actually is just as uncertain as the opposite. Either way the community has lost money if the forecast is wrong.

**Liquidity**—A combination of uncertainty and liquidity problems—ability to obtain the needed $2,500,000—began to develop around the BOH expansion, and the Bureau staff noted a substantial drop in enthusiasm while the analysis was being conducted. Finances might be a problem for BMC, but this group had the largest public support and as a result, the best opportunity to raise funds. The overall liquidity issue—deferring any investment until more funds are available or more alternatives are investigated—did not exist. The State Health Department was insistent upon steady progress because it viewed three facilities as inadequate (both BMC buildings and SAM).

A complex liquidity issue was involved in the SAM renovation. First, SAM was unable to get as good an interest rate as BMC. Its borrowing would be at eight percent, when 6.75 was quoted for BMC. This would raise the annual cost, as noted under the capital cost discussion. Second, in order to reduce the immediate payment burden, a "balloon" terminal principal payment was contemplated rather than the usual mortgage amortization schedule. (This preserved more of the operating cost advantage SAM claimed as justification for its renovation, but created a deferred obligation.) Finally, when the possibility of denial of support under Public Law 92-603, the Social Security Amendments of 1972, was raised, the hospital declared that it would not claim Medicare reimbursement for the renovation. Data showed that thirty-eight percent of the patient days were Medicare reimbursed. The remaining patients would have to bear over fifty percent more capital costs each if this decision were implemented. These plans were unappealing to many committee members. The result was a substantial intangible liquidity burden for alternatives (1) and (3).

**Control**—As the data were collected and analyzed and, more important, understood by the policy makers, the control and equity issues became increasingly visible. Resolution clearly depended on the presentation of credible organization constraints to assure equal access and evenhanded public management free of domination from any one group. The Bureau proposed many specific steps toward this end. These divided into two groups: first, recommendations for representative control (trustee membership, selection procedures and the like); and second, recommendations for specific changeover provisions, such as guarantees of staff membership for physicians and employment for other staff.

A subtle control issue centers around two quite separate considerations. First, about a twenty percent reduction in the use rate is included in the construction alternatives. Equitable application would call for changes in practice among all doctors as indicated by uniform peer review. Second, the hospitals are currently organized so that one group of DOs dominates that staff of one hospital. The combination suggests a potential inequity, and becomes an intangible cost of all the alternatives under formal consideration. The same argument can be extended with the MDs to the group using SAM. This issue favors single management and a combined medical staff for all hospitals as a way to insure equitable distribution of hospital access among doctors.

**Amenities**—These were largely irrelevant to the Bay City negotiations. A reduced convenience of design was noted in connection with the SAM renovation.

**Equity**—Three institutions started the study protecting their "rights" and traditions. In the final recommendations, these considerations had substantially diminished from the original positions. Access, uncertainty, and liquidity issues had been raised which BOH supporters could not successfully overcome to justify their expansion. SAM's claims were also attacked. On the other hand, control concessions were made to protect the rights of all patients and staff. These allayed some fears. A final concession to SAM was a recommendation that its trustees both have seats on the board of BMC and be allowed to operate the original facility until completion of the new facility (but without renovating their building).

## Outcome

Community leaders report that SAM will proceed with construction, but may accept merger later. BOH will not expand. Thus, a decision has been reached for alternative 1 of table II.4.6. The new BMC will be at its old site, not at the BOH site. Obstetrics and pediatrics mergers are now being considered. The Samaritan renovation was against the advice of the regional planning council, but construction was begun before the implementation date of the Medicare payment restrictions.

## Discussion

This illustration is of interest principally because of the complex and fluid SAM situation and the reliance on intangibles. Differences of opinion regarding the value of these intangibles were reflected in the outcomes. There were three decisions, and consensus was reached on two: the location of BMC and the size of BOH. The intangibles (control, access, and equity) were the sole determinant of the first; no tangible cost difference was ever suggested. Uncertainty, liquidity, and the access of MDs versus DOs to beds determined the second, overcoming an estimated tangible difference over $2,000,000 ($146,000 per year at forty years, 6.75 percent, table II.4.6).

There was considerable dispute over the tangible cost of the SAM renovation. Capital costs for those seventy beds were agreed: $1,200,000 for renovation, $2,900,000 for replacement. The annual cost was in dispute, because of the project life assumption. See table II.4.8.

**TABLE II.4.8**
Costs of SAM renovation

| | *Proponents of Renovation $/year* | *Opponents of Renovation $/year* |
|---|---|---|
| Annual cost of new construction (40 years, 6.75%) | $209,000 | $209,000 |
| Annual cost of renovation (8%) | $107,000 or less (30-year life or more) | $179,000 or more (10-year life or less) |
| Net savings from renovation | $102,000 or more | $30,000 or less |

Proponents claimed an operating cost difference of over $500,000 per year, which was denied in entirety by opponents.

The opportunity cost was not accepted as a tangible cost, but was known to be about $100,000 per year in favor of new construction. It clearly outweighed the modest savings from renovation, $30,000 per year, in the eyes of opponents, but not the proponents' claim of $102,000 per year or more.

The other intangibles were not needed by the proponents, although they clearly put a high value on them. They included nontechnical quality, equity, and control issues.

The convictions were strongly held, and the debate and strategic maneuvering were intense. What was contributed by the technical analysis, in such a situation? Precisely this: that the SAM renovation was the correct issue to debate, because there were valid cases on both sides. Had the tangible costs indicated a more extreme condition—for example either no renovation needs at SAM or a renovation cost of twice the $1,200,000—it is likely that the issue would have been settled by those findings.

The greatest weakness of this illustration is the out-of-hand rejection of SAM's claim that they did the job cheaper in terms of operating costs. A survey of costs by diagnosis at the three hospitals was feasible and probably should have been done. If it supported SAM's claim after adjustment for costs of renovation and opportunity costs, only technical quality issues would remain. A consultant could have been obtained to comment upon the kinds of patients who could be treated as well at SAM as at BMC. The total operating cost saving claimed by SAM was over $500,000 per year. The estimates of annual capital and opportunity costs, although crude, were only half this amount. The argument against SAM's continuation thus rests solely on the untested assumption that more than half the operating cost differential was due to patient mix.

## Summary

In this chapter a method for dealing with complex centralization questions has been described and illustrated. The method depends on the careful identification of a list of feasible alternatives, the division of the issues into cost elements, the estimation of as many elements as possible in tangible dollar terms, and the description of the remaining elements as intangibles. The applications of this method have indicated the following conclusions.

### Data Collection

Data collection for this method is relatively expensive and open-ended as to cost. The two illustrations each required from two to three man-months of professional time and an approximately equal amount of clerical support. In each case there were other studies which could have been done which would have increased that cost. Political processes have their own momentum, and this generates time pressures on the data collection and analysis. These pressures add to the cost of data gathering, limiting the depth and precision which can be obtained. Under these constraints, it is important that the investigation be wisely divided among the elements. Excessive precision in some elements at the expense of others must be avoided. Large elements tend to dominate the final outcome. Thus it is critical that all these elements are identified and estimated. Precision of measurement of other elements can be limited to that achieved by the least precise tangible estimate for the major elements.

A number of judgments are involved in the data collection and cost estimation. These include assumptions regarding conditional feasibilities, interest rates, project lives, renovation possibilities and requirements, and the evaluation of the precision of estimates. It is important that these decisions be undertaken by skilled and neutral analysts. The supervising analysts should be employed by a body capable of selecting any alternative, not by a body with a vested interest. This does not mean that local professionals have no role, as the Jackson obstetrics study indicates. Even if they have distinct interests, they are frequently reliable, inexpensive sources of specific information. In major elements, multiple independent analysts can be employed. The capital cost estimates, for example, could be obtained from two or more architects. The analysts should have professional training and experience. Although many specialists can be involved, the supervising analyst must coordinate their diverse and sometimes conflicting views.

### Critical Nature of Initial Steps

The most frightening possibility in this method is the omission of the best solution in step one, or its deletion in step two, when the alternatives for detailed investigation are determined. The cost of an error may be very high, but there are few data available to indicate this cost when these decisions are made.

Capable representatives of special interests will move forcefully at these points to delete alternatives distasteful to their group. Protection lies only in the neutrality of the analysts, the requirements for comprehensive presentation of alternatives and conditional feasibilities, and the existence of a broadly representative decision making body.

## Dominance of Certain Elements

It is our experience that a large difference must be available to cause people to leave the status quo. These large differences are most likely to be contributed by either capital costs or opportunity costs. Even projects with very promising operating cost savings and intangible benefits have difficulty winning acceptance on this ground alone. Capital and opportunity costs occur at specific intervals in time, and then disappear from consideration. Replacement or expansion capital becomes necessary, or new activities are desired. When these things occur, the capital investments are liquid and opportunities are present. After the capital has been put in place, the liquidity and the opportunity are lost. Thus a generally desirable project can be destroyed by too hasty investment in replacement, which commits the community to one alternative. Similarly, opportunity cost savings can be created by integrating several different revisions at once, and lost by failing to identify conditional feasibilities in time to do anything about them. This condition leads to developing a strategy of interrelating several projects in various areas over a fairly long planning horizon. Projects may be deferred on two contingencies: to await the need to replace capital investment in a specific location, and to be reviewed for opportunity cost advantages in connection with other proposals. The former is more or less predictable. The latter calls for continuous monitoring as the local situation changes. In effect, the latter is what resulted with the Jackson OB merger proposal and it occurred essentially because no clear capital advantage could be demonstrated, and the control and equity intangibles offset one another.

## Weaknesses in the Method

The methodology remains cumbersome at best. The decisions become very complex and tedious as the number of alternatives which survive the second step increase. It is possible to accommodate three or four possibilities in a decision making process of this kind, but more than this becomes quite difficult. For five alternatives, there will be ten pairs, which is probably more than a reasonably motivated board can hold in its mind. It is this difficulty which represents the primary weakness of the method, in our opinion. Practicality forces too many alternatives out at step two.

The other arguments which might be cited against the method, its tedious complexity, large data requirements, and emphasis on difficult-to-evaluate intangible considerations, appear to the Bureau to be inherent in the complexity and difficulty of the problems to be faced. We believe that the strength of the method lies in its attention to comprehensiveness in the review of both the alternatives and the costs of each alternative.

## NOTES

[1]*Cf.* J. O. McClain and V. R. Rao, "Trade-Offs and Conflicts in Evaluation of Health System Alternatives: Methodology for Analysis." *Health Services Research,* Spring 1974, pp. 35-52. This paper develops a sophisticated, but untested method of dealing with the values of decision makers, an element of the problem largely ignored in the following discussion.

[2]D. B. Starkweather, "Hospital Organization Performance and Size." *Inquiry,* Vol. 10, No. 3, September 1973, pp. 10-18.

[3]"Guidelines for Hospital Obstetrics Departments and Newborn Nurseries." Lansing: Bureau of Health Facilities, Michigan Department of Health, 1972.

[4]"Optimal Criteria for Care of Heart Disease Patient." *Journal of the American Medical Association,* Vol. 226, No. 11, December 10, 1972, pp. 1340-1344.

"Renal Disease Plan for Michigan." Lansing: Office of Health and Medical Affairs, Michigan Department of Health, October 25, 1973.

[5]These data are subject to a number of problems of validity and reliability, particularly when they are considered as standards or goals. The point here is that the actual performance of large hospitals does not uniformly reflect the expected economies of scale.

[6]T. Y. Holper, *Administrative Review of Shared and Consolidated Services.* Chicago: The American Hospital Association, 1973.

[7]John R. Griffith, *Quantitative Techniques for Hospital Planning and Control.* Lexington, MA: D.C. Heath & Co., 1972, chapter 9.

[8]In 1973 when the Bureau was presenting the Jackson obstetrics study, the faculty member in charge decided to ignore interest rate considerations, because he felt it would confuse his unsophisticated audience of consumers and physicians. He was promptly challenged by the president of one of the boards of trustees for using an inadequate and inaccurate method. It is well to remember that present value methods are taught in business schools and are increasingly common in capital decision making in industry. They have been used in the banking business for centuries.

[9]An interesting case is presented by donated capital. Whether general or designated, the gift would be treated as increasing the endowment and surplus position of the institution and would be costed in the operation including interest at an appropriate rate. The annual payment would be made back to endowment or surplus and would be available for reinvestment in the continuation or expansion of the initial activity or in other opportunities.

[10]William L. Dowling and Howard S. Zuckerman, "Analysis of Obstetric Facilities and Services: Foote and Mercy Hospitals." Ann Arbor: Bureau of Hospital Administration, The University of Michigan, 1972.

[11]*Ibid.* Feasibility study by H. W. Rucfrok, AIA, of Harley, Ellington, Pierce, Yee Associates, Southfield, MI, p. 21h.

[12]The interest rate is predicated on access to tax-free state supported bonds.

[13]Dowling and Zuckerman, "Analysis of Obstetric Services," p. 24.

[14]*Ibid.*, p. 25.

[15]*Ibid.*, pp. 28-29.

[16]Eric Helt and John R. Griffith, "A Study of Health Facility and Service Needs, Bay City, Michigan." Ann Arbor: Bureau of Hospital Administration, The University of Michigan, 1968.

[17]Alan C. Foose and John R. Griffith, "A Comprehensive Study of Health Facilities and Service Needs, 1973, Bay City, Michigan." Ann Arbor: Bureau of Hospital Administration, The University of Michigan, 1973.

[18]*Ibid.*, p. 96.

[19]*Ibid.*, p. 87.

# Section III

# Cost Oriented Control Systems in Hospitals

This section contains the descriptions and the results of the authors' efforts to develop and implement operational systems in hospitals. Common themes throughout the papers are the need to determine the appropriate amount of resources needed to perform an activity, to control the use of the activity through proper scheduling systems, and to establish budgets so that the probability of having sufficient resources is at a predetermined level.

The papers are a reflection of the authors' opinions concerning the operational systems that should have the highest priority from a cost saving viewpoint. Wherever possible, specific examples of the cost saving are included to provide the reader with as much information as possible concerning the relative value of the systems.

# III.1

# Dynamics of Hospital Operational Control Systems

*by Walton M. Hancock*

## Introduction

In any hospital or organization performing services repetitively, management must give considerable attention to "operating disciplines," the guidelines of ongoing operation. Operating disciplines specify procedures for such functions as admitting a patient, billing, and scheduling nursing personnel, and if they are correctly established they have builtin evaluation and control mechanisms. These permit management to determine whether various systems are functioning according to the overall objectives of the organization.

Unfortunately, operating disciplines can be established haphazardly and function for long periods of time without any controls at all. The admission system can function but still result in unfilled beds, unnecessary transfers, and surgical cancellations. Bills can be rendered without all charges recorded. Nursing personnel can be scheduled with excess personnel on slack days or insufficient staff on peak days. The most common indication of inefficient operating disciplines is management engaging in repetitive "fire fighting." Developing efficient control systems entails, in many hospitals, a major shift in the style of management.[1] This new style consists of:

- Explicit goals publicized and explained to all affected personnel
- Predictive rather than reactive management
- Control systems encouraging close tolerance operation
- Increased decision making at lower levels

## What is Control?

An operational control system is a system that causes certain expectations to be attained. A budget, for example, is said to be "under control" if actual expenditures are close to those predicted. For a control system to operate properly, the following must exist in at least rudimentary form:

- A prediction of future events—"an expectation"
- A method of measurement in the same units as the expectation
- A method of determining if exceptions exist
- A procedure for reporting exceptions
- Corrective actions to remove exceptions so that expectation can be achieved

Many control systems are present in hospitals. Examples are readily discovered governing output (admission lab work, bills issued to Blue Cross), resources (number of nursing personnel on a given floor, raw food cost per meal), quality (surgical tissue committees, laboratory unknown results), and efficiency (percent occupancy, pounds of laundry per manhour). When compared to the above list of necessary characteristics, however, many control systems are seen to be poorly designed. Uncertain expectations, poor measurement, unreliable detection of exceptions, and incomplete corrections cause control systems to lose effectiveness; yet at least some of these problems are present in any complex organization. As a result, control systems must be periodically evaluated. The purpose of this section is to provide evaluators with a useful background in the establishment and evaluation of control systems in hospital operations. The comments here are general in nature and draw from experience in both industry and hospitals. Later sections deal with specific and often sophisticated control systems.

## The Relation of Control to Objectives

Objectives may be set in many ways. Frequently they are proposed by middle management, reviewed for consistency and feasibility by the administrator, and then formalized. They may be based on improving past performance levels or more adequately meeting new needs. They may be qualitative or quantitative in nature; however, qualitative objectives should be adopted with caution, as there will be no measure of whether or not the objective is accomplished.

An objective is constrained principally by the need for an appropriate measure. Hence, most control systems are quantitatively based, and the development of controls parallels the development of measurement systems which often exist for other purposes. In hospitals, the most developed control systems are usually based on payroll, other accounts payable, accounts receivable, and quantitative medical records systems such as PAS (Professional Activities Study). Additional control systems can always be established using separate data collection systems rather than those already in existence, but the cost of doing this is high and to be avoided if at all possible.

A second consideration in developing controls is the perceived value of the objective. If the perceived value is high, emphasis is placed on the establishment of controls. For example, the increase in the number of malpractice lawsuits has stimulated the need for medical quality controls, and the increase in cost of care has stimulated the establishment of PSROs (professional standards review organizations). If the perceived value is low, controls are not justified. Examples are use of disposable supplies by low volume users, telephone expense, and the [illegible]personnel needs of small departments. Perceived values can change over time and necessitate the development of new controls and the deletion or modification of others.

A third consideration is the interdependence between various aspects of the hospital system. For example, stabilizing occupancy reduces the need for more elaborate daily controls of nursing staff, food purchases, and laboratory and radiology staffs, because the stabilized demand stabilizes needed resources also.

The interdependence of control systems is important to understand also, because the accomplishment of one objective may lead to an out-of-control situation in another. As an example, if a hospital controls nursing staff at the budgeted level but fails to control number of patients, the situation may be "in control" according to budget expectations, but out of control with respect to cost per patient. Nursing hours and cost per patient are interdependent, and if the decision maker strives to achieve control over both, conflicts can occur. A preferred procedure is to establish compatible objectives so that the behavior of the decision maker is more consistent. In the above example, the establishment of controls on the budgeted levels of nursing personnel and the stabilization of the occupancy rate are compatible goals. If the nursing supervisor can be expected to stay within the budget and the admissions department can be expected to attain the stated occupancy goal, the establishment of goal priorities and internal conflicts are minimized. It may be difficult to stabilize occupancy, particularly if an excess of inpatient beds exists. Under these conditions, the stabilization of occupancy will require delaying elective admissions even though there are beds available. This situation may be in conflict with the goals of many physicians, who want patients admitted without delay if beds are available. Major conflicts are likely to occur, making it difficult to stabilize occupancy and keep nursing hours per patient day within limits.

Goals are also interdependent in another sense; care must be taken not to overemphasize certain aspects of hospital goals simply because they are measurable. Specifically, it is charged that control systems on efficiency impair quality. This charge has a sensible ring to it but must be interpreted with care. Control on efficiency need not impair quality, either

**FIGURE III.1.1**
An example of organizational levels

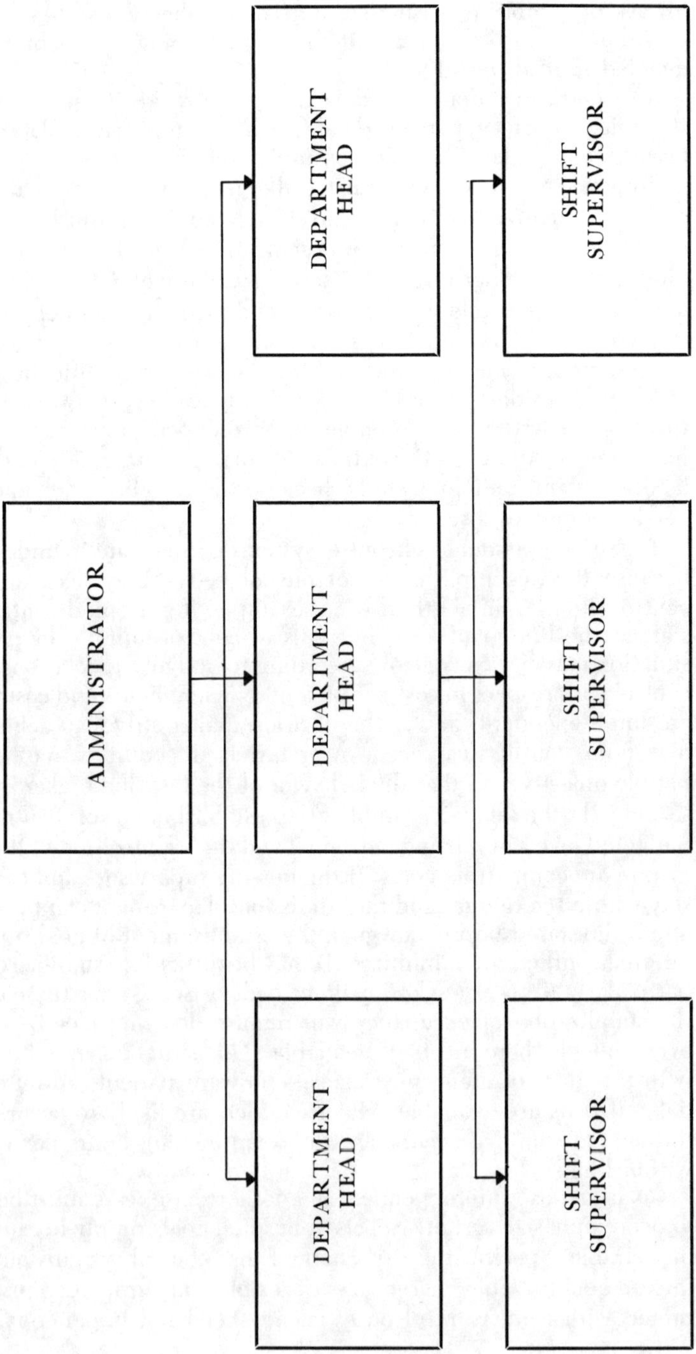

because slack is present or because the two are consistent. Moreover, quality levels are maintained in many cases by internalized control systems. Experience indicates that internalized systems do not disappear with the establishment of measurable goals. If there are conflicts, their resolution under mature management usually achieves both quality and efficiency goals. When conflicts cannot be resolved, the accomplishment of both goals may require goal modification.

The effects of operational controls in hospitals, therefore, start with the functions to be controlled and are restricted by the quantitative information routinely available, the perceived value of the aspects to be controlled, and the interactions between control objectives. If control is obtained, the behavior of the participants will be affected in desirable, i.e., "expected," ways.

## The Concept of Primary, Secondary, and Super Controls

In most operational control systems, it is desirable to consider several levels of control. The reason is that different types of decisions are appropriate for different levels in an organization. Figure III.1.1 is a three-level organization that might be found in a hospital. The labels shown in figure III.1.1 are unimportant; the levels of management are the focus of attention. The question is, "Who should do what?" (The Board of Trustees will not be considered here.) Suppose, as an example, that the objective is to maintain a certain level of service on each of three shifts. The primary control of the situation is at the shift supervisor level. It is his job to make whatever decisions are necessary to provide a staff that will maintain the appropriate level of service. If an employee is ill, the shift supervisor has primary responsibility for finding a replacement. Part-time help, the use of people from other areas, and overtime are possible solutions. This formulation of the responsibilities is quite different from that envisioned in static systems such as position control. Primary control assumes a policy level decision on the amount of service and the delegation of implementation to the primary supervisor or primary controller. In this sense, it is a decentralized system because it increases the responsibility and authority of first line management. This approach also facilitates more flexible control, capable of working in a variety of conditions of occupancy. Finally, it can achieve these ends without damaging the authority of the upper levels. Proper reporting of exceptions from the policy decision will permit upper management to retain control of the final outcome and even improve its control.

The responsibilities of level two (secondary control) are to help shift supervisors by being responsive to repeated unsuccessful attempts to meet the desired objectives. For example, suppose a shift supervisor encounters repeated absenteeism and cannot maintain the service level even though he has attempted the possible solutions that are within his sphere of influence. The primary loop, the shift supervisor decision process, is then failing to function and the secondary control loop is activated. In this instance, the need is to provide the shift supervisor with feasible solutions. The first step is to see if the absenteeism can be reduced. If it cannot, then a pool of people shared between department heads might be established to help the situation. Another solution might be to cross-train people from each department so that an excess of personnel in one department could be used to cover a shortage in another. Each of these possibilities requires the active involvement of the department heads, the secondary control level. The data needed in the secondary control loop are related to the number of repeated failures in the primary loop. Thus, the type of information required at the secondary control loop is different and usually substantially less than at the primary loop.

The third control level is a super control loop which, in figure III.1.1 is at the administrator level. It is a control on the department heads to signal when, after sufficient time has elapsed, they are unable to maintain the feasible solutions needed for the primary loop to function. Therefore, the existence of problems escalates over time to successively higher levels of management until a level is notified that can cause the system to perform according to expectation.

Suppose, in this example, the department head tries to establish a program to train people from different areas so that an excess in one area can be used in another and does not receive the cooperation of the other department heads. Also, he attempts to establish a pool of people that can be cross-trained and used for resource-short areas but is unsuccessful. If he exhausts his possible solutions without obtaining a satisfactory one, the primary and secondary loops will continue not to function correctly, and after an appropriate period of time, the administrator will be notified that the problem exists. The timing, of course, depends on the situation, but generally each level would have two or three reporting periods in which to achieve solutions before the activity advances to the next level. The rate at which the next higher control loop is triggered is heavily dependent upon the time it takes to solve the particular problems at hand and the perceived criticalness of the service.

It is worth reiterating that each level of management is given ample time to solve its own problems before calling in the higher levels. This is one of the strong points of operational exception systems because it promotes the delegation of authority to the lower levels. Each level is expected to solve its own problems insofar as possible, and if it cannot, it is in the best position to assist the next higher level. The so-called "principle of no surprises" applies here. When each successive level of management is brought into a problem, the lower levels are not surprised that their supervisors are involved.[2] Not only are they not surprised—or sometimes more appropriately, not embarrassed—but they have been attempting to solve their problem themselves, thereby saving their superiors' time and enabling all parties to participate in getting the out-of-control situation resolved. The result is that the shift supervisor becomes a much more active and productive part of the management system.

## The Stability of Control Systems

In order to be effective, operational control systems must minimize the deviation of the actual from the expected. Instability is a condition where instead of minimizing the deviation, the controls cause the deviation to increase over time. Several conditions are likely to cause this to happen.

### Too Much Information Getting to Higher Levels

In the previous description of the primary, secondary, and super control systems, the information to the secondary and super levels has to do only with the repeated failure to maintain the service expectation at the primary level. For example, the department head should be interested, if, over a two-week period, there were two or more instances where the service level was not maintained. At the super control level, the administrator might be interested in becoming involved if the service level was not maintained four or more times during a one-month period. The normal information flow, then, allows time lags to occur that enable the lower control levels to function. Suppose, on the other hand, the administrator receives word of the nonachievement of a service level as soon as the shift supervisor does. The presence of information concerning nonperformance may cause the administrator to become inappropriately involved before his subordinates have had an opportunity to correct the nonperformance. Therefore, it is important not to give the administrator this information. Repeated instances of premature super control intervention will result in the lower management levels ceasing to function, overloading of the higher levels, and reduced quality of decisions.

Perhaps it is not completely clear at this point why the inappropriate involvement of the administrator will cause instability. A simple but common cause is that the administrator has many things to do during the course of the day and may on some occasions become involved because he has a chance to look at the data and on other days he will not. This situation will make it extremely difficult for the lower levels to anticipate what he will do and in many cases will cause them to hesitate to initiate action on their own because of the increased uncertainty as to whether or not they are responsible for the solution of the problem. Therefore, the transmission of too much data to higher levels causes a random involvement, less assumption of responsibility by the lower levels, and confusion as to primary responsibility. The chances of instability are therefore increased. Although this concept is simple, it is frequently violated in hospitals. Several control levels get identical data at the same time and allegedly use it for control. The results are usually: everyone ignores it; randomly selected bits are investigated; or several people investigate the same thing, causing confusion and inefficiency. Examples can be found using financial reports, census reports, and PAS and HAS data.

## Bad Data

Since in any management control system there is a method of measuring whether or not the expected result is achieved, incorrect information can decrease the stability of the system by causing incorrect control reactions. Bad data have two forms: where the data are valid but delivered after they are needed; and where the data themselves are incorrect. A typical example of the former case is where an employee telephones and asks the operator to tell the shift supervisor that he will be a half-hour late. If the information is not transmitted within a reasonable period of time, the shift supervisor will make changes in personnel based on the assumption that the employee is not coming. The result will be that changes will be made to allow for the absenteeism of the employee which, after one half-hour, will cause an inappropriate service level. An example of the latter case is where an employee does not report his time correctly. For example, if an employee is to work in department X today but then is asked to shift to department Y at 1:00 P.M. in order to cover a shortage, and fails to record the shift from department X to Y; then, the information feedback system reflects the failure to shift and will show too much resource in department X and too little in department Y. This will trigger an erroneous report to the shift supervisor saying that the service level was not obtained and may result in an inappropriate decision.

Eventually, poor information affects the credibility of the entire process. Since the purpose of management information systems is to cause people to behave in desirable ways, credibility of the information reported bcomes paramount because mistrust will cause people to disregard the signals of out-of-control situations. This form of error often results from the overspecification of detail. The relative size of the error is much larger if the information system is carried to too fine a level. Data should be reported only at the minimum level of detail necessary for the primary controller to make a reasonable diagnosis of what has gone wrong. Even if more detailed information is available, it should be filed for special studies rather than routinely reported. Secondary controllers, as noted above, get even less.

### Lack of Properly Trained Supervisors

In the absenteeism problem above, the range of feasible solutions for the shift supervisor was seen to be drawing from a pool, using excesses from another department, and/or overtime. The shift supervisor must have the flexibility to use at the appropriate time one or more oı the feasible solutions. This presumes that he knows what the feasible solutions are and is given the authority to act. Unfortunately, many management systems are established so that supervisors have to learn too much by experience. Formal training in the range of decisions available to them and what they are expected to do in any particular case is given in a haphazard manner. This causes the control systems to be unstable because, while the supervisors are learning by experience, many functions will be out of control, thereby involving the higher levels of control. The secondary or super control loops become overloaded with problems, making expectation very difficult to attain because the problem solving processes are being conducted with insufficient time to obtain the necessary information.

## Traditional Hospital Control Systems

Most hospitals have a few formal control systems. For example, accounts receivable trial balances or laboratory unknown values are commonly used. These scattered systems are of limited value because they do not cover major aspects of hospital operation. Integrated systems covering large quantities of expenditures, demand, or quality are rare. Those that routinely operate to close tolerances are rarer still.

In many hospitals, the concept of management control centers primarily around manpower and materials budgets. In general, great attention is paid by the administrator to the budget because of its importance in pricing, cash flow, and the perceived necessity of controlling the rate of dollar expenditure. In order to determine appropriate charges, previous activity levels, such as the number of patient days and the number of lab tests run, are often used directly as a forecast for the future year. The forecast expenditures for labor and materials are also historically based.[3] It is assumed that the level of expenditure in the previous year(s) was satisfactory and that future expenditures will be at the same rate (with adjustments for inflation) and that the activity base will be as in the past. The basic result of this type of control process is that everything is done as it was last year with minor adjustments for foreseeable changes.

Many hospital administrators brag about keeping their institutions in control, and when pressed as to what they mean, they explain that they are able to achieve their yearly budgets within one or two percent. Figure III.1.2 is an example of the results of a nursing budget that was in control in this sense.[4] This is a plot of the average number of nursing hours per patient day (N.H./P.D.) for a medical-surgical ward in a hospital. The administrator and the director of nurses had budgeted 4.2 hours per patient day over the year for this particular area. This figure was obtained by taking the previous year's data and dividing the number of hours worked by the forecast number of patient days. The budget expectation for the present year was achieved over the twelve months. However, several problems arise: (1) The number of hours per patient day shows high variability. If one assumes that a certain number of hours per patient day are necessary to provide the service at prescribed quality levels, then was quality service given throughout the year? (2) If quality service was given throughout the year and if the variability was minimized around the low number of hours per patient day (3.5), wouldn't the result be a substantial reduction in the cost of providing the service? (3) The hours per patient day were low during the first four months and then increased sharply. Later, it appears that an effort was made to reduce the amount of labor in the second part of the year in order to attain the budget. If the quality of service was maintained, this indicates that there was too much resource available in the middle of the year, which further indicates that too much resource was budgeted for the area.

A conclusion is that the control system was operating on an annual basis, which is far too long a period to minimize and stabilize the use of the resource.

Another example is the controlling of service departments such as the laboratory. Budgets are established presuming a certain level of activity consistent with the previous year. Since laboratories cannot control the demands placed on them by physicians, this procedure seems to be the best that one can follow. But what about the rate of accomplishment of work in the laboratory? For example, if the lab meets its budget but takes two days to get the results back to the physician, is it providing the same level of service as one that meets the budget and gets the results back in one day? The length of time it takes for the laboratory to get the test back to the physician may affect the patient's length of stay. Also, the longer the turnaround time of laboratory work, the easier it is to meet the budget because the peaks and valleys of demand can be smoother. Perhaps a more appropriate control system would be to see to it that the laboratory maintains a budgeted level of expenditure but at the same time meets a stipulated service requirement. Service requirements are not evident in data normally collected by hospitals. Therefore, additional information has to be generated in order to meet the higher level objectives. The establishment of the service objective may initially increase the budget because of increased volumes (assuming laboratory results affect the

**FIGURE III.1.2**
Average nursing hours per patient day for each week of 1969

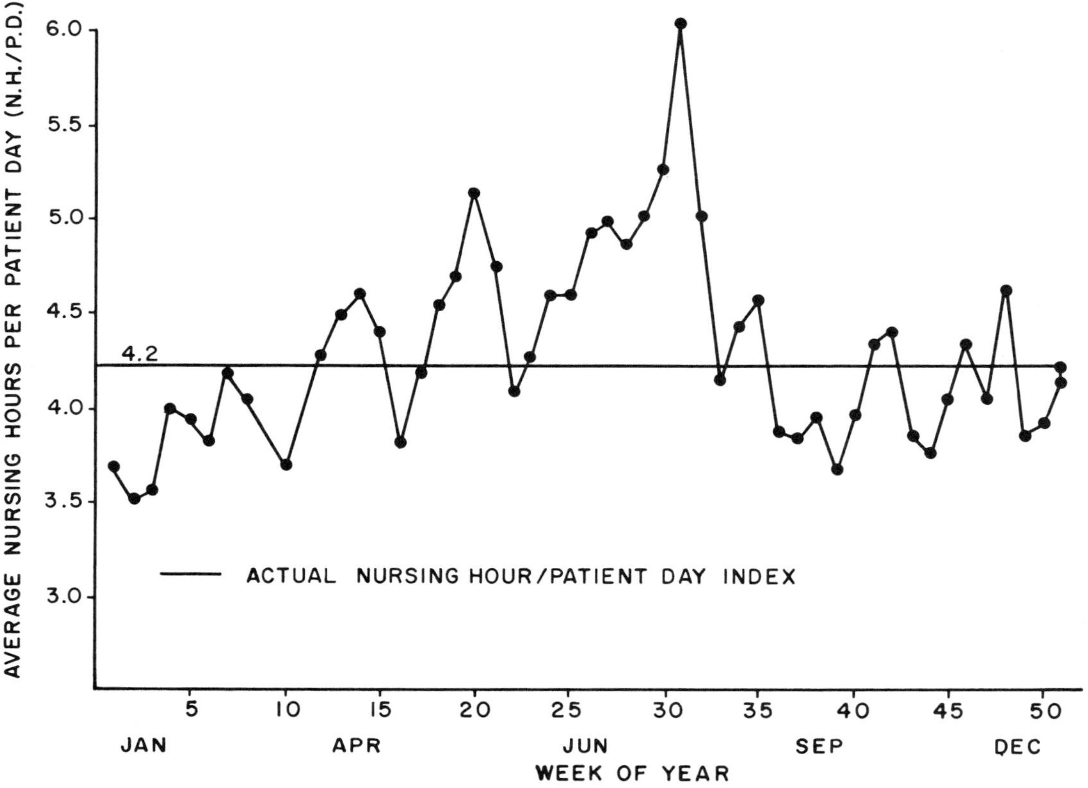

length of stay and the hospital occupancy is maintained). The establishment of a service objective will also cause an intensive investigation of the flow of work from the physician to the laboratory and then back to the medical record. The high time delay aspects of the flow will be identified and corrected. The budget can then be reestablished using the new procedures and activity levels. The primary control loop will then consist of two measures: budget and services. Either or both can cause an out-of-control situation to occur. The maintenance of two goals simultaneously is characteristic of complex control systems and is a job well trained managers can do. Despite this, one sometimes hears the comment that such a dual goal is impossible, that quality of care must come first. It is difficult to accept these arguments in light of the fact that one key element in quality—how long it takes to return information to the doctor—is rarely measured.

## Using Improved Control Systems

The examples presented in this chapter are typical of the types of changes in controls that are needed if hospital systems are to advance. If costs are to be controlled, the essential components are the ability and incentive to investigate more carefully the expenditure of resources, the appropriate amount of resource necessary to perform a function, and the true objective of the expenditure. Variation in the cost of an activity provides important clues as to where significant savings in costs can be achieved.

Examination of the resources consumed per unit of activity may also be important for supplying a quality service. It is conceivable that the amount of resource for an activity can be too little and the quality can suffer without the administration becoming aware of the situation. On the other hand, without proper controls, the desire for quality can result in costs being inflated by resources provided to ensure a very low probability of insufficient resources at any point in time. This is typically what happens using traditional control systems in hospitals which have an excess of beds. In these situations, there will be infrequent times when the hospital will be full, causing a need for higher than average resources. Usually, these higher resources are budgeted on a full time basis to take care of this situation. The result is that the hospital has excess resources a large percentage of the time. Traditional budget-based control systems are also used in other organizations with the same disadvantages just described. These have been overcome by not only looking at last year's performance, but by attempting to determine the possible sources of excess costs and what can be done to control them. For example, figure III.1.3 contains the same data plotted in figure III.1.2, but in addition, a dashed line is plotted which gives the number of nursing hours per patient

**FIGURE III.1.3**
Average actual nursing hours per patient day and nursing hours per patient day assuming a fixed staff

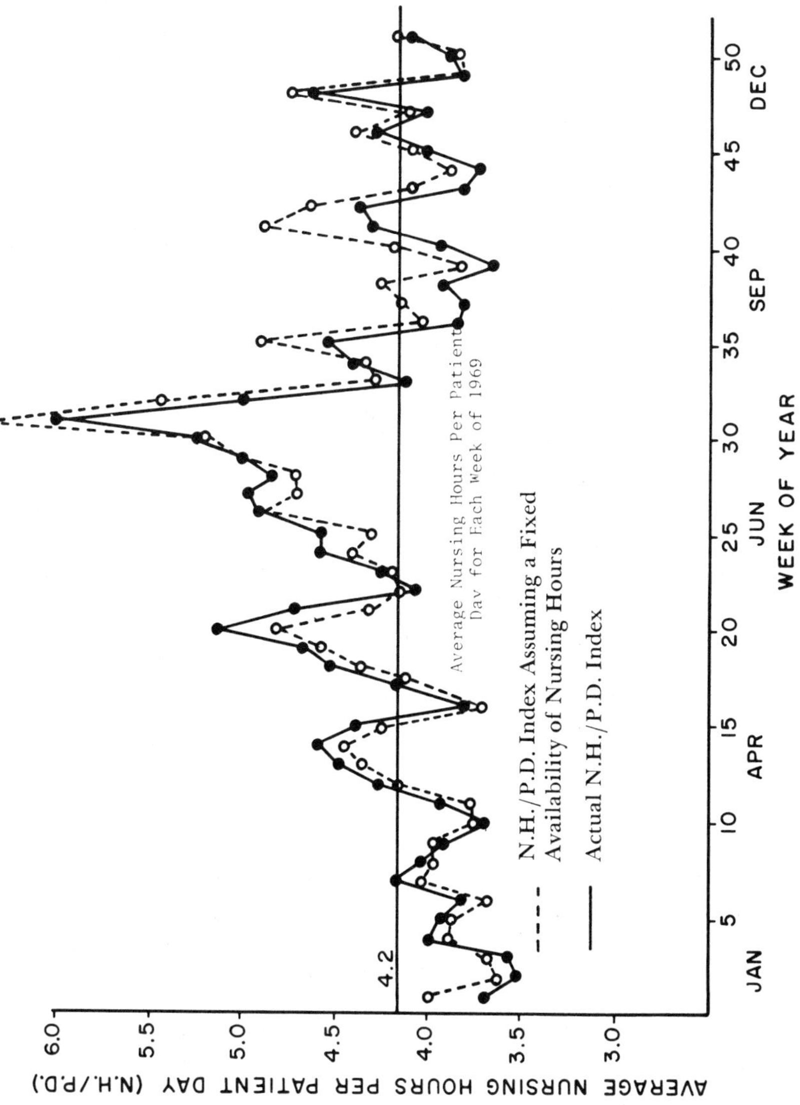

day that would be available if a fixed staff were employed. Since the curves are almost identical, the evidence is clear that the nursing supervisor has used the control mechanisms given to her by the budget officers. She has maintained a constant work force. Figure III.1.4 is a plot of the census during the period. Lows in census correspond to the highs in N.H./P.D. The conclusion is that the variation in census is the main contributor to the wide swings in N.H./P.D. index, and if the variation were reduced, the nursing budget could be reduced without going below 3.5 N.H./P.D. If we assume that the census can be stabilized, we can now pose the question: If we could control the census perfectly and staffed at 3.5 N.H./P.D., what would be the savings? Since the present budget is $2,200,000, the savings would be (.70/4.2) x ($2,200,000) or $366,667, which is a 16.7 percent improvement. This is the maximum we can save, assuming the 3.5 N.H./P.D. is constrained by quality of care considerations. What procedures are most appropriate?

The following are worthy of consideration: 1. *The census repeatedly drops in the summer months in the hospital.* Since the drop is substantial, two possibilities exist: (a) Schedule vacations for the nursing staff in June, July, and August, thereby reducing the nursing hours available consistent with the census. (b) Using an admission scheduling program, actively encourage a higher rate of elective surgery during this period, thereby increasing the census. 2. *The census during the rest of the year varies randomly around 120.* Variance from week to week is high, indicating that no controls exist to reduce variation.

Since the census has such wide variation from week to week, it should be realistically possible to keep the census below 125 by stabilizing the amount of elective surgery with more careful scheduling in fifteen of the fifty-two weeks. The savings can be calculated as follows:

• The highest census (136) corresponds to 3.5 N.H./P.D. If the maximum census were reduced to 125, then (136 x 3.5) ÷ 125 = 3.81 N.H./P.D.

• Since our lower bound of 3.5 N.H./P.D. is always to be achieved, the average requirement of 4.2 N.H./P.D. can be reduced by 3.81 − 3.5 or .31. 3.89 would then be the budgeted figure. The savings would be (.31 ÷ 4.2) x $2,200,000 or $162,381/year. This would be a savings of 7.4 percent.[5]

It is important to point out that most budget officers do not generally examine the causes of cost and, therefore, are not in a position to encourage much more than the status quo. Because of this, the procedure that is widely used in many organizations is that the annual budget, after being adjusted for salary increases, is reduced by a fixed percentage, usually five percent. The philosophy is that the operating people have as one of their major responsibilities the goal of continually improving the

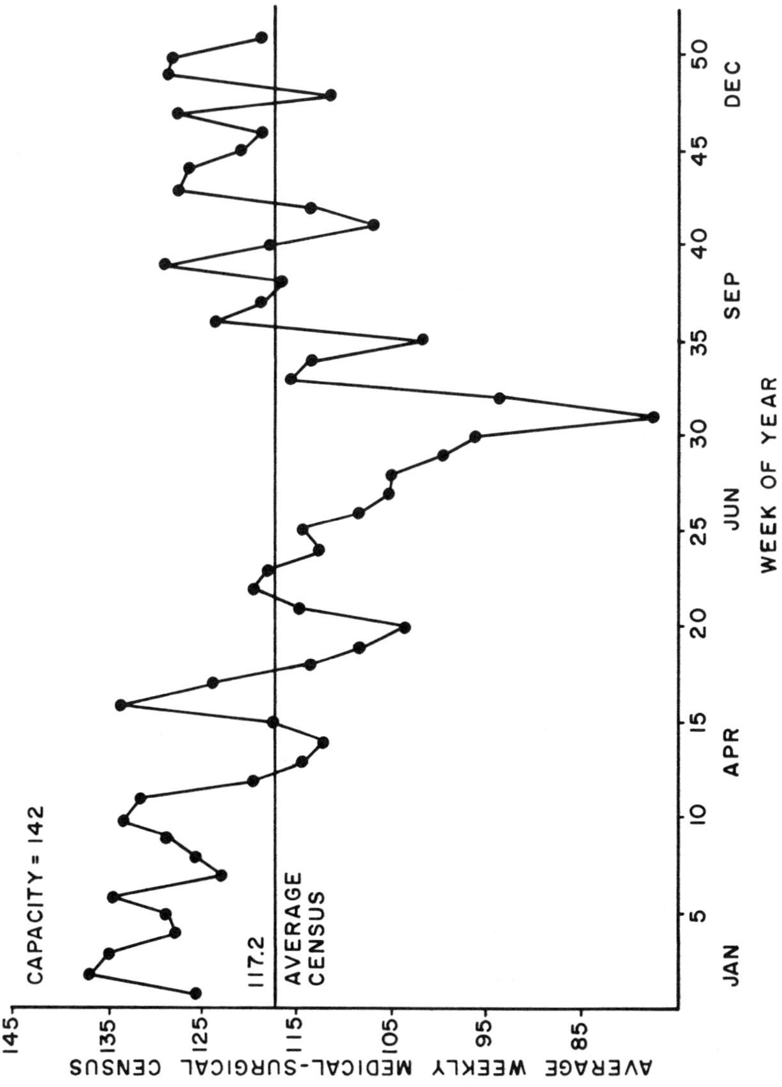


**FIGURE III.1.4**
Average census for each week of 1969

cost of the operation. It is their job to initiate the investigations and install the control systems that will enable the cost reduction objective to be accomplished.

The purpose of the arbitrary reduction is to encourage the improvement of performance. It is worth noting that such an improvement appears possible without reducing quality of care below levels currently in effect (i.e., 3.5 N.H./P.D.). To achieve it, however, would require a concerted effort of administration and nursing, as well as the acceptance of the medical staff. Such a complex operation is not likely to be undertaken in the absence of clear incentives.

## Data Base Requirements

As mentioned previously, one of the constraints in the establishment of a control system is the availability of measures of objective achievement. In many situations this is not a serious restriction. For example, the analysis done in the previous section was done using existing information. The variables to be controlled could be successfully implemented using existing data. The development of the N.H./P.D. required the merging of data collected from payroll and the census. Since this will be on a weekly basis, the merging can be done by hand without affecting the quality of the control process because the time required to reduce the data is not critical.

In most successful control systems, the data base has to be in such a form that appropriate reduction and analysis can be made in sufficient time to enable the control process to function. Work routines have to be established to assure accomplishment. The establishment of these routines takes considerable effort over long periods of time. This is one of the main reasons why existing data systems should be used if possible. Also, the implementation of the control system is quicker, the acceptance of the integrity of the data is higher, and the cost of implementation and operation is kept at a minimum. The routine systems of payroll, accounts receivable, general accounting, and medical records are of such importance in many hospitals that their proper functioning is the major responsibility of someone in the organization. He makes sure the data are received when needed and that there are a minimum of errors.

With the rise in internal and external needs for routine data reduced to specified formats and the increasing availability of computer service companies and relatively inexpensive computer systems, many hospitals are transforming their data systems to computers. In most cases, the decision to use a computer is based on the fact that the computer is a more cost-effective method of processing payrolls, accounts receivable, and budgets. The philosophy adopted by many administrators is that if the introduction of a computer for the "bread and butter" operations is no more costly than hand systems, the hospital can have access to many secondary advantages of great potential. These are as follows:

• *A substantial decrease in the error rate (ten to 100 times).*

• *The ability to merge data bases more readily.* For example, most control systems involving calculations of resources/activity require merging.

• *The ability to reduce information from the same base for the specific needs of different management levels.* For example, in the control system discussion three management levels are involved, each requiring a different reduction of data. Also, information is only given when exceptions exist. This type of reporting is best done by computer.

• *The ability to interrogate the data base for additional information.* For example, if one wanted to check the feasibility of reducing the nursing hours per patient day in the example already given, by scheduling summer vacations only, the number of weeks of vacation to be taken could be retrieved and compared with the expected excess nursing hours. Internal programming capability is usually required to perform extraordinary interrogations in reasonable times.

• *The ability to perform extensive calculations quickly and accurately in minimum time.* For example, in section III.3 Warner describes a nurse scheduling scheme, and in section III.4 Trivedi discusses a daily nurse allocation model. Both of these systems are infeasible without computer resources. In Warner's case, the calculations are too extensive to be done reliably by hand, and in Trivedi's situation, numerous calculations have to be done between 7:00 A.M. and 7:15 A.M. that can only be done by computer. Even the basic payroll data reports suggested by Lipson in section III.7 are difficult to achieve manually.

The initiative for attempting to cost-justify the computer system should be the desire on the part of the administrator to get more timely and more properly reduced data for control purposes even though it is wise to constrain or eliminate any planned increases in expenditures. Unfortunately, the introduction of the computer does not automatically solve the administrator's problems. His problems change from information underload to information overload. Considerable maturity in terms of who should get what information and in what form becomes a necessary requirement in realizing the full benefits of the computer system. Since data in many forms and in large quantities can be obtained just by pushing a button (or hiring a programmer), the following problems are usually experienced by the administrator with a new computer system:

• *Everyone is provided with a full copy of the output.* The result is that the information is not used because no one has time to reduce the data for his specific needs. Eventually, the more able managers will specify exactly what information they need and in what format.

• *People will be encouraged to discard their existing data systems because the computer is faster and better.* This situation, if it occurs, usually results in chaos. The existence of information that is not properly reduced and that people do not know how to use will cause a deterioration in hospital operations. Alternatively, the new system is treated as redundant and ignored, while the old one is continued indefinitely. Ideally, people should be encouraged to retain their existing control systems until they feel comfortable with the new ones and then become weaned to the new systems. A particular point to make here is that informal communications between people are in practically all cases faster than computer systems. Since the primary control loops depend heavily on rapid communication of out-of-control situations, the informal communications are to be encouraged—not discouraged. Another reason for the encouragement is that formal control systems provide signals that an out-of-control condition exists, but the control system is not designed to communicate *why* the system is out of control. The informal communication links are absolutely necessary to supply this information.

## Organizational Changes Resulting From Improved Operational Control Systems

The purpose of this section is to discuss the changes in organizational behavior that are facilitated as one moves toward better control systems. Experience indicates that the following changes occur.

### Reactive Administration to Leadership Through Prediction and Planning

Reactive administration is "putting out fires." Little previous planning is usually involved and the decision maker relies heavily on previous experience to make appropriate decisions at any given time. Because little effort is invested in planning, which is the development of desirable expectations, decisions tend to be past, not future, oriented. Administrators who allow themselves to get into this position find that over a period of time they have survived, but they have not made significant improvements in their operations. The main reason is that their decisions are not consistent with a plan or with each other. Control systems place on the decision maker the necessity of making plans about future expectations. Under these situations, the appropriate decisions for particular types of problems that will occur can be made in advance. The staffing level control example above is typical of the type of leadership brought about by the development of proper management information systems. Acceptable variation, alternative solutions, and criteria for their use are all established in advance in a well-designed staffing system. The transition in management styles is not limited to nonclinical areas, but extends to problems involving the medical staff and its leadership as well.

### Reactive Position to Leadership Position of the Medical Staff

It is repeatedly observed that the administrator can be at a serious disadvantage in proposing constructive programs to the medical staff. The reasons are many, but they include lack of planned objectives for the medical staff, lack of measures of institutional performance (such as turnaround time of laboratory and x-ray reports) that directly affect medical performance, and inability to operate hospital systems to close tolerances (such as ninety-five percent adult medical and surgical occupancy). The proper improvement of hospital systems is rarely contrary to legitimate medical staff goals and is frequently complementary to them. This is particularly true in the newer responsibilities of the medical staff, such as those implied in PSRO legislation.

## Operational Objectives and Their Measurement Rather Than Status Quo Cost Control

Examples have been given where traditional budgeting approaches result in doing as well as last year with adjustments for inflation. Operational objectives, on the other hand, center around the amount of resources used for a given activity with the basic assumption that if the resources for a given activity are used correctly, the budget will be within control. Under the former, budgetary procedures are established at the super control level to tolerances so broad that secondary and primary controls do not have to exist for budgetary procedures to be followed. This means that there can be little incentive and no mechanism for operational improvement. Distortions occur which are not consistent with quality medical care at minimum cost. Unnecessary admissions, excessive lengths of stay, overstaffing, low occupancies, and slow turnaround times of service departments can occur at the same level as in the past and go undetected. Many of these elements reflect as much on quality as they do on cost. This point should not be overlooked—the protection of quality is one of the defenses used by special interest groups who wish to avoid close tolerance operations.

## Determining Why Systems Go Out of Control

With the use of operational control systems, there will be occasions when out-of-control situations exist. Frequently, the problem is that someone does not know what to do. The role of the secondary and super control levels is in many cases primarily that of a teacher, informing people of the latitude they have in the decision making process and at the same time making sure that they understand how to perform correctly. This is consistent with the findings of behavioral scientists concerning the methods of achieving maximum productivity of social groups.[6] The information system identifies that the system is failing but allows each group time to solve its own problems, thereby utilizing the problem solving resources efficiently. This procedure minimizes the probability of the system failing for the same reasons in the future.

## Enhancement of Lower Level Management Within Hospitals

If the primary and secondary loops are caused to function by the management information system, the lower managerial levels, like the shift supervisor and department heads, are expected to make the appropriate decisions. Their jobs are enhanced as a result. The people occupying these jobs generally respond more favorably toward their responsibilities because they feel that they have more control over the factors affecting them.

Perhaps this section should be concluded by saying that the function of the management in operational systems is to have a plan and to try to cause things to go according to plan as smoothly as possible. The way to do this is to set high goals, provide the technical support for accomplishing them, and then concentrate on those areas which need further support in order to achieve the goals. Improved information systems are consistent with these objectives. Managements that have attempted them have found that the number of problems that occur on a daily basis is much smaller than heretofore thought possible, because considerable attention is paid to solving problems of a general nature so that they will no longer continue to recur. The result is that in the long run, the higher levels of objectives can be achieved with the same amount of management resource and in the short run a higher level of management resource is needed to implement the new system.

## NOTES

[1]Three levels of control systems are frequently discussed: strategic planning; management control; and operational control. This section deals with operational control, which is primarily concerned with the accomplishment of specific objectives.

[2]It is worth a passing note that the primary controller is rarely "surprised" by the first formal or written report of exception. Good primary controllers work directly with their own observations and realities and the abstractions of quantitative data merely confirm these. It is an important point of systems design that this capability of primary controllers be enhanced, not interfered with, by the system.

[3]The forecasts are sometimes improved by statistical analysis, but the point is that they assume the relevance of previous history.

[4]Figures III.1.2, III.1.3, and III.1.4 are modifications of figures found in "Inpatient Admissions Scheduling: An Application to a Nursing Service," a doctoral dissertation by Galen P. Briggs, Jr., The University of Michigan, 1971.

[5]In this instance, 3.5 N.H./P.D. appeared to be a satisfactory level, providing it was not exceeded (in a negative sense). Since there are no universally agreed upon ratios, each hospital has to be analyzed using its perception of the quality of nursing care. Also, a separate budget exists for vacations. The budget was found to be inflated by the vacations taken during low census periods. Substantial savings could have been made by more carefully scheduling vacations and then reducing

the staff budget for time worked. Although the data are not available at this writing, estimates made of the potential savings were one-third to one-half of the vacation accrual budget.

[6]Peter F. Drucker, *The Practice of Management*. New York: Harper and Brothers, 1954.

Rensis Likert, *The Human Organization*. New York: McGraw-Hill, 1967.

# III.2

# Admission Scheduling and Control Systems

*by Walton M. Hancock, D. Michael Warner, Shyam Heda, and Paul Fuhs*

## Introduction

The process of admitting a patient is the primary act which commits the resources of the hospital for the present and for a number of days into the future. Consequently, a thorough examination of the admissions process is an inescapable aspect of any major study in controlling the costs of hospital operation. Because hospitals differ in the rate and type of incoming patients and in internal operating policies, the admissions procedure for one hospital might not be appropriate for another. A general procedure, therefore, must be adaptable to a range of conditions. The one presented below is tailored to medium-sized community hospitals but may be extended to other conditions with caution. The procedure is oriented to adult medical-surgical patients but may be extended to any other group of patients where a significant fraction are elective.

## The Goals of the Admissions Process

It is important to state the objectives of an admission procedure explicitly. The overall objective of the Bureau team was to demonstrate methods to minimize the cost of running a hospital subject to the constraint that quality of service be maintained. This overall objective dictates the objectives of the admissions process, which are in general cost minimization subject to satisfactory service of demand. However, the specific objectives differ depending on whether the hospital is generally overbedded or underbedded. An overbedded hospital is a facility where demand for beds is normally less than capacity. An underbedded hospital is taken as any other condition, including those hospitals where demand equals capacity.

For the overbedded hospital, the admissions objectives should be to minimize variations in census and to schedule as many patients as possible, subject to the following constraints:

- Minimum acceptable nursing hours per patient day are maintained.
- Admission delays are within policy levels. Frequently these have to be established during the implementation of the system.
- Weekend census policies are maintained.

A scheduling system serving these goals was used in the adult medical-surgical unit of Able Hospital. The following potential to reduce costs was found: When twenty percent of the patients were scheduled instead of admitted immediately, the census variance was substantially reduced. The average delay in admission for that twenty percent was approximately two days. Nursing staff could be reduced approximately seven percent with a resultant payroll saving of approximately $39,000 per year if the probability of .008 that the nursing hours per patient day going below 3.2 was acceptable. This saving allows the actual scheduling of nursing personnel where any need less than a full time person was provided for by assigning an additional person.

This example is given to illustrate the importance of the constraints on the main objective of minimizing census variations. The smaller the census variation, the more closely the nursing resources can be fit to the nursing demand. Of course, savings may also be realized in other departments because the level of peak demands will be lower. Dietary, housekeeping, laboratory, and operating rooms are potential areas.

The scheduling of elective patients enables as much diagnosis and care as possible to be undertaken prior to admission. Preadmission testing and/or preadmission orders scheduling patients for services more quickly after admission can result in future savings through length of stay reductions.

An underbedded hospital is a facility where demand generally equals or exceeds the resources available. Occupancies of ninety percent or more on the medical-surgical units are generally indicative of this condition. The objectives for an underbedded hospital are different from those for overbedded facilities because in an underbedded hospital it becomes possible to minimize cost by maintaining maximum use of beds. Therefore, the objectives are as follows:

Maximize census and schedule as many patients as possible subject to the following constraints:

- Cancellations do not exceed an acceptable number.
- Turnaways do not exceed an acceptable number.
- Weekend census does not exceed policy.

Cancellations are defined as patients that have been scheduled for admission who cannot be admitted due to lack of beds. Turnaways are unscheduled patients arriving at the hospital (usually emergencies) who cannot be accommodated.

Cancellations and turnaways have different significance in different hospitals. One hospital considered ten cancellations per week normal. Another considered two per month to be the limit. The same is true of turnaways. In one hospital, a portion of emergency patients, after verification of the nature of their emergency, were routinely sent to another hospital in the local area, whereas a second hospital had a policy of admitting all emergencies even if scheduled patients had to be cancelled. (The policy was influenced by the fact that the second hospital was the only facility within fifty miles.) Also, turnaways frequently have a different connotation than the literal interpretation. A turnaway is sometimes accommodated by putting a bed in the hall, thus temporarily increasing capacity. This solution is still less than ideal, and therefore it is called a turnaway to control the frequency of its occurrence.

A weekend policy constraint is included because some hospitals have policies such as every other weekend off for their nursing staffs, which mean that weekend census is constrained by the availability of nurses. The constraint must be stated explicitly in terms of maximum permissible occupancy.

The scheduling of patients is included as part of the objective in the underbedded case for the same reason as in the overbedded situation. The ability to implement procedures to reduce length of stay is much greater because the scheduling of patients and delayed admissions are more readily accepted by physicians under high occupancy conditions. Also, there is more motivation to reduce length of stay in order to increase the throughput of patients.

Baker Hospital, where much of the system development and testing occurred, is an underbedded facility. Prior to the decision of hospital authorities to increase the throughput, average occupancy was eighty-eight percent in the adult medical-surgical unit, with long queues of patients waiting for admission. The admission procedures used (no scheduling for medical patients, erratic surgical scheduling, lack of control of emergency admissions, calling medical patients in the late afternoon to restore census after surgicals had arrived) did not permit the facility to be used to the fullest extent. The new administrator, appointed with the explicit directive to increase occupancy, ordered admission personnel to fill every bed every evening. The result was that more surgical patients were scheduled, emergencies were more carefully scrutinized by the medical utilization review committee, and call-in procedures were improved. The census increased to ninety-four to ninety-five percent. However, the cancellations and turnaways increased to five to ten per week for many weeks, a level intolerable to the medical staff. The admission scheduling system described later in this chapter was then introduced. The results for the first twenty weeks after implementation were:

• The average census was 94.1 percent.

• There were no emergency turnaways.

• There were no ICU/CCU turnaways.

• The cancellation rate was less than one per week.

• All elective surgery was scheduled. As a byproduct, use of the operating rooms was stabilized.

• The amount of management attention necessary on a daily basis was reduced (and was easily within tolerable levels).

• Approximately half of the elective medical patients and all of the elective surgical patients were scheduled. Early testing on the day of admission and preadmission testing were actively being considered.

• The estimated revenue increase due to increased occupancy (eighty-eight to ninety-four percent) was $560,000 per year with only minor additions to the admissions department staff and variable costs of care.

The methodologies presented in following parts of this chapter suggest even better results than achieved in this initial trial because the technology has since been improved.

## A Brief History of the Development of the Admission Scheduling System

The initial attempt to schedule the admissions process was in an overbedded facility. The implementation problems are discussed in section IV.3 of this book. The system consisted of elective surgical and medical scheduling allowances for each day of the week and a call-in procedure to fill beds that were open because of the differences between scheduled admissions and discharges on any given day. The admissions officer, comptroller, director of nursing, and administrator were supportive of the efforts at all times. However, when elective admissions were delayed even as much as one or two days, the medical staff reacted negatively. The situation was compounded by the Bureau's attempts to minimize variance in discharge estimates by introducing a physician-supplied estimate of discharge, by the decision of hospital authorities to install a new computer system with insufficient internal staff, by the proximity of another overbedded hospital, and by the need to develop technology during the implementation process.[1]

The Bureau team concluded that the overbedded situation was a great deterrent to minimizing costs because of the difficulty of convincing physicians that admissions should be delayed when there were empty beds. This difficulty persisted even when it was made clear to the physicians that if the patients were admitted there would be inadequate nursing care available. The only solution to this dilemma was to shut down a wing of the hospital. The administrator and trustees were not willing to do this.

As the result, the Bureau team started to work intensively in an underbedded facility. A real-time computer-aided admissions system was designed with an improved physician-based discharge estimating system. Difficulty was experienced in getting the on-line system operational, and a manual system was installed as an interim step that did not require physician discharge estimates. The manual system produced the results presented earlier in this chapter. These were so satisfactory that even though the computer system would enable the scheduling of practically all of the elective medical patients, the cost of its operation in the absence of an internal computer capability for accounting operations could not be justified. The result was that further work was directed to the manual system. The improved manual system is described in the next section.

## The Scheduling System

An admission scheduling system is a set of rules for controlling the flow of patients into a hospital where the rules are designed to meet certain goals concerning the flow and placement of patients. The overbedded hospital scheduling system has the following specific goals:

- Maximize occupancy on all units.
- Give all nonemergency surgical patients a firm date of admission and maximize the number of medical patients given firm dates of admission.
- Hold the expected number of cancellations per week to an acceptable low level.
- Hold the expected number of emergency (ER) turnaways, ICU/CCU turnaways, and OB turnaways to acceptable low levels.
- The system (or set of rules) should be easy enough to understand and follow that admissions office personnel can apply it without aid of special calculations or a computer.

It is easily seen that many of the above goals directly conflict with one another. The design of the system must, therefore, meet the goals by maintaining a proper balance among them to the extent that they conflict.

The scheduling environment is summarized in figure III.2.1. Patients entering the hospital are classified into six service types (left of figure III.2.1) and the units into which patients flow into four types (right side of figure III.2.1). Notice that some patients can go to more than one unit, although usually there exists a preference for the unit in which the patient should be placed. Thus, ER patients usually go directly to the medical-surgical unit, but if that is full, they may be temporarily held in an ER holding area (if one exists). If the holding area, too, is full, some hopsitals will temporarily place an ER patient in the ICU/CCU unit. Similarly, some GYN patients may be placed in the OB unit in some hospitals, although usually this is limited to some maximum number. (Although not shown in figure III.2.1, in some hospitals ICU/CCU patients may also be held temporarily on the medical-surgical unit or in the ER holding area.) The scheduling system is designed around the environment of a particular hospital, conforming to present policies and facilities. The system is also, of course, designed around a particular hopsital's arrival rates of different types of patients (on different days of the week) and the capacities of the different units.

The remainder of this section describes the structure of the scheduling system, and the following section develops methods of establishing appropriate parameters for the system for a particular hospital.

The system consists of a set of policy rules, called "allowances."

**The Surgical Allowance**—All nonemergency surgical patients are given fixed dates of admission in the future. The surgical allowance specifies the maximum number of surgical patients to schedule on any particular day.

**FIGURE III.2.1**
Flow of patient types

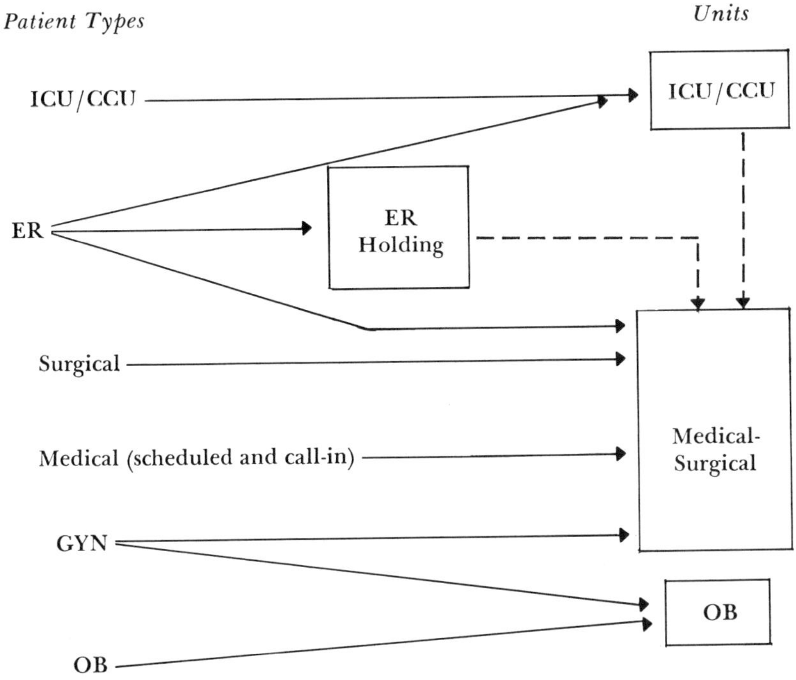

Example: Schedule no more than the following surgical patients:

| SUN | MON | TUES | WED | THURS | FRI | SAT |
|---|---|---|---|---|---|---|
| 16 | 14 | 14 | 12 | 12 | 0 | 0 |

**The GYN Allowance**—(Optional. Used by those hospitals who schedule GYN patients separately from general surgery. For other hospitals, the GYN are included in the surgical allowance.) The GYN allowance is applied in the same manner as the surgical allowance.

Example: Schedule no more than the following GYN patients:

| SUN | MON | TUES | WED | THURS | FRI | SAT |
|---|---|---|---|---|---|---|
| 2 | 2 | 3 | 3 | 3 | 0 | 0 |

**The Medical Allowance**—Applied in the same manner as the surgical allowance.

Example: Schedule no more than the following medical patients:

| SUN | MON | TUES | WED | THURS | FRI | SAT |
|---|---|---|---|---|---|---|
| 2 | 2 | 1 | 1 | 1 | 7 | 7 |

**The Census Reduction Allowance**—This is formed by combining the following two allowances:

*The Emergency (ER) Allowance:* Sometime in the afternoon (say 1:00 P.M.) after all discharges and scheduled patient arrivals are known, medical patients on a waiting list ("call-ins") may be called in to fill empty beds. Care must be taken, however, that some beds are left empty to accommodate ER patients who will arrive between then and (say) 9:00 A.M. the next day (when discharges begin). The ER allowance is the number of beds to leave empty to accommodate such ER arrivals.

Example: Leave six empty beds each day for ER arrivals.

*Weekend Allowance:* Because surgery is typically performed only on weekdays, discharges on Sunday, Monday, and Tuesday are the lowest of the week, while admissions on these three days are the highest. Thus, some provision must be made to leave an appropriate number of beds empty on Saturday, Sunday, and Monday (and perhaps other) nights to accommodate the excess of admissions over discharges on the next day. Thus a weekend allowance, *in addition to the ER allowance,* must be left empty.

Example: In addition to the ER allowance, leave the following number of beds empty:

| SUN | MON | TUES | WED | THURS | FRI | SAT |
|---|---|---|---|---|---|---|
| 7 | 3 | 0 | 0 | 0 | 0 | 12 |

These two allowances are combined to form the *census reduction allowance:* the total number of beds to leave empty each day.

Example: At 1:00 P.M., call in medical patients from the waiting list until the following number of beds is left empty:

| SUN | MON | TUES | WED | THURS | FRI | SAT |
|---|---|---|---|---|---|---|
| 13 | 9 | 6 | 6 | 6 | 6 | 18 |

**Med/Max Call-In Limit**—In addition to the census reduction allowance, the number of medical call-ins is subject to daily maximums in order not to disturb the balance of available beds necessary to accommodate patients already scheduled for the next few days.

Example: Do not call in more than the following waiting line patients:

| SUN | MON | TUES | WED | THURS | FRI | SAT |
|---|---|---|---|---|---|---|
| 10 | 8 | 6 | 8 | 8 | 10 | 10 |

**The Cancellation Allowance**—This allowance is the number of beds that must be left empty for arriving emergency patients *even if scheduled patients must be cancelled to do so.*

Example: At 1:00 P.M., leave the following beds empty even if scheduled patients must be cancelled:

| SUN | MON | TUES | WED | THURS | FRI | SAT |
|---|---|---|---|---|---|---|
| 4 | 4 | 4 | 4 | 4 | 4 | 4 |

The above rules handle the six different patient types as follows:

*ICU/CCU patients:* Admit immediately to the ICU/CCU unit (or hold temporarily as policy and space permit, in the ER holding area or the medical-surgical unit).

*ER patients:* Admit immediately to the medical-surgical unit, or if full, to the ER holding area (if one exists), or if full, to the ICU/CCU unit, as policy and space permit.

*OB patients:* Admit immediately to the OB unit.

*Surgical patients:* Give firm dates of admission up to allowance maximums and admit as those dates arrive to the medical-surgical unit, but cancel if number of beds falls below cancellation allowance.

*Medical patients:* Give firm date of admission to all so desiring, and maintain list of patients wanting admission as soon as possible (patients may be both scheduled and on the waiting list). Admit scheduled patients as their dates arrive to the medical-surgical unit (subject to cancellation allowance), and call in from waiting list up to the census reduction allowance (or med/max call-in limit).

*GYN patients:* Give firm dates of admission (either according to the GYN allowance, or include as part of the surgical allowance). Admit to either the OB unit or the medical-surgical unit, as policy and space permit.

There are, of course, many other patient flow decisions made each day by the admitting office, mostly concerning the transfer of patients among units. Policies governing such decisions are considered as part of the scheduling environment of a particular hospital, and the scheduling system is designed around them.

The question remains of how to set allowances so that the hospital maintains proper balance among conflicting goals. Occupancy, cancellations, turnaways, and the medical-surgical balance are very sensitive to specific values for the allowances. In addition, the relationships between, say, the census reduction allowance, cancellations, and turnaways are extremely complex. To be able to evaluate how a particular "schedule," or set of values for all the allowances, meets and balances the goals, a computer model has been developed to simulate the operation of the above scheduling system for a particular hospital. By systematically evaluating many potential schedules on the computer simulator, the one that best meets the objectives can be identified.

## Identifying the Best Schedule for the Admission Scheduling System

The computer simulator is able to "operate" a given hospital as if it were using a particular schedule and to generate performance information relating to the goals to be met, such as number of cancellations a week and the average occupancy experienced over 200 or more weeks of simulated time. An initial schedule, however, must be provided as a starting point for the search for the best schedule. Thus, the search has two phases: identifying a "good" initial schedule; and making changes in that schedule and evaluating the new one, repeating this process until the best schedule is identified.

In order to set an initial schedule and simulate the operation of a particular hospital, a fair amount of data describing the operation of the hospital must be available. These data include arrival distributions by day of week, and length of stay distributions by day of week of admission, for:

- ICU/CCU patients
- OB patients
- GYN patients
- Surgical patients
- Medical patients
- Emergency patients

In addition, priorities of admission to the medical-surgical unit among scheduled medical, scheduled surgical, scheduled emergency (both direct and from the emergency holding area), and ICU/CCU transfers must be specified to reflect hospital policy. Other priorities are also specified, such as the preferred placement of ICU/CCU patients, if the ICU/CCU unit is full.

Table III.2.1 displays admissions data from Baker Hospital for 1971. No data were available concerning the actual demand on the hospital except that on several occasions during 1971 elective surgeries were scheduled six weeks in advance. Therefore, the patient arrival rate was exceeding the admission rate for substantial portions of the year. Figure III.2.2 displays the capacities and patient flows at Baker (not shown is the possibility of holding ICU/CCU patients briefly on the medical-surgical floor or in the ER holding area if ICU/CCU is full). Figure III.2.3 lists the specific objectives to be met by the scheduling system.

The strategy for identifying the best schedule for Baker is the following:

- Set surgical allowance, census reduction allowance, cancellation allowance, and med/max call-in limit to initial values (the "initial schedule").

**TABLE III.2.1**
Average admissions, transfers, and discharges by day of week Baker Hospital 1971

| | SU | MO | TU | WE | TH | FR | SA | TOT |
|---|---|---|---|---|---|---|---|---|
| Non-ER Surg Admissions | 15.0 | 13.7 | 12.0 | 11.9 | 12.0 | 1.0 | 1.2 | 66.8 |
| ER (Med + Surg) Admissions | 7.0 | 7.0 | 7.0 | 7.0 | 7.0 | 7.0 | 7.0 | 49.0 |
| ICU/CCU Transfers to Med-Surg | 2.0 | 2.0 | 2.0 | 2.0 | 2.0 | 2.0 | 2.0 | 14.0 |
| Non-ER Med Admissions | 1.8 | 2.5 | 4.0 | 3.3 | 3.5 | 6.6 | 5.9 | 27.6 |
| Total Med-Surg Admissions | 25.8 | 25.2 | 25.0 | 24.2 | 24.5 | 16.6 | 16.1 | 157.4 |
| Total Med-Surg Discharges | 18.3 | 12.0 | 21.6 | 26.2 | 23.3 | 23.7 | 32.3 | 157.4 |

Occupancy about ninety-three percent on medical-surgical unit.

• Make simulation runs, adjusting above, until cancellations and turn-aways are near zero. This is the "intermediate schedule."

• Set medical allowance.

• Make simulation runs, again adjusting all above, until system is acceptable.

The initial surgical allowance is set to reflect current nonemergency surgical admissions at Baker:

| | SU | MO | TU | WE | TH | FR | SA | Total |
|---|---|---|---|---|---|---|---|---|
| Current Admissions: | 15 | 13.7 | 12. | 11.9 | 12 | 1 | 1 | 66.6 |
| Initial Schedule: | 16 | 14 | 12 | 12 | 13 | 0 | 0 | 67 |

**FIGURE III.2.2**
Scheduling environment for Baker Hospital

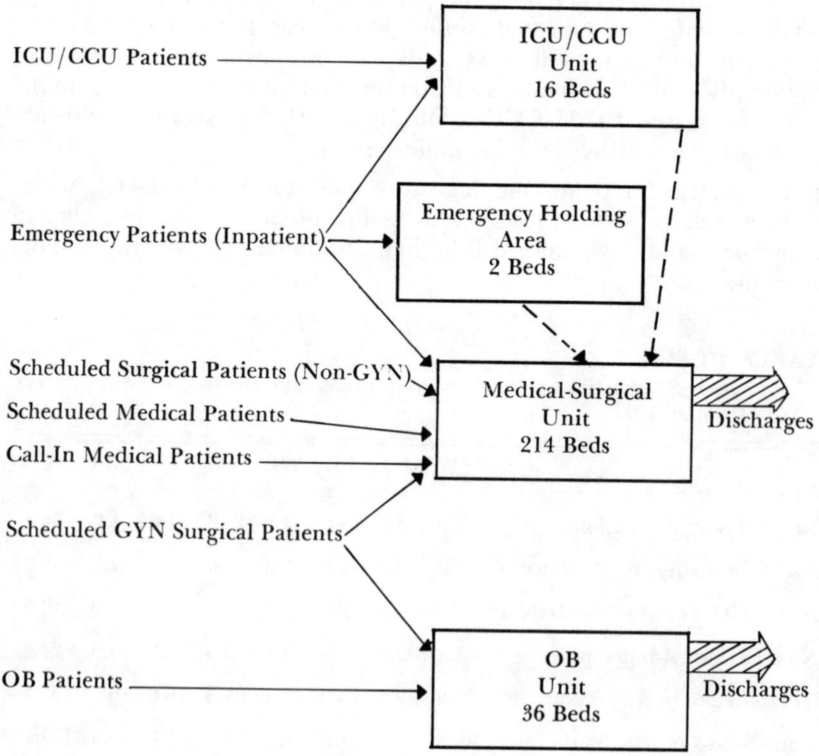

The census reduction allowance is a combination of the emergency allowance and the weekend allowance. The initial emergency allowance is set at the ninety-fifth percentile of the emergency arrival distribution (patients arriving between 1:00 P.M. and 9:00 A.M.). This is eleven each day for Baker.

The initial weekend allowance is set based on 1971 daily average arrivals and discharges:

| | SU | MO | TU | WE | TH | FR | SA |
|---|---|---|---|---|---|---|---|
| Arrivals: | 26 | 25 | 25 | 24 | 25 | 17 | 16 |
| Discharges: | 18 | 12 | 22 | 26 | 23 | 24 | 32 |

The initial values are set beginning with Thursday and working backwards. Since discharges are greater than admissions on Friday, we need leave no empty beds open on Thursday night. However, we need to leave two beds empty on Wednesday night to cover the difference between arrivals and discharges on Thursday. These beds are provided by the excess of discharges over admissions on Wednesday so that no beds are needed Tuesday. On Monday we must leave three beds for Tuesday. This logic results in the following allowance:

| SU | MO | TU | WE | TH | FR | SA |
|---|---|---|---|---|---|---|
| 13 | 3 | 0 | 2 | 0 | 0 | 8 |

**FIGURE III.2.3**
Objectives of the scheduling system

Average no more than

.5 Cancellations per week

.5 ER turnaways per week

.2 ICU turnaways per week

2 Failed ICU transfers per week

.2 OB turnaways per week

And

Maintain current number of surgical patients per week

Maximize occupancy

Maximize number of scheduled medical patients

The initial ER allowance and weekend allowance are combined to form the initial census reduction allowance as follows. For those days (Monday through Friday) that the initial weekend allowance is small, the two are simply added. For the other days, only the *mean* ER arrival rate (=7 for Baker) is added to the weekend allowance, since ninety-five percent protection is not needed. Thus, our initial census reduction allowance is:

| SU | MO | TU | WE | TH | FR | SA |
|---|---|---|---|---|---|---|
| 20 | 14 | 11 | 13 | 11 | 11 | 15 |

The initial cancellation allowance is set to the average ER arrival rate: seven each day.

The initial maximum call-in allowance is set, from past experience with the system, to eight for each day.

Thus, our initial schedule (no scheduled medicals) is:

| | SU | MO | TU | WE | TH | FR | SA |
|---|---|---|---|---|---|---|---|
| Census Reduction Allowance | 20 | 14 | 11 | 13 | 11 | 11 | 15 |
| Med/Max Call-In Limit | 8 | 8 | 8 | 8 | 8 | 8 | 8 |
| Cancellation Allowance | 7 | 7 | 7 | 7 | 7 | 7 | 7 |
| Surgical Allowance | 16 | 14 | 12 | 12 | 13 | 0 | 0 |

The results of a 200-week simulation run of Baker using this schedule are displayed in table III.2.2. While the cancellation rate (.20 per week) and ER turnaway rate (.17 per week) are within acceptable levels as specified in the goals, they will increase when medical patients are scheduled. These rates and the census can be improved by making slight changes in the initial allowances, and this is done by noting on which days cancellations and ER turnaways are occurring, on which days census is low, and adjusting the allowances to improve those days. Our search strategy calls for adjusting this schedule, evaluating the change with a simulation run, and repeating this process until the best schedule without scheduled medical patients is found. The result of this first search (involving eight simulation runs) is the intermediate schedule, displayed in table III.2.3. The results of this schedule (200-week simulation) are displayed in table III.2.4.

The third step of the search strategy is to set an intermediate medical allowance, such that the *increase* in risk of cancellation is $\leq .05$ and the *increase* in risk of violating the census reduction allowance is $\leq .10$. (These two numbers are based on current experience with the system.) These increases are reflected in the distribution of the number of useable beds at 1:00 P.M. generated by the intermediate schedule simulation—table III.2.5 displays this distribution for Thursday. If the number of empty beds is less than four (the cancellation allowance), patients must be cancelled. Thus for Thursday, there was one day when four patients had to be cancelled (the "0" row) and one day when three patients had to be cancelled (the "1" row). If one medical patient had been promised admission on Thursday, the percentage of days on which cancellations occurred would have increased by 1.5. Thus, five medical patients may be scheduled on Thursday without increasing the risk of cancellation by more than .05. However, only two may be scheduled without increasing the risk of violating the census reduction allowance (eleven) by more than .10.

Similarly, the other days of the week are analyzed to produce the following intermediate medical allowance:

| SU | MO | TU | WE | TH | FR | SA |
|---|---|---|---|---|---|---|
| 2 | 2 | 1 | 1 | 2 | 7 | 4 |

Step four of the search strategy leads (after approximately twelve 200-week simulation runs) to the final schedule shown in table III.2.6. The results of this schedule are displayed in table III.2.7.

The final schedule operated the medical-surgical unit at ninety-six percent occupancy, while holding cancellations, ER turnaways, and ICU turnaways below the goals stated in figure III.2.3. OB turnaways were also held below the constraints of figure III.2.3 and occupancy was sixty-three percent. (These are controlled by the limit on the number of GYN patients allowed on OB, set either by hospital policy or considered as a decision variable in the simulation analysis.) On the ICU unit, forced transfers (forcing an ICU patient to the medical-surgical unit one day prematurely to allow another ICU patient into the ICU unit) were held to .96 a week, and on the average, .63 ICU patients per week were kept in the ICU unit one day longer than was necessary—a delayed transfer. The ICU occupancy was seventy-two percent.

The occupancy can be increased slightly above the final results but only by suffering unacceptable increases in cancellations and turnaways. Cancellations may be decreased by allowing more ER patients to be delayed in the ER holding area or the ICU unit, but this was also felt to be an undesirable trade-off. Many similar trade-offs were evaluated in arriving at the final schedule, and the understanding of such trade-offs must be considered one of the major outputs of the analysis.

Each simulation run (of 200 weeks) takes approximately twenty seconds of CPU time on an IBM 360/67. (This corresponds to approximately $5.00 on this machine.)

## TABLE III.2.2
### Results from initial schedule

MS FLOOR SUMMARY STATISTICS

| TOT | SUN | MON | TUE | WED | THU | FRI | SAT | |
|---|---|---|---|---|---|---|---|---|
| 0.20 | 0.00 | 0.05 | 0.03 | 0.08 | 0.03 | 0.00 | 0.00 | AVG # OF CANCELLATIONS |
| 0.17 | 0.00 | 0.04 | 0.03 | 0.05 | 0.04 | 0.00 | 0.00 | AVG # OF EMG TURNAWAYS |
| 0.01 | 0.00 | 0.00 | 0.00 | 0.00 | 0.00 | 0.00 | 0.00 | AVG # OF ICU TURNAWAYS |
| 0.00 | 0.00 | 0.00 | 0.00 | 0.00 | 0.00 | 0.00 | 0.00 | AVG # OF GYN PTS. ADMITTED |
| 36.48 | 4.23 | 5.05 | 4.52 | 4.57 | 4.27 | 7.70 | 6.13 | AVG # OF CALL-IN PTS. ADMITTED |
| 159.61 | 27.94 | 26.54 | 23.92 | 24.04 | 25.05 | 16.91 | 15.21 | AVG # OF ADMISSIONS |
| 159.62 | 16.93 | 16.30 | 23.38 | 24.03 | 24.19 | 28.38 | 26.40 | AVG # OF DISCHARGES |
| 200.20 | 195.50 | 205.70 | 206.30 | 206.30 | 207.10 | 195.70 | 184.50 | AVG # OF BEDS OCCUPIED |
| 94 | 91 | 96 | 96 | 96 | 97 | 91 | 86 | AVG % OF OCCUPANCY |

OB FLOOR SUMMARY STATISTICS

| TOT | SUN | MON | TUE | WED | THU | FRI | SAT | |
|---|---|---|---|---|---|---|---|---|
| 0.05 | 0.00 | 0.00 | 0.01 | 0.01 | 0.02 | 0.00 | 0.00 | AVG # OF OB TURNAWAYS |
| 0.00 | 0.00 | 0.00 | 0.00 | 0.00 | 0.00 | 0.00 | 0.00 | AVG # OF GYNS TO MED-SURG |
| 42.37 | 6.70 | 6.77 | 6.27 | 6.60 | 6.13 | 4.85 | 5.05 | AVG # OF ADMISSIONS |
| 42.40 | 5.85 | 5.63 | 5.94 | 6.10 | 6.24 | 6.36 | 6.27 | AVG # OF DISCHARGES |
| 22.90 | 22.00 | 23.10 | 23.50 | 24.00 | 23.90 | 22.40 | 21.20 | AVG # OF BEDS OCCUPIED |
| 63 | 61 | 64 | 65 | 67 | 66 | 62 | 59 | AVG % OCCUPANCY |

ICU FLOOR SUMMARY STATISTICS

| TOT | SUN | MON | TUE | WED | THU | FRI | SAT | |
|---|---|---|---|---|---|---|---|---|
| 0.01 | 0.00 | 0.00 | 0.00 | 0.00 | 0.00 | 0.00 | 0.00 | AVG # OF ICU TURNAWAYS |
| 1.55 | 0.20 | 0.19 | 0.25 | 0.25 | 0.23 | 0.20 | 0.22 | AVG # OF FORCED TRANSFERS |
| 0.43 | 0.00 | 0.08 | 0.07 | 0.14 | 0.13 | 0.00 | 0.00 | AVG # OF DELAY TRANSFERS TO MED-SUR |
| 0.30 | 0.05 | 0.05 | 0.04 | 0.04 | 0.02 | 0.03 | 0.05 | AVG # OF DELAY ADMITTANCES |
| 0.27 | 0.04 | 0.04 | 0.04 | 0.04 | 0.04 | 0.02 | 0.04 | DELAYED IN EMERGENCY HOLDING AREA |
| 0.03 | 0.01 | 0.01 | 0.00 | 0.00 | 0.01 | 0.01 | 0.01 | DELAYED ON MED-SURG UNIT |
| 14.59 | 2.33 | 2.21 | 2.07 | 2.07 | 2.00 | 1.98 | 1.93 | AVG # OF ADMISSIONS |
| 13.09 | 2.01 | 1.86 | 1.76 | 1.85 | 1.84 | 1.95 | 1.80 | AVG # OF TRANSFERS |
| 11.01 | 10.92 | 11.09 | 11.15 | 11.14 | 11.07 | 10.90 | 10.81 | AVG # OF BEDS OCCUPIED |
| 69 | 68 | 69 | 70 | 70 | 69 | 68 | 68 | AVG % OCCUPANCY |

EHA FLOOR SUMMARY STATISTICS

| TOT | SUN | MON | TUE | WED | THU | FRI | SAT | |
|---|---|---|---|---|---|---|---|---|
| 0.09 | 0.04 | 0.09 | 0.14 | 0.13 | 0.17 | 0.02 | 0.04 | AVG # OF BEDS OCCUPIED -- TOTAL |
| 5 | 2 | 4 | 7 | 6 | 9 | 1 | 2 | AVG % OCCUPANCY -- TOTAL |
| 0.05 | 0.00 | 0.05 | 0.10 | 0.08 | 0.13 | 0.00 | 0.00 | AVG # OF BEDS OCCUPIED BY EMERGENCY PTS. |
| 3 | 0 | 2 | 5 | 4 | 7 | 0 | 0 | AVG % OF BEDS OCCUPIED BY EMERGENCY PTS. |
| 0.04 | 0.04 | 0.04 | 0.04 | 0.04 | 0.04 | 0.02 | 0.04 | AVG # OF BEDS OCCUPIED BY ICU PTS. |
| 2 | 2 | 2 | 2 | 2 | 2 | 1 | 2 | AVG % OF BEDS OCCUPIED BY ICU PTS. |

DISTRIBUTION OF EHA CENSUS

| ZERO | ONE | >TWO |
|---|---|---|
| 0.94 | 0.02 | 0.03 |

MED PATIENT TYPE SUMMARY STATISTICS

| TOT | SUN | MON | TUE | WED | THU | FRI | SAT | |
|---|---|---|---|---|---|---|---|---|
| 0.00 | 0.00 | 0.00 | 0.00 | 0.00 | 0.00 | 0.00 | 0.00 | AVG # OF CANCELLATIONS |
| 66.54 | 8.61 | 9.39 | 8.70 | 8.77 | 8.52 | 12.04 | 10.50 | AVG # OF ADMITTANCES |
| 0.00 | 0.00 | 0.00 | 0.00 | 0.00 | 0.00 | 0.00 | 0.00 | AVG # OF SCHEDULED MED ADMITTED |
| 36.48 | 4.23 | 5.05 | 4.52 | 4.57 | 4.27 | 7.70 | 6.13 | AVG # OF CALL-INS ADMITTED |
| 24.09 | 3.45 | 3.48 | 3.39 | 3.31 | 3.44 | 3.45 | 3.55 | AVG # OF MED EMG ADMITTED |
| 5.97 | 0.93 | 0.85 | 0.79 | 0.89 | 0.80 | 0.89 | 0.81 | AVG # OF MED ICU ADMITTED |
| 66.60 | 6.54 | 8.57 | 9.73 | 9.86 | 10.15 | 12.91 | 8.83 | AVG # OF DISCHARGES |
| 97.90 | 99.20 | 100.00 | 99.00 | 97.90 | 96.30 | 95.40 | 97.10 | AVG # OF BEDS OCCUPIED |

SURG PATIENT TYPE SUMMARY STATISTICS

| TOT | SUN | MON | TUE | WED | THU | FRI | SAT | |
|---|---|---|---|---|---|---|---|---|
| 0.20 | 0.00 | 0.05 | 0.03 | 0.08 | 0.03 | 0.00 | 0.00 | AVG # OF CANCELLATIONS |
| 93.07 | 19.33 | 17.15 | 15.22 | 15.26 | 16.53 | 4.86 | 4.71 | AVG # OF ADMITTANCES |
| 59.46 | 14.41 | 12.40 | 10.53 | 10.44 | 11.66 | 0.00 | 0.00 | AVG # OF SCH SURG ADMITTED |
| 0.00 | 0.00 | 0.00 | 0.00 | 0.00 | 0.00 | 0.00 | 0.00 | AVG # OF GYN ADMITTED |
| 24.93 | 3.62 | 3.55 | 3.45 | 3.61 | 3.58 | 3.60 | 3.50 | AVG # OF SUR EMG ADMITTED |
| 8.67 | 1.29 | 1.19 | 1.23 | 1.21 | 1.28 | 1.26 | 1.20 | AVG # OF SURG ICU ADMITTED |
| 93.02 | 10.39 | 7.73 | 13.65 | 14.17 | 14.03 | 15.46 | 17.57 | AVG # OF DISCHARGES |
| 97.30 | 91.20 | 100.70 | 102.20 | 103.30 | 105.80 | 95.20 | 82.30 | AVG # OF BEDS OCCUPIED |

**TABLE III.2.2 Cont.**

GYN PATIENT TYPE SUMMARY STATISTICS

| TOT | SUN | MON | TUE | WED | THU | FRI | SAT | |
|---|---|---|---|---|---|---|---|---|
| 0.00 | 0.00 | 0.00 | 0.00 | 0.00 | 0.00 | 0.00 | 0.00 | AVG # OF CANCELLATIONS |
| 0.00 | 0.00 | 0.00 | 0.00 | 0.00 | 0.00 | 0.00 | 0.00 | AVG # OF GYN ADMITTED TO M-S |
| 7.33 | 1.58 | 1.54 | 1.43 | 1.47 | 1.30 | 00.00 | 0.00 | AVG # OF GYN ADMITTED TO OB |
| 7.33 | 0.97 | 0.73 | 0.91 | 1.00 | 1.20 | 1.28 | 1.23 | AVG # OF GYN DIS FROM OB |
| 3.70 | 2.80 | 3.60 | 4.20 | 4.60 | 4.70 | 3.40 | 2.20 | AVG # OF BEDS OCC ON OB |

EMG PATIENT TYPE SUMMARY STATISTICS

| TOT | SUN | MON | TUE | WED | THU | FRI | SAT | |
|---|---|---|---|---|---|---|---|---|
| 0.17 | 0.00 | 0.04 | 0.03 | 0.05 | 0.04 | 0.00 | 0.00 | AVG # OF TURNAWAYS |
| 0.46 | 0.00 | 0.06 | 0.11 | 0.12 | 0.16 | 0.00 | 0.00 | AVG # OF DELAY ADMITTANCES |
| 0.37 | 0.00 | 0.05 | 0.10 | 0.08 | 0.13 | 0.00 | 0.00 | AVG # OF DELAYED IN EHA |
| 0.08 | 0.00 | 0.01 | 0.01 | 0.03 | 0.03 | 0.00 | 0.00 | AVG # OF DELAYED ON ICU |

OB PATIENT TYPE SUMMARY STATISTICS

| TOT | SUN | MON | TUE | WED | THU | FRI | SAT | |
|---|---|---|---|---|---|---|---|---|
| 0.05 | 0.00 | 0.00 | 0.01 | 0.01 | 0.02 | 0.00 | 0.00 | AVG # OF TURNAWAYS |
| 35.04 | 5.11 | 5.23 | 4.84 | 5.12 | 4.82 | 4.85 | 5.05 | AVG # OF ADMITTANCES |
| 35.06 | 4.87 | 4.90 | 5.03 | 5.10 | 5.04 | 5.08 | 5.04 | AVG # OF DISCHARGES |
| 19.20 | 19.20 | 19.50 | 19.30 | 19.30 | 19.10 | 18.90 | 18.90 | AVG # OF BEDS OCCUPIED |

The results of the final schedule may also be compared with the results achieved in Baker Hospital. These comparisons are shown in table III.2.8.

## Sensitivity Analysis

When using the simulator to develop schedules, questions have arisen concerning the sensitivity of results to characteristics of the input parameters. Specifically, questions have been raised concerning the sensitivity of the simulation output parameters to the following:

- Variations in average length of stay
- Variations in the shape of the length of stay distributions
- The effect of different values of med/max call-in limit

### Variations in Length of Stay (LOS)

Figure III.2.4 is a plot of the mean length of stay of elective surgical patients of a thirty-four bed unit of a hospital (not Baker). The mean of this distribution is 4.77 days.[2] The dashed lines are confidence limits to determine if the length of stay (LOS) is varying randomly. The two points outside the limits (2/73 and 3/73) were quickly identified by hospital personnel to be the result of a flu epidemic among the staff which disrupted operations. The rest of the data are within the limits with no trends of significant length. This means that LOS on a monthly basis is a random variable around a stable mean. A modified form of the simulator (utilizing a different method of obtaining the census reduction allowance) was run where the number of scheduled surgeries was held constant but different LOS were used. The LOS chosen were 4.288 days, 4.77 days, and 5.252

**TABLE III.2.3**
Initial and intermediate schedule: Baker Hospital

| | | SU | MO | TU | WE | TH | FR | SA |
|---|---|---|---|---|---|---|---|---|
| Census | | | | | | | | |
| Reduction | Initial | 23 | 12 | 11 | 12 | 12 | 15 | 31 |
| Allowance | Intermediate | 20 | 11 | 11 | 11 | 11 | 13 | 26 |
| Med/Max | Initial | 8 | 8 | 8 | 8 | 8 | 8 | 8 |
| Call-In Limit | Intermediate | 8 | 8 | 8 | 8 | 8 | 8 | 8 |
| Cancellation | Initial | 7 | 7 | 7 | 7 | 7 | 7 | 7 |
| Allowance | Intermediate | 4 | 4 | 4 | 4 | 4 | 4 | 4 |
| Surgical | Initial | 16 | 14 | 12 | 12 | 13 | 0 | 0 |
| Allowance | Intermediate | 17 | 13 | 12 | 12 | 13 | 0 | 0 |

**FIGURE III.2.4**
Average length of stay by month

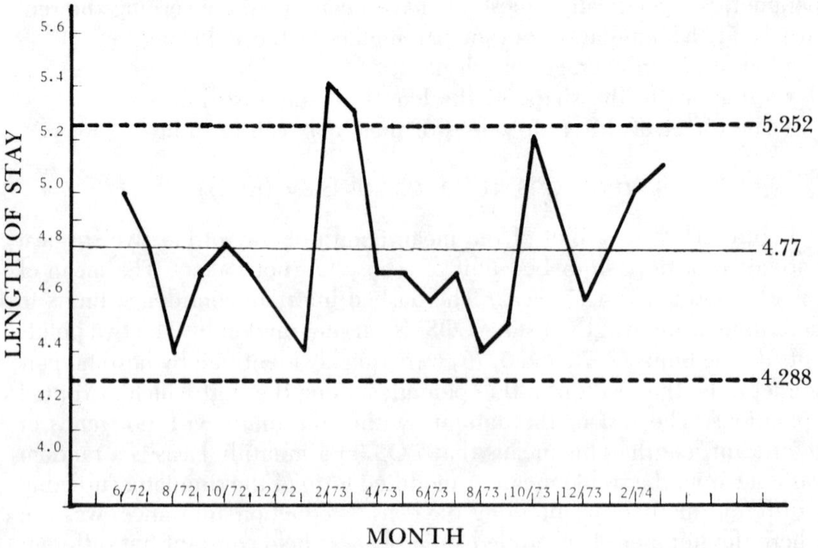

## TABLE III.2.4
Results from intermediate schedule

MS FLOOR SUMMARY STATISTICS

| TOT | SUN | MON | TUE | WED | THU | FRI | SAT | |
|---|---|---|---|---|---|---|---|---|
| 0.05 | 0.00 | 0.03 | 0.00 | 0.01 | 0.01 | 0.00 | 0.00 | AVG # OF CANCELLATIONS |
| 0.15 | 0.00 | 0.05 | 0.03 | 0.04 | 0.02 | 0.00 | 0.00 | AVG # OF EMG TURNAWAYS |
| 0.01 | 0.00 | 0.00 | 0.00 | 0.01 | 0.00 | 0.00 | 0.00 | AVG # OF ICU TURNAWAYS |
| 0.00 | 0.00 | 0.00 | 0.00 | 0.00 | 0.00 | 0.00 | 0.00 | AVG # OF GYN PTS. ADMITTED |
| 38.81 | 4.98 | 5.10 | 4.74 | 4.45 | 4.47 | 7.84 | 7.21 | AVG # OF CALL-IN PTS. ADMITTED |
| 161.87 | 29.84 | 25.33 | 24.13 | 23.84 | 24.99 | 17.52 | 16.21 | AVG # OF ADMISSIONS |
| 161.87 | 17.64 | 16.87 | 23.99 | 23.45 | 24.58 | 28.47 | 26.85 | AVG # OF DISCHARGES |
| 200.40 | 197.20 | 205.70 | 205.90 | 206.20 | 206.70 | 195.70 | 185.00 | AVG # OF BEDS OCCUPIED |
| 94 | 92 | 96 | 96 | 96 | 97 | 91 | 86 | AVG % OCCUPANCY |

OB FLOOR SUMMARY STATISTICS

| TOT | SUN | MON | TUE | WED | THU | FRI | SAT | |
|---|---|---|---|---|---|---|---|---|
| 0.10 | 0.00 | 0.00 | 0.03 | 0.01 | 0.02 | 0.03 | 0.00 | AVG # OF OB TURNAWAYS |
| 0.00 | 0.00 | 0.00 | 0.00 | 0.00 | 0.00 | 0.00 | 0.00 | AVG # OF GYNS TO MED-SURG |
| 42.33 | 6.16 | 6.62 | 6.60 | 6.11 | 6.56 | 4.94 | 5.33 | AVG # OF ADMISSIONS |
| 42.35 | 5.87 | 6.04 | 5.82 | 6.16 | 5.88 | 6.28 | 6.28 | AVG # OF DISCHARGES |
| 22.90 | 22.10 | 22.70 | 23.50 | 23.40 | 24.10 | 22.70 | 21.80 | AVG # OF BEDS OCCUPIED |
| 64 | 61 | 63 | 65 | 65 | 67 | 63 | 61 | AVG % OCCUPANCY |

ICU FLOOR SUMMARY STATISTICS

| TOT | SUN | MON | TUE | WED | THU | FRI | SAT | |
|---|---|---|---|---|---|---|---|---|
| 0.01 | 0.00 | 0.00 | 0.00 | 0.01 | 0.00 | 0.00 | 0.00 | AVG # OF ICU TURNAWAYS |
| 0.51 | 0.09 | 0.09 | 0.05 | 0.05 | 0.06 | 0.06 | 0.10 | AVG # OF FORCED TRANSFERS |
| 0.16 | 0.00 | 0.07 | 0.01 | 0.05 | 0.03 | 0.00 | 0.00 | AVG # OF DELAY TRANSFERS TO MED-SURG |
| 0.01 | 0.00 | 0.01 | 0.00 | 0.00 | 0.00 | 0.00 | 0.00 | AVG # OF DELAY ADMITTANCES |
| 0.01 | 0.00 | 0.01 | 0.00 | 0.00 | 0.00 | 0.00 | 0.00 | DELAYED IN EMERGENCY HOLDING AREA |
| 0.00 | 0.00 | 0.00 | 0.00 | 0.00 | 0.00 | 0.00 | 0.00 | DELAYED ON MED-SURG UNIT |
| 13.93 | 1.91 | 1.90 | 2.02 | 2.12 | 2.03 | 2.01 | 1.94 | AVG # OF ADMISSIONS |
| 13.60 | 1.97 | 1.76 | 2.03 | 1.85 | 2.03 | 2.00 | 1.94 | AVG # OF TRANSFERS |
| 9.70 | 9.56 | 9.61 | 9.56 | 9.84 | 9.84 | 9.79 | 9.71 | AVG # OF BEDS OCCUPIED |
| 61 | 60 | 60 | 60 | 61 | 52 | 61 | 61 | AVG % OF OCCUPANCY |

EHA FLOOR SUMMARY STATISTICS

| TOT | SUN | MON | TUE | WED | THU | FRI | SAT | |
|---|---|---|---|---|---|---|---|---|
| 0.07 | 0.02 | 0.09 | 0.10 | 0.11 | 0.16 | 0.00 | 0.00 | AVG # OF BEDS OCCUPIED -- TOTAL |
| 3 | 1 | 5 | 5 | 5 | 8 | 0 | 0 | AVG % OF OCCUPANCY -- TOTAL |
| 0.06 | 0.01 | 0.08 | 0.09 | 0.10 | 0.06 | 0.00 | 0.00 | AVG # OF BEDS OCCUPIED BY EMERGENCY PTS. |
| 3 | 1 | 4 | 4 | 5 | 8 | 0 | 0 | AVG % OF BEDS OCCUPIED BY EMERGENCY PTS. |
| 0.01 | 0.00 | 0.01 | 0.01 | 0.01 | 0.00 | 0.00 | 0.00 | AVG # OF BEDS OCCUPIED BY ICU PTS. |
| 0 | 0 | 1 | 0 | 0 | 0 | 0 | 0 | AVG % OF BEDS OCCUPIED BY ICU PTS. |

DISTRIBUTION OF EHA CENSUS

| ZERO | ONE | >TWO |
|---|---|---|
| 0.96 | 0.02 | 0.30 |

**TABLE III.2.5**

Distribution of useable beds at 1:00 P.M. including scheduled patients, but no call-ins or cancellations

| | NUMBER | INCIDENCE | PERCENT | |
|---|---|---|---|---|
| | 0 | 1 | .5 | |
| | 1 | 1 | .5 | |
| | 2 | 0 | 0.0 | |
| | 3 | 0 | 0.0 | |
| Cancellation Allowance → | 4 | 3 | 1.5 | ≤ 5% (4–8) |
| | 5 | 0 | 0.0 | |
| | 6 | 3 | 1.5 | |
| | 7 | 0 | 0.0 | |
| | 8 | 4 | 2.0 | |
| | 9 | 4 | 2.0 | |
| | 10 | 9 | 4.5 | ≤10% (10–12) |
| Census Reduction Allowance → | 11 | 5 | 2.5 | |
| | 12 | 9 | 4.5 | |
| | 13 | 11 | 5.5 | |
| | 14 | 12 | 6.0 | |
| | 15 | 5 | 2.5 | |
| | 16 | 12 | 6.0 | |
| | 17 | 13 | 6.5 | |
| | 18 | 11 | 5.5 | |
| | 19 | 17 | 8.5 | |
| | 20 | 10 | 5.0 | |
| | 21 | 12 | 6.0 | |
| | 22 | 13 | 6.5 | |
| | 23 | 9 | 4.5 | |
| | 24 | 8 | 4.0 | |
| | 25 | 8 | 4.0 | |
| | 26 | 5 | 2.5 | |
| | 27 | 2 | 1.0 | |
| | 28 | 1 | .5 | |
| | 29 | 3 | 1.5 | |
| | 30 | 2 | 1.0 | |
| | 31 | 0 | 0.0 | |
| | 32 | 2 | 1.0 | |
| | 33 | 0 | 0.0 | |
| | 34 | 3 | 1.5 | |
| | 35 | 0 | 0.0 | |
| | 36 | 1 | .5 | |
| | 37 | 0 | 0.0 | |
| | 38 | 0 | 0.0 | |
| | 39 | 1 | .5 | |

**TABLE III.2.6**
Initial and final schedule for medical-surgical unit

| | | SU | MO | TU | WE | TH | FR | SA |
|---|---|---|---|---|---|---|---|---|
| Census Reduction Allowance | Initial | 23 | 12 | 11 | 11 | 11 | 14 | 31 |
| | Final | 20 | 11 | 11 | 11 | 11 | 13 | 26 |
| Med/Max Call-In Limit | Initial | 8 | 8 | 8 | 8 | 8 | 8 | 8 |
| | Final | 10 | 10 | 10 | 10 | 10 | 10 | 10 |
| Cancellation Allowance | Initial | 7 | 7 | 7 | 7 | 7 | 7 | 7 |
| | Final | 3 | 3 | 3 | 3 | 3 | 3 | 3 |
| Surgical Allowance | Initial | 16 | 14 | 12 | 12 | 13 | 0 | 0 |
| | Final | 17 | 13 | 12 | 12 | 13 | 0 | 0 |
| Medical Allowance | Initial | 2 | 2 | 1 | 1 | 2 | 7 | 4 |
| | Final | 2 | 2 | 2 | 2 | 2 | 7 | 4 |

days. These correspond to the confidence limits and overall mean LOS as depicted in figure III.2.4. The results are shown in table III.2.9. With increasing LOS the results are as follows:

- The number of called-in medical patients decreases
- The cancellation rate increases
- The patient throughput decreases

The conclusions are that the simulation results are sensitive to the variations in the mean LOS and that because of this sensitivity, control charts such as presented in figure III.2.4 would appear to be highly desirable in order to quickly detect nonrandom variations in LOS.

The simulation output, however, is usually within the acceptable range, as long as LOS is varying randomly around a fixed mean. Note that random variations affect primarily the number of call-ins, which are handled by the routine decision processes. If seasonal trends in mean LOS are known, then, of course, the schedules should be reexamined.

## Variations in the Shape of LOS Distribution

Figure III.2.5 is a plot of two distributions: one titled "Actual," which is the distribution of surgical LOS for Sunday at Baker Hospital, and the Poisson distribution with the same mean. The Poisson is used for comparison purposes because it is frequently assumed where the actual distribution is not available.[3] Obviously, there are substantial differences in the shape of the distributions, even though they have the same means.

**TABLE III.2.7**
Results from final schedule

MS FLOOR SUMMARY STATISTICS

| TOT | SUN | MON | TUE | WED | THU | FRI | SAT | |
|---|---|---|---|---|---|---|---|---|
| 0.23 | 0.00 | 0.06 | 0.03 | 0.01 | 0.13 | 0.00 | 0.00 | AVG # OF CANCELLATIONS |
| 0.43 | 0.00 | 0.11 | 0.05 | 0.13 | 0.13 | 0.00 | 0.00 | AVG # OF EMG TURNAWAYS |
| 0.02 | 0.00 | 0.00 | 0.00 | 0.01 | 0.00 | 0.01 | 0.00 | AVG # OF ICU TURNAWAYS |
| 0.00 | 0.00 | 0.00 | 0.00 | 0.00 | 0.00 | 0.00 | 0.00 | AVG # OF GYN PTS. ADMITTED |
| 24.22 | 1.08 | 2.42 | 2.82 | 3.30 | 2.79 | 7.45 | 4.35 | AVG # OF CALL-IN PTS. ADMITTED |
| 166.74 | 27.50 | 23.95 | 24.20 | 25.05 | 25.04 | 23.98 | 16.99 | AVG # OF ADMISSIONS |
| 166.73 | 17.43 | 18.09 | 24.37 | 24.93 | 24.98 | 29.45 | 27.46 | AVG # OF DISCHARGES |
| 204.70 | 202.70 | 208.60 | 208.40 | 208.60 | 208.60 | 203.10 | 192.70 | AVG # OF BEDS OCCUPIED |
| 96 | 95 | 97 | 97 | 97 | 97 | 95 | 90 | AVG % OCCUPANCY |

OB FLOOR SUMMARY STATISTICS

| TOT | SUN | MON | TUE | WED | THU | FRI | SAT | |
|---|---|---|---|---|---|---|---|---|
| 0.05 | 0.01 | 0.00 | 0.00 | 0.01 | 0.01 | 0.01 | 0.00 | AVG # OF OB TURNAWAYS |
| 0.00 | 0.00 | 0.00 | 0.00 | 0.00 | 0.00 | 0.00 | 0.00 | AVG # OF GYNS TO MED-SURG |
| 42.15 | 6.61 | 6.29 | 6.22 | 6.37 | 6.56 | 4.97 | 5.11 | AVG # OF ADMISSIONS |
| 42.17 | 5.68 | 5.89 | 5.69 | 6.25 | 5.98 | 6.24 | 6.42 | AVG # OF DISCHARGES |
| 22.60 | 22.10 | 22.50 | 23.00 | 23.20 | 23.70 | 22.50 | 21.20 | AVG # OF BEDS OCCUPIED |
| 63 | 61 | 63 | 64 | 64 | 66 | 62 | 59 | AVG % OCCUPANCY |

ICU FLOOR SUMMARY STATISTICS

| TOT | SUN | MON | TUE | WED | THU | FRI | SAT | |
|---|---|---|---|---|---|---|---|---|
| 0.02 | 0.00 | 0.00 | 0.00 | 0.01 | 0.00 | 0.01 | 0.00 | AVG # OF ICU TURNAWAYS |
| 0.96 | 0.16 | 0.18 | 0.09 | 0.11 | 0.13 | 0.13 | 0.16 | AVG # OF FORCED TRANSFERS |
| 0.63 | 0.00 | 0.13 | 0.13 | 0.15 | 0.21 | 0.00 | 0.00 | AVG # OF DELAY TRANSFERS TO MED-SURG |
| 0.00 | 0.00 | 0.00 | 0.00 | 0.00 | 0.00 | 0.00 | 0.00 | AVG # OF DELAY ADMITTANCES |
| 0.00 | 0.00 | 0.00 | 0.00 | 0.00 | 0.00 | 0.00 | 0.00 | DELAYED IN EMERGENCY HOLDING AREA |
| 0.00 | 0.00 | 0.00 | 0.00 | 0.00 | 0.00 | 0.00 | 0.00 | DELAYED ON MED-SURG UNIT |
| 13.76 | 2.02 | 1.76 | 1.91 | 1.99 | 2.08 | 1.97 | 2.01 | AVG # OF ADMISSIONS |
| 13.57 | 1.83 | 1.79 | 1.97 | 2.17 | 1.85 | 2.15 | 1.80 | AVG # OF TRANSFERS |
| 11.55 | 11.57 | 11.50 | 11.61 | 11.47 | 11.76 | 11.45 | 11.50 | AVG # OF BEDS OCCUPIED |
| 72 | 72 | 72 | 73 | 72 | 73 | 72 | 72 | AVG % OCCUPANCY |

EHA FLOOR SUMMARY STATISTICS

| TOT | SUN | MON | TUE | WED | THU | FRI | SAT | |
|---|---|---|---|---|---|---|---|---|
| 0.21 | 0.07 | 0.31 | 0.35 | 0.31 | 0.42 | 0.01 | 0.00 | AVG # OF BEDS OCCUPIED -- TOTAL |
| 11 | 3 | 15 | 8 | 5 | 21 | 0 | 0 | AVG % OCCUPANCY -- TOTAL |
| 0.21 | 0.07 | 0.30 | 0.35 | 0.30 | 0.41 | 0.01 | 0.00 | AVG # OF BEDS OCCUPIED BY EMERGENCY PTS. |
| 10 | 3 | 15 | 18 | 15 | 21 | 0 | 0 | AVG % OF BEDS OCCUPIED BY EMERGENCY PTS. |
| 0.00 | 0.00 | 0.00 | 0.00 | 0.00 | 0.00 | 0.00 | 0.00 | AVG # OF BEDS OCCUPIED BY ICU PTS. |
| 0 | 0 | 0 | 0 | 0 | 0 | 0 | 0 | AVG % OF BEDS OCCUPIED BY ICU PTS. |

DISTRIBUTION OF EHA CENSUS

| ZERO | ONE | >TWO |
|---|---|---|
| 0.88 | 0.03 | 0.09 |

Table III.2.10 contains the simulation outputs of the medical-surgical unit at Baker using the two distributions. A comparison of the data reveals that there is a radical change in the daily discharge rate (circled in the figure) which in turn has changed the simulation results significantly (cancellations from .61 to .26 per week, turnaways from .04 to .20 per week, and the number of patients called in from 23.23 to 26.05 per week). These differences would lead to the establishment of different allowances for a hospital—ones that would not correspond to the actual situation—thus, the actual LOS distributions are highly desirable.

**TABLE III.2.8**
Results from final schedule: medical-surgical

| | *Actual Figure* | *Simulation Result* |
|---|---|---|
| Med-Surg occupancy (weekly average) | 94.1% | 96.0% |
| OB turnaways/week | 0 | .05 |
| ICU/CCU turnaways/week | 0 | .02 |
| Surgical cancellations/week | Less than 1/week | .21 |

**TABLE III.2.9**
A comparison of simulation outputs for different lengths of stay

| | *4.288 Days* | *4.77 Days* | *5.252 Days* |
|---|---|---|---|
| Scheduled patients | 32 | 32 | 32 |
| Called-in patients | 12.37 | 9.46 | 7.05 |
| | 44.37 | 41.46 | 39.05 |
| Less cancellations (patients/day) | .04 | .14 | .18 |
| | 44.33 | 41.32 | 38.87 |

## Effect of Different Values of Med/Max Call-In Limit

The function of the med/max call-in limit is to limit the number of call-ins on any given day. The final solution for Baker Hospital has a med/max of ten. To observe the effect of changes in med/max on the simulation output parameters, the optimal solution was rerun with med/max set at four and twelve. A comparison of the results (table III.2.11) indicates the following:

- The expected occupancy is lower with med/max = 4 (.94 vs. .96).
- The cancellation rate is much lower with med/max = 4 (.31 vs. .70).
- Patient admissions are fewer with med/max = 4 (161.34 vs. 165.61).
- The differences in admissions are primarily due to the number of medical call-ins, which are less with med/max = 4 (17.61 vs. 22.74).

The observations are consistent with the argument that the higher the med/max, the more quickly census will be restored if high discharges occur. This results in an increase in occupancy. However, the higher med/max is, the more risk of cancellation on days following the admission

## TABLE III.2.10

### Simulation outputs for differing length of stay distributions

MS FLOOR SUMMARY STATISTICS

| TOT | SUN | MON | TUE | WED | THU | FRI | SAT | |
|---|---|---|---|---|---|---|---|---|
| 0.61 | 0.00 | 0.25 | 0.14 | 0.07 | 0.13 | 0.00 | 0.00 | AVG # OF CANCELLATIONS |
| 0.04 | 0.00 | 0.00 | 0.01 | 0.00 | 0.02 | 0.00 | 0.00 | AVG # OF EMG TURNAWAYS |
| 0.00 | 0.00 | 0.00 | 0.00 | 0.00 | 0.00 | 0.00 | 0.00 | AVG # OF ICU TURNAWAYS |
| 0.01 | 0.00 | 0.00 | 0.01 | 0.00 | 0.00 | 0.00 | 0.00 | AVG # OF GYN PTS. ADMITTED |
| 23.23 | 1.13 | 2.10 | 2.79 | 2.87 | 2.73 | 7.41 | 4.18 | AVG # OF CALL-IN PTS. ADMITTED |
| 166.65 | 26.56 | 24.35 | 24.24 | 24.64 | 25.34 | 24.29 | 17.22 | AVG # OF ADMISSIONS |
| 166.72 | 17.76 | 17.56 | 24.07 | 25.38 | 25.02 | 29.59 | 27.33 | AVG # OF DISCHARGES |
| 204.70 | 202.00 | 208.70 | 208.90 | 208.20 | 208.50 | 203.20 | 193.20 | AVG # OF BEDS OCCUPIED |
| 96 | 94 | 98 | 98 | 97 | 97 | 95 | 90 | AVG % OCCUPANCY |

Simulation Output for Baker Final Schedule Using the

Actual Length of Stay Distribution

MS FLOOR SUMMARY STATISTICS

| TOT | SUN | MON | TUE | WED | THU | FRI | SAT | |
|---|---|---|---|---|---|---|---|---|
| 0.26 | 0.00 | 0.00 | 0.03 | 0.07 | 0.15 | 0.00 | 0.00 | AVG # OF CANCELLATIONS |
| 0.20 | 0.00 | 0.00 | 0.01 | 0.09 | 0.10 | 0.00 | 0.00 | AVG # OF EMG TURNAWAYS |
| 0.03 | 0.01 | 0.00 | 0.00 | 0.02 | 0.00 | 0.00 | 0.00 | AVG # OF ICU TURNAWAYS |
| 0.01 | 0.00 | 0.00 | 0.00 | 0.00 | 0.00 | 0.00 | 0.00 | AVG # OF GYN PTS. ADMITTED |
| 26.05 | 4.28 | 7.03 | 4.49 | 2.93 | 1.99 | 3.61 | 1.70 | AVG # OF CALL-IN PTS. ADMITTED |
| 68.58 | 29.73 | 30.47 | 25.67 | 23.88 | 23.60 | 20.24 | 14.98 | AVG # OF ADMISSIONS |
| 68.58 | 26.10 | 23.88 | 24.05 | 23.15 | 22.65 | 23.24 | 25.51 | AVG # OF DISCHARGES |
| 204.30 | 199.00 | 205.60 | 207.30 | 208.00 | 208.90 | 205.90 | 195.40 | AVG # OF BEDS OCCUPIED |
| 95 | 93 | 96 | 97 | 97 | 98 | 96 | 91 | AVG % OCCUPANCY |

Simulation Output for Baker Final Schedule Where the

Length of Stay Distributions are Assumed to be Poisson

## TABLE III.2.11

### Simulation outputs of the optimal solution with med/max = 4 and 12: Baker final

MS FLOOR SUMMARY STATISTICS

| TOT | SUN | MON | TUE | WED | THU | FRI | SAT | |
|---|---|---|---|---|---|---|---|---|
| 0.31 | 0.00 | 0.22 | 0.03 | 0.02 | 0.02 | 0.00 | 0.00 | AVG # OF CANCELLATIONS |
| 0.42 | 0.00 | 0.09 | 0.11 | 0.12 | 0.09 | 0.00 | 0.00 | AVG # OF EMG TURNAWAYS |
| 0.01 | 0.00 | 0.00 | 0.01 | 0.00 | 0.00 | 0.00 | 0.00 | AVG # OF ICU TURNAWAYS |
| 0.03 | 0.00 | 0.00 | 0.01 | 0.00 | 0.01 | 0.00 | 0.00 | AVG # OF GYN PTS. ADMITTED |
| 17.61 | 2.07 | 1.98 | 2.25 | 2.45 | 2.15 | 3.55 | 3.16 | AVG # OF CALL-IN PTS. ADMITTED |
| 161.34 | 27.59 | 24.75 | 23.69 | 23.93 | 24.86 | 20.01 | 16.49 | AVG # OF ADMISSIONS |
| 161.39 | 17.57 | 16.58 | 23.94 | 24.22 | 23.98 | 28.13 | 26.96 | AVG # OF DISCHARGES |
| 200.80 | 197.50 | 205.70 | 205.50 | 205.20 | 206.10 | 198.00 | 187.50 | AVG # OF BEDS OCCUPIED |
| 94 | 92 | 96 | 96 | 96 | 96 | 93 | 88 | AVG % OCCUPANCY |

Optimal Solution with Med/Max = 4

Baker Final

MS FLOOR SUMMARY STATISTICS

| TOT | SUN | MON | TUE | WED | THU | FRI | SAT | |
|---|---|---|---|---|---|---|---|---|
| 0.70 | 0.00 | 0.26 | 0.21 | 0.11 | 0.10 | 0.00 | 0.00 | AVG # OF CANCELLATIONS |
| 0.39 | 0.00 | 0.11 | 0.13 | 0.09 | 0.06 | 0.00 | 0.00 | AVG # OF EMG TURNAWAYS |
| 0.00 | 0.00 | 0.00 | 0.00 | 0.00 | 0.00 | 0.00 | 0.10 | AVG # OF ICU TURNAWAYS |
| 0.00 | 0.00 | 0.00 | 0.00 | 0.00 | 0.00 | 0.00 | 0.00 | AVG # OF GYN PTS. ADMITTED |
| 22.74 | 0.90 | 2.27 | 2.56 | 2.71 | 2.35 | 8.25 | 3.70 | AVG # OF CALL-IN PTS. ADMITTED |
| 165.61 | 26.50 | 24.44 | 24.10 | 24.13 | 24.66 | 24.94 | 16.83 | AVG # OF ADMISSIONS |
| 165.59 | 17.90 | 17.64 | 24.06 | 24.51 | 24.38 | 29.67 | 27.41 | AVG # OF DISCHARGES |
| 205.00 | 202.10 | 208.90 | 209.00 | 208.60 | 208.80 | 204.10 | 193.50 | AVG # OF BEDS OCCUPIED |
| 96 | 94 | 98 | 98 | 97 | 98 | 95 | 90 | AVG % OCCUPANCY |

Optimal Solution with Med/Max = 12

**FIGURE III.2.5**
Comparison of an actual length of stay with a Poisson distribution

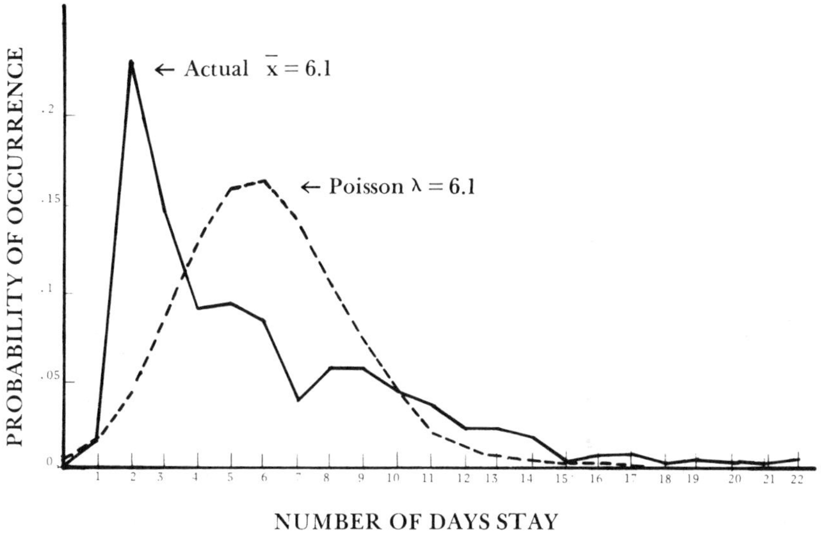


of higher medical call-ins. Table III.2.12 gives a graphical picture of the distribution of available beds at 1:00 P.M. Note that the variance of available beds is much less for med/max = 12 and that the distribution is concentrated on the lower end of the scale. The result is higher occupancy through quicker response to lower census. There is also less capability for scheduled medicals because the marginal probabilities are higher in the census reduction allowance and cancellation allowance regions. (These data are for Sunday using the Baker final solution where the census reduction allowance was set at twenty and the cancellation allowance was four.)

## Simulation Error

The last consideration of sensitivity is the amount of simulation error associated with 200-week simulation runs using different random number generator seeds. Our experience with over fifty such runs indicates the range of error for the key outputs are:

| *Output* | *Error* |
|---|---|
| Avg. cancellations/week | ± .2 |
| Avg. ER turnaways/week | ± .2 |
| Avg. ICU turnaways/week | ± .01 |
| Avg. occupancy | ± .005% |

**TABLE III.2.12**

Distribution of available beds at 1:00 P.M. for med/max = 4 and med/max = 12: Baker final schedules used

| | % OCCURRENCE (MED/MAX = 4) | FREQUENCY (MED/MAX = 4) | | % OCCURRENCE (MED/MAX = 12) | FREQUENCY (MED/MAX = 12) | |
|---|---|---|---|---|---|---|
| 3.0000 | | | | .5 | 1 | +X |
| 4.0000 | | | | .5 | 1 | +X |
| 5.0000 | .5 | 1 | +X | 1.0 | 2 | +XX |
| 6.0000 | 0. | 0 | + | 0. | 0 | + |
| 7.0000 | 0. | 0 | + | .5 | 1 | +X |
| 8.0000 | 0. | 0 | + | .5 | 1 | +X |
| 9.0000 | 1.0 | 2 | +XX | .5 | 1 | +X |
| 10.000 | 1.0 | 2 | +XX | 1.5 | 3 | +XXX |
| 11.000 | .5 | 1 | +X | 2.0 | 4 | +XXXX |
| 12.000 | 2.0 | 4 | +XXXX | 1.0 | 2 | +XX |
| 13.000 | 0. | 0 | + | 5.0 | 10 | +XXXXXXXXXX |
| 14.000 | 4.5 | 9 | +XXXXXXXXX | 6.0 | 12 | +XXXXXXXXXXXX |
| 15.000 | 3.0 | 6 | +XXXXXX | 5.5 | 11 | +XXXXXXXXXXX |
| 16.000 | 2.0 | 4 | +XXXX | 5.0 | 10 | +XXXXXXXXXX |
| 17.000 | 5.0 | 10 | +XXXXXXXXXX | 10.0 | 20 | +XXXXXXXXXXXXXXXXXXXX |
| 18.000 | 1.5 | 3 | +XXX | 6.0 | 12 | +XXXXXXXXXXXX |
| 19.000 | 4.5 | 9 | +XXXXXXXXX | 9.5 | 19 | +XXXXXXXXXXXXXXXXXXX |
| 20.000 | 3.0 | 6 | +XXXXXX | 4.0 | 8 | +XXXXXXXX |
| 21.000 | 8.5 | 17 | +XXXXXXXXXXXXXXXXX | 4.5 | 9 | +XXXXXXXXX |
| 22.000 | 4.5 | 9 | +XXXXXXXXX | 7.5 | 15 | +XXXXXXXXXXXXXXX |
| 23.000 | 3.0 | 6 | +XXXXXX | 9.0 | 18 | +XXXXXXXXXXXXXXXXXX |
| 24.000 | 5.0 | 10 | +XXXXXXXXXX | 6.0 | 12 | +XXXXXXXXXXXX |
| 25.000 | 7.0 | 14 | +XXXXXXXXXXXXXX | 5.5 | 11 | +XXXXXXXXXXX |
| 26.000 | 6.5 | 13 | +XXXXXXXXXXXXX | 4.0 | 8 | +XXXXXXXX |
| 27.000 | 3.5 | 7 | +XXXXXXX | 1.0 | 2 | +XX |
| 28.000 | 5.5 | 11 | +XXXXXXXXXXX | 1.0 | 2 | +XX |
| 29.000 | 4.5 | 9 | +XXXXXXXXX | 1.0 | 2 | +XX |
| 30.000 | 1.5 | 3 | +XXX | 0. | 0 | + |
| 31.000 | 2.0 | 4 | +XXXX | .5 | 1 | +X |
| 32.000 | 2.5 | 5 | +XXXXX | 0. | 0 | + |
| 33.000 | 2.0 | 4 | +XXXX | 0. | 0 | + |
| 34.000 | 2.5 | 5 | +XXXXX | .5 | 1 | +X |
| 35.000 | 2.5 | 5 | +XXXXX | 0. | 0 | + |
| 36.000 | 1.5 | 3 | +XXX | 0. | 0 | + |
| 37.000 | 1.5 | 3 | +XXX | 0. | 0 | + |
| 38.000 | 1.0 | 2 | +XX | 0. | 0 | + |
| 39.000 | 1.5 | 3 | +XXX | .5 | 1 | +X |
| 40.000 | 1.0 | 2 | +XX | | | |
| 41.000 | .5 | 1 | +X | | | |
| 42.000 | .5 | 1 | +X | | | |
| 43.000 | .5 | 1 | +X | | | |
| 44.000 | .5 | 1 | +X | | | |
| 45.000 | 0. | 0 | + | | | |
| 46.000 | .5 | 1 | +X | | | |
| 47.000 | 0. | 0 | + | | | |
| 48.000 | 1.0 | 2 | +XX | | | |
| 49.000 | 0. | 0 | + | | | |
| 50.000 | 0. | 0 | + | | | |
| 51.000 | .5 | 1 | +X | | | |

MED/MAX = 4      MED/MAX = 12

## The Admissions Simulation Game

### Introduction

In an effort to disseminate the concepts of the manual system to as many hospitals as possible with a minimum expenditure of resources, an admissions game is used to help educate hospital personnel. The admissions simulation game is an interactive computer program where the operator runs many simulated days and makes "real life" kinds of admissions decisions. The game was designed to teach admitting supervisors the mechanics of the admission system and to teach them to make decisions while keeping certain objectives in mind.

The mechanics of the system include the various allowances explained previously under the heading "Scheduling System" and a set of decision rules using the allowances to make the correct decisions.

### Scheduling Environment of the Game

The game simulated the admitting operations of Baker Hospital. The capacities of each unit and the patient flows are the same as those shown in figure III.2.2. When playing the simulation game, it is also important to realize the time of day each type of patient arrives and when each decision is made. When running the game, a day is broken into four time intervals: 12:00 midnight to 9:00 A.M., 9:00 A.M. to 11:00 A.M., 11:00 A.M. to 1:00 P.M., and 1:00 P.M. to 12:00 midnight. Figure III.2.6 shows the decision times and the patient flows during the four time intervals. From 12:00 midnight until 9:00 A.M., emergency, OB, and ICU/CCU patients arrive and are admitted. At 9:00 A.M., a decision concerning ICU/CCU transfers is made if there are any patients awaiting transfer. Between 9:00 A.M. and 11:00 A.M., about eighty percent of the discharges from the medical-surgical unit and OB unit occur. At 11:00 A.M., decisions concerning ICU/CCU transfers (if any), cancellation of scheduled patients, and call-in medical patients are made. The rest of the discharges occur between 11:00 A.M. and 1:00 P.M. At 1:00 P.M., a decision concerning how many GYN surgical patients (if there are any) to admit to the OB unit has to be made. Also, decisions concerning remaining ICU/CCU transfers, cancellations, and call-ins have to be made. From 1:00 P.M. to 12:00 midnight, emergency, OB, and ICU/CCU patients are admitted as they arrive.

Figure III.2.7 is an example of the data sheet produced at the beginning of each run of the game. It shows distributions of unuseable beds, patient arrivals, and discharges for each unit. This information is important not only to show the number of patients that arrive and are discharged each day at Baker, but also to show that certain decisions should be based on the arrivals or discharges expected to occur. For example, a distribution of

**FIGURE III.2.6**
Chronological patient flow in Baker Hospital

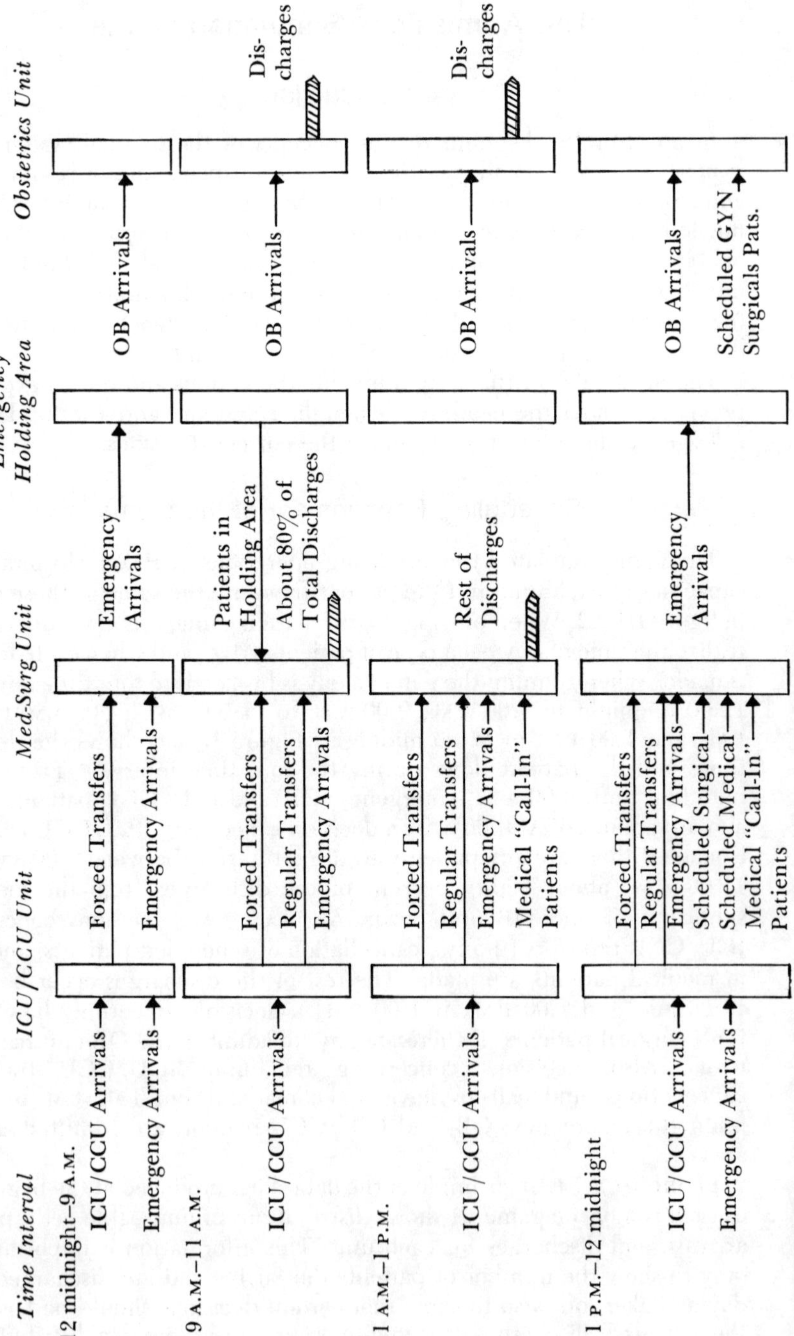

**FIGURE III.2.7**
Example of game's data sheet

| | | SU | MO | TU | WE | TH | FR | SA |
|---|---|---|---|---|---|---|---|---|
| Total OB Arrivals | (Avg.) | 5 | 5 | 5 | 5 | 5 | 5 | 5 |
| | ( 5%) | 2 | 2 | 2 | 2 | 2 | 2 | 2 |
| | (95%) | 9 | 9 | 9 | 9 | 9 | 9 | 9 |
| OB Arrivals (1–11) | (Avg.) | 4 | 4 | 4 | 4 | 4 | 4 | 4 |
| | ( 5%) | 2 | 2 | 2 | 2 | 2 | 2 | 2 |
| | (95%) | 6 | 6 | 6 | 6 | 6 | 6 | 6 |
| Discharges | (Avg.) | 5 | 6 | 6 | 7 | 6 | 7 | 6 |
| | ( 5%) | 2 | 2 | 2 | 2 | 2 | 3 | 2 |
| | (95%) | 9 | 10 | 10 | 11 | 10 | 11 | 10 |
| GYN Surgery | (Avg.) | 1 | 1 | 1 | 1 | 1 | 0 | 0 |
| | ( 5%) | 0 | 0 | 0 | 0 | 0 | 0 | 0 |
| | (95%) | 4 | 4 | 4 | 4 | 4 | 0 | 0 |

Med–Surg Unit: Capacity = 214

Unuseable M-S Beds (Avg.) = 2 (5%) = 0 (95%) = 5

| | | SU | MO | TU | WE | TH | FR | SA |
|---|---|---|---|---|---|---|---|---|
| Total Emergency Arr. | (Avg.) | 7 | 7 | 7 | 7 | 7 | 7 | 7 |
| | ( 5%) | 3 | 3 | 3 | 3 | 3 | 3 | 3 |
| | (95%) | 12 | 12 | 12 | 12 | 12 | 12 | 12 |
| Emer. Arr. (1–11) | (Avg.) | 7 | 7 | 7 | 7 | 7 | 7 | 7 |
| | ( 5%) | 3 | 3 | 3 | 3 | 3 | 3 | 3 |
| | (95%) | 11 | 11 | 11 | 11 | 11 | 11 | 11 |
| Discharges | (Avg.) | 19 | 17 | 22 | 23 | 24 | 25 | 26 |
| | ( 5%) | 13 | 10 | 16 | 15 | 15 | 19 | 18 |
| | (95%) | 25 | 24 | 28 | 31 | 34 | 31 | 34 |
| Scheduled Surgery | | 16 | 14 | 12 | 12 | 13 | 0 | 0 |
| Scheduled Medical | | 2 | 2 | 2 | 2 | 2 | 7 | 4 |

ICU/CCU Unit: Capacity = 16

| | | SU | MO | TU | WE | TH | FR | SA |
|---|---|---|---|---|---|---|---|---|
| ICU/CCU Arr. | (Avg.) | 2 | 2 | 2 | 2 | 2 | 2 | 2 |
| | ( 5%) | 0 | 0 | 0 | 0 | 0 | 0 | 0 |
| | (95%) | 5 | 5 | 5 | 5 | 5 | 5 | 5 |

Relevant Data:
OB Unit: Capacity = 36 (of which 22 are reserved for OB patients)
Unuseable OB Beds (Avg.) = 1 (5%) = 0 (95%) = 3

emergency arrivals between 1:00 P.M. and 11:00 A.M. the next day is given. The average of this distribution is 7, the fifth percentile point is 3, and the ninety-fifth percentile point is 11. This distribution is important in certain decisions because 1:00 P.M. is the last decision time of the day, and 11:00 A.M. is when discharges begin the next day.

## Baker Hospital Admissions Objectives

The admissions objectives that hospital personnel are asked to use when running the game are those displayed in figure III.2.3. To help evaluate how well the objectives are met, an objective function is built into the game, consisting of various performance measures concerning admissions. Attached to each term is a relative weighting factor. The following simple equation shows how the value of the objective function is calculated.

**Objective function = (Term No. 1)(Weight No. 1) + (Term No. 2)(Weight No. 2) + · · · + (Term No. 8)(Weight No. 8)**

A definition of each term and the initial weighting factor for each term appear in figure III.2.8.

**FIGURE III.2.8**
Relative weighting factors

| *Term* | *Definition* | *Relative Weighting Factor for Baker* |
|---|---|---|
| EMPTY | Average number of empty med-surg beds per day (excluding any useable beds) | 1.0 |
| SCAN | Average number of surgical cancellations per day | 4.0 |
| MCAN | Average number of medical cancellations per day | 4.0 |
| ERTURN | Average number of emergency patients turned away per day | 8.0 |
| OBTURN | Average number of OB patients turned away per day | 10.0 |
| ICUTURN | Average number of ICU/CCU patients turned away per day | 10.0 |
| FORCED | Average number of ICU/CCU patients forced to med-surg unit because unit census is at capacity and an ICU/CCU arrival occurs | 2.0 |
| DELAY | Change in the ratio of surgical delay time to medical delay time | 1.0 |

An inspection of the weighting factors of the objective function gives the best indication of the objectives to strive for when running the game. ICU/CCU turnaways and OB turnaways have the highest weights and thus the greatest importance. In fact, ten empty beds has the same value as one OB or ICU/CCU turnaway.

## Simulation Game Decision Strategy

The following is a set of decision rules to use when making each decision in the game. These decision rules incorporate both the various allowances and the admissions objectives for Baker Hospital. It is important to point out that if objectives are used other than those chosen for Baker Hospital, the decision rules would change—especially the use of the five and ninety-five percent points of the distributions. These rules assume that emergency patients will be admitted to the ICU/CCU unit if need be and that ICU/CCU patients will be force transferred to the medical-surgical unit if the ICU/CCU unit is full and an ICU/CCU patient arrives.

The value of each term in the decision rules can be obtained either from the computer output immedicately preceding the decision or from the game's data sheet (figure III.2.7).

*9:00* A.M.

a. How many ICU/CCU patients do you wish to transfer?

*Maximum No. of Transfers* = Present empty useable medical-surgical beds + 5% medical-surgical discharges + Capacity of emergency holding area − Scheduled non-GYN surgery − Scheduled medical − 95% emergency arrivals today.

*11:00* A.M.

a. How many ICU/CCU patients do you wish to transfer?

**Maximum No. of Transfers** = Present empty useable medical-surgical beds+ Additional medical-surgical discharges expected (¼ of known discharges) + Capacity of emergency holding area − Scheduled non-GYN surgery − Scheduled medical −95% emergency arrivals today.

b. How many scheduled medical or surgical patients do you wish to cancel?

**No. To Cancel** = 0. (The number to cancel is always zero at 11:00 A.M. because we do not have complete discharge data yet. However, the following formula gives an indication of the number that might have to be cancelled later.)

**No. Which Will Be Cancelled** = Scheduled non-GYN surgery + Scheduled medical + Cancellation allowance − Present empty useable medical-surgical beds − Additional medical-surgical discharges expected (¼ of known discharges) − Capacity of emergency holding area.

c. How many medical patients do you wish to call in?

**Maximum No. to Call In** = Present empty useable medical-surgical beds + Capacity of emergency holding area – Scheduled non-GYN surgery – Scheduled medical – Census reduction allowance.(Do not exceed med/max call-in limit.)

*1:00 P.M.*

a. How many scheduled GYN surgeries do you wish to admit to the OB unit?

**Maximum No. of GYN Surgeries to Admit to OB Unit** = Present useable empty OB beds – 95% OB arrivals (1:00 P.M. -11:00 A.M.).

b. How many ICU/CCU patients do you wish to transfer?

**Maximum No. of Transfers** = Present empty useable medical-surgical beds + Capacity of emergency holding area – Scheduled non-GYN surgery – Scheduled medical – 95% Emergency arrivals (1:00 P.M. -11:00 A.M.).

c. How many scheduled medical or surgical patients do you wish to cancel?

**No. To Cancel** = Scheduled non-GYN surgery + Scheduled medical + Cancellation allowance + No. called in at 11:00 A.M. – Present empty useable medical-surgical beds –Capacity of emergency holding area.

d. How many medical patients do you wish to call in?

**Maximum No. To Call In** = Present empty useable medical-surgical beds + Capacity of emergency holding area — Scheduled non-GYN surgery –Scheduled medical – Census reduction allowance –No. called in at 11:00 A.M. (Do not exceed med/max call-in limit.)

## Simulation Game Decision Example

To help understand how to make decisions using the allowances and decision rules, an example of a Wednesday's output of the game, including decisions, will be presented. In review, the Baker Hospital allowances to use for Wednesday are:

| | | |
|---|---|---|
| Census Reduction Allowance | = | 11 |
| Cancellation Allowance | = | 4 |
| Med/Max Call-In Limit | = | 10 |
| Surgical Allowance | = | 12 |
| Medical Allowance | = | 2 |
| GYN Allowance | = | 0 |

A day in the game begins at 12:00 midnight by printing the useable capacity and census of each unit (see figure III.2.9). The first decision point concerns ICU/CCU transfers at 9:00 A.M. Using the decision rule:

**a. Maximum No. To Transfer** (9:00 A.M.) = Present empty useable medical-surgical beds (213—207 = 6) + 5% Medical-surgical discharges (=15, obtained from relevant data sheet, figure III.2.7) + Capacity of emergency holding area (2) – Scheduled non-GYN surgery (12–1 = 11)

− Scheduled medical (2) − 95% emergency arrivals today (12) =

$$6 + 15 + 2 - 11 - 2 - 12 = -2 = 0.$$

Thus, none were transferred at 9:00 A.M.

At 11:00 A.M., there were still ICU/CCU patients awaiting transfer since they were not transferred at 9:00 A.M. Using the decision rule:

**b. Maximum No. To Transfer** (11:00 A.M.) = Present empty useable medical-surgical beds (213−186 = 27) + Additional medical-surgical disharges expected (¼ of 21 = 5) + Capacity of emergency holding area (2) − Scheduled non-GYN surgery (12−1 = 11) − Scheduled medical (2) − 95% emergency arrivals today (12) =

$$27 + 5 + 2 - 11 - 2 - 12 = 9.$$

Thus, the two transfers were completed.

Next is the 11:00 A.M. cancellation decision. From the decision rule, no patient is ever cancelled at 11:00 A.M. However, an indication of the number which will be cancelled is:

**c. No. Which Will Be Cancelled** = Scheduled non-GYN surgery (12−5 = 7) + Scheduled medical (2) + Cancellation allowance (4) − Present empty useable medical-surgical beds (213−186−2 = 25) − Additional medical-surgical discharges expected (¼ of 21 = 5) − Capacity of emergency holding area (2) =

$$7 + 2 + 4 - 25 - 5 - 2 = -19 = 0.$$

Thus, there is a strong indication that no patients will have to be cancelled. Note that this equation now includes the exact number of non-GYN scheduled surgeries (19−5 = 7), where in previous equations, the expected number of non-GYN surgeries (12−1 = 11) was used.

The next decision is the 11:00 A.M. call-in decision:

**d. Maximum No. To Call In** (11:00 A.M.) = Present empty useable medical-surgical beds (213−186−2 = 25) + Capacity of emergency holding area (2) − Scheduled non-GYN surgery (12−5 = 7) − Scheduled medical (2) − Census reduction allowance (11) =

$$25 + 2 - 7 - 2 - 11 = 7.$$

Thus, seven medical patients were called in.

The last three decisions were at 1:00 P.M. All were made according to the correct decision rules:

**e. Maximum No. of GYN Surgeries To Admit to OB Unit** = Present empty useable OB beds (12) − 85% OB arrivals (6) =

$$12 - 6 = 6.$$

Thus, all five were admitted.

**f.** (There were no ICU/CCU patients left awaiting transfer.)

**g. No. To Cancel** (1:00 P.M.) = Scheduled non-GYN surgery (7) + Scheduled medical (2) + Cancellation allowance (4) + No. called in at 11:00 A.M. (7) − Present empty useable medical-surgical beds (34) −

**FIGURE III.2.9**
Examples of a Wednesday output including decisions

```
                WEDNESDAY MORNING MIDNIGHT

USEABLE CAPACITIES . . . .

MED-SURG = 213
OB = 34
ICU/CCU = 16
EMER. HOLDING AREA = 2

CENSUS . . . .

MED-SURG UNIT:  204 {OF WHICH 129 ARE MED AND 75 ARE SURG}
OB UNIT:  21 {OF WHICH 16 ARE OB AND 5 ARE GYN}
ICU:  8
EMER. HOLDING AREA:  0

                    9:00 A.M. WEDNESDAY

TOTAL EMER. ARRIVALS {MIDNIGHT TO 9 A.M.}:  3
  NUMBER ADMITTED:  3

NUMBER OB ADMISSIONS {MIDNIGHT TO 9 A.M.}:  2

ICU ARRIVALS {MIDNIGHT TO 9 A.M.}:  1
  REGULAR ICU ADMISSIONS:  1

CENSUS:
  MED-SURG:  207
  ICU/CCU UNIT:  9
  OB UNIT:  23 {OF WHICH 5 ARE GYN}
  EMER. HOLDING AREA:  0

PATIENTS AWAITING TRANSFER FROM ICU:  2
HOW MANY TRANSFERS NOW?

0

                    11:00 A.M. WEDNESDAY

MED-SURG DISCHARGES UNTIL 11 A.M.:  21
EMER. ARRIVALS {9-11}:  3

OB DISCHARGES UNTIL 11 A.M.:  4 {OF WHICH 0 ARE GYN}
OB ADMISSIONS {9-11}:  3

ICU ARRIVALS {9 A.M. TO 11 A.M.}:  1
  REGULAR ICU ADMISSIONS:  1

CENSUS:
  MED-SURG:  186
  ICU/CCU UNIT:  10
  OB UNIT:  22 {OF WHICH 5 ARE GYN}
  EMER. HOLDING AREA:  0

PATIENTS AWAITING TRANSFER FROM ICU:  2
HOW MANY TRANSFERS NOW?

2
```

**FIGURE III.2.9 Cont.**

```
SCHEDULED MEDICAL:  2
SCHEDULED SURGICAL:  12 {OF WHICH % ARE GYN}

IF YOU WISH TO CANCEL ANY SCHEDULED PATIENTS, ENTER BELOW.

                           MED    SUR
                            0      0

HOW MANY MEDICAL PATIENTS DO YOU WANT TO CALL IN?
  WAITING LINE HAS 32 PATIENTS.

7

# OF PATIENTS ATTEMPTED TO CALL IN:  7
# OF PATIENTS COMING IN:  7

                     1:00 P.M. WEDNESDAY

OB UNIT . . . .

UNUSEABLE BEDS:  2
DISCHARGES:  1 {OF WHICH 0 ARE GYN}
OB ADMISSIONS {11-1}:  1
CENSUS:  22 {OF WHICH 5 ARE GYN}
# OF USEABLE EMPTY OB BEDS = 12
SCHEDULED GYN SURGICAL PATIENTS:  5

HOW MANY GYN SCHEDULED SURGERIES DO YOU WANT TO ADMIT TO OB UNIT?

5

MED-SURG UNIT . . . .

UNUSEABLE BEDS:  0
DISCHARGES {11-1}:  8 {TOTAL DISHCARGES TODAY:  29}
EMER. ADMITTED.  {11-1}:  0
#  OF USEABLE EMPTY MED-SURG BEDS = 34

ICU ARRIVALS {11 A.M. TO 1 P.M.}:  0

IF YOU WISH TO CANCEL ANY ADDITIONAL SCHEDULED PATIENTS, ENTER BELOW.

                           MED    SUR
                            0      0

HOW MANY ADDITIONAL MEDICAL PATIENTS DO YOU WANT TO CALL IN?
# OF PATIENTS ON WAITING LINE NOT YET CALLED:  16
# OF PATIENTS COMING IN ALREADY:  7

3

TOTAL # OF PATIENTS ATTEMPTED TO CALL IN:  10
TOTAL # OF PATIENTS COMING IN:  10

ICU ARRIVALS {1 P.M. TO MIDNIGHT}:  2
  REGULAR ICU ADMISSIONS:  2

TOTAL EMER. ARRIVALS {1 P.M. TO MIDNIGHT}:  2
  NUMBER ADMITTED:  2

OB ADMISSIONS {1 P.M. TO MIDNIGHT}:  0
```

Capacity of emergency holding area (2) =

$$7 + 2 + 4 + 7 - 34 - 2 = -16 = 0.$$

**h. No. To Call In** (1:00 P.M.) = Present empty useable medical-surgical beds (34) + Capacity of emergency holding area (2) − Scheduled non-GYN surgery (7) − Scheduled medical (2) − Census reduction allowance (11) − No. Called in at 11:00 A.M. (7) =

$$34 + 2 - 7 - 2 - 11 - 7 = 9.$$

However, since the med/max call-in limit is ten and seven patients were called in at 11:00 A.M., only three more patients should be called in.

## Incremental Learning Process

The game was designed to be used as part of a four-stage incremental learning process. Admitting supervisors are asked to make three slightly different runs of the game with each run emphasizing different facets of the system. When running the game, many times it was difficult to see the effect that a particular decision had on the system. Because of this, the game was designed so it could be run in a "nonrandom" mode. Nonrandom means that discharges and nonscheduled arrivals (emergency, OB, and ICU/CCU) are set at their day of week averages. This removed the random factor in the game and seemed to help hospital personnel gain an initial understanding of the system and also see the effects of their decisions.

The specific goals of each of the four stages are:

a. *Run No. 1 (nonrandom mode)*

(1) Learn to operate and become at ease with the computer terminal.

(2) Learn and understand the scheduling allowances (surgical, medical, and GYN).

(3) Become familiar with admissions objectives.

b. *Run No. 2 (nonrandom mode)*

(1) Learn and understand the census reduction allowance, cancellation allowance, and med/max call-in limit.

(2) Use all of the allowances to make correct decisions (learn how to use the decision rules).

c. *Run No. 3 (random mode)*

(1) Further increase the understanding of the mechanics of the game by running it with emergency, OB, and ICU/CCU arrivals randomly occurring.

(2) Observe that the system can adapt to random arrival and discharge patterns while maintaining the admitting objectives.

d. *Have the admitting supervisors discuss the application of the system (objectives, allowances, and decision rules) in relation to their own hospitals.* Implementing the system is usually part of this discussion.

## Conclusions and Extensions

The system that has been described needs to stand the test of time by being implemented and evaluated in an increasing number of hospitals. Extensions and modifications will have to be made to the simulation and/or to the decision algorithms in order to accommodate the different hospital characteristics. In addition, the manual system that has been described is limited in its ability to schedule as many medical patients as possible. A real-time computer-aided system, which would predict discharges more accurately, would improve this capability. Most of the technology is available for such a system and plans are being made to implement one in the future.

The manual system will be a useful tool for many hospitals for the foreseeable future. It does not require an on-site or real-time computer, and the decision rules are stable and relatively easily taught to admissions personnel especially with the availability of the game.

A number of hospitals are in the process of collecting data and establishing admission procedures with the methodologies presented in this paper. With practically every new application, small changes are made in the simulator to reflect the conditions of the particular situation. The main problem experienced by hospitals attempting to use the simulator is that the data required, especially LOS distributions, are not readily available. In response to this problem, the Greater Detroit Area Hospital Council, Detroit, Michigan has contracted with the Commission on Professional and Hospital Activities of Ann Arbor, Michigan to obtain the data needed for the simulator directly from the Professional Activities Study computer tapes. They will not only provide the data more quickly but with more accuracy.

### NOTES

[1]Galen P. Briggs, Jr., "Inpatient Admissions Scheduling: An Application to a Nursing Service." Doctoral dissertation, The University of Michigan, 1971.

[2]Peter Yannitelli, Walton M. Hancock, and John Fleming, "The Development of a Scheduling System for a Surgical Wing of El Camino Hospital." Richmond, Virginia: National Co-operative Services Center for Hospital Management Engineering, November 1974.

[3]The Poisson assumption is made because the mean is the only statistic known. Since the variance of a Poisson distribution equals the mean, an estimate of the variance can be made. Also, length of stay distributions tend to become more symmetric as the mean increases, which is a property of the distribution.

# III.3

# Computer-Aided System for Nurse Scheduling

*by D. Michael Warner*

## Introduction

The nurse scheduling decision is one of three interrelated nursing manpower decisions. Annually, the staffing decision is negotiated between hospital administration and nursing administration, establishing the number of full time equivalent personnel positions, by skill, to be funded to each nursing unit for the year.[1] From this decision, nursing personnel are hired into the positions and are scheduled each four-week (or similar) period to be on or off duty each day and shift of the period. Finally, in some hospitals, a shift-by-shift reallocation of "float" nurses between units is made to account both for changes in the demand of nursing services on the units and for absenteeism of nursing personnel.[2] Although the three are interrelated, we will treat the scheduling decision separately by noting that a part of the input to the scheduling decision is supplied by the staffing decision, and that the scheduling decision in turn supplies input to the reallocation decision. The scheduling decision is normally made independently for each nursing unit.

Specifically, a schedule (see figure III.3.1 for example) specifies when each registered nurse (RN: the first sixteen nurses of figure III.3.1), licensed practical nurse (LPN: the next nine), and nurse's aide (AIDE: the last seven) will be on the day (D), evening (E), or night (N) shift for each day in the scheduling horizon with consideration for both coverage and quality.

**Coverage** is the minimum number of RNs, RNs+LPNs, and TOTAL (RNs+LPNs+AIDEs) provided each day and each shift of the scheduling horizon (the bottom rows of figure III.3.1).

**Quality** includes certain staffing policies, such as minimizing the assignment of long work stretches, giving every other weekend off, and granting requests for particular days off or on.

The scheduling system described below maximizes an expression of the quality of the schedules, quantified as to how well the nurses like the schedules they will work, subject to the constraint that minimum coverage is met. In those cases where it is not possible to meet coverage, the seriousness of the coverage violation is minimized.

The scheduling decision is usually made by the head nurse of the unit, a nursing supervisor, or another nursing administrator. According to Murray, the scheduling decision can take one hour per bed per month of primarily nursing supervisor time (160 hours per month for a 167 bed hospital).[3] Schuette found the time at The University of Michigan Hospital to be an average of forty-five minutes per nurse per month, but without including some clerical tasks associated with the decision.[4]

While the most tangible justification for improving the decision process is in reducing the amount of time needed to develop schedules, the most significant justification is that better quality schedules can be produced. Melbin, for instance, has shown that there is a relation between the schedules that nurses work and turnover, absenteeism, and lateness.[5]

The following part of this chapter describes the computer-aided scheduling system. The next describes the implementation and evaluation of the system over a two-year period for several units in one of the implementation hospitals. A brief description of the mathematical programming formulation is included in the appendix.

## The Computer-Aided System

There are two parts to the scheduling system. A set of four policy decisions are made initially for each unit. Then, for each scheduling period (four or six weeks), certain period-specific input such as restrictions on the days a particular nurse may work during this period is specified. These two elements are then used to formulate a mathematical programming model whose solution is a schedule. The policy decisions are stored, along with other data, on a computer disk file and changed only when the policies themselves change.

The four policy decisions are:

**Coverage** (see figure III.3.2)—In addition to minimum levels of RN, RN+LPN, and TOTAL personnel, maximum additional nurses are specified to evenly distribute extra ·(over minimum) personnel, if any. Finally, days and shifts which can most easily sustain a shortage of one nurse are ranked, as well as days on which extra nurses are desired, if there are extra.

**Weekend**—Each nurse is assigned a cyclical weekend pattern such that weekend coverage for the unit as a whole is met. For some units (or hospitals), this may be every other weekend off, while for others it may be every third weekend off, or a specific two of five off. Although a fixed weekend policy is felt to be an important benefit of the system—incorporating fairness and stability into the schedules produced—the system can accommodate units without fixed schedules. In addition, the weekend policy may be temporarily violated if necessary (at Christmas, or if two nurses want to "trade" weekends, etc.).

**Rotation**—(A nurse "rotates" to duty on another shift. For example, a nurse may be hired to work mostly on the day shift but also to rotate to the evening shift.) Nurses are specified as fixed schedule, permanent shift, or rotator. A fixed schedule nurse works exactly the same schedule each week (or each two-week cycle, etc.). A permanent shift nurse works only one shift, but not a fixed schedule. A rotator is identified as a day to evening (DE), day to night (DN), day to both evening and night (DR), or EN or

**FIGURE III.3.1**

Output of computer scheduler

SUR SCHEDULE FOR PERIOD BEGINNING JUN 10 1973

| | | 10 | 11 | 12 | 13 | 14 | 15 | 16 | 17 | 18 | 19 | 20 | 21 | 22 | 23 | 24 | 25 | 26 | 27 | 28 | 29 | 30 | 1 | 2 | 3 | 4 | 5 | 6 | 7 | PERCENTAGES TO DATE | | | | |
|---|---|---|---|---|---|---|---|---|---|---|---|---|---|---|---|---|---|---|---|---|---|---|---|---|---|---|---|---|---|---|---|---|---|---|
| | | SU | MO | TU | WE | TH | FR | SA | SU | MO | TU | WE | TH | FR | SA | SU | MO | TU | WE | TH | FR | SA | SU | MO | TU | WE | TH | FR | SA | RO/%N | WE | RG | RM | #W |
| 1 HAKE | D | D | D | | D | D | D | | | D | D | D | | D | D | D | D | | D | D | D | | | D | D | D | | D | D | | 50 | 0 | 0 | 28 |
| 2 FRANK | D | | D | D | D | D | | D | D | D | | D | D | D | | | D | D | D | D | | D | D | D | D | D | D | | | | 50 | 0 | 0 | 12 |
| 4 BRAUN | N | - | - | - | | N | N | | N | N | N | N | N | | | | N | N | N | | N | N | N | N | N | | N | N | | | 51 | 0 | 0 | 28 |
| 5 BOYD | N | N | | | N | N | N | N | B | | | - | - | - | - | - | | | N | N | N | N | N | | | N | N | N | N | | | 0 | 0 | 28 |
| 6 HAMMER | N | N | N | | | | | | | N | N | | | | N | N | N | N | | # | # | # | # | # | N | N | | | | | 51 | 40 | 40 | 28 |
| 7 COLLINS | DE | D | | E | E | E | E | | | E | E | | D | D | D | D | | D | D | | D | D | D | D | | D | D | D | # | 26 | 48 | 5 | 5 | 28 |
| 8 REID | DN | | N | N | | D | D | D | # | - | - | C | | N | N | N | N | | | N | D | D | D | D | | D | D | D | | 27 | 48 | 5 | 5 | 28 |
| 9 CHESLIK | DN | # | - | - | - | - | # | D | D | D | | N | N | N | | | D | D | D | D | | D | D | D | D | | D | D | | 23 | 50 | 12 | 12 | 28 |
| 10 MENIFEE | DR | D | | N | N | D | D | | | D | D | D | D | | D | D | | E | C | C | C | | | E | E | E | E | | D | 27/10 | 50 | 0 | 0 | 28 |
| 12 TURNEY | DR | | D | D | D | D | | N | N | D | D | | D | D | | | D | D | E | E | | E | E | E | E | | D | D | | 28/ 9 | 50 | 0 | 0 | 28 |
| 14 SCHMITZ | DR | | D | D | D | | D | E | E | E | | D | D | D | | | D | D | C | C | C | | | N | D | D | D | | N | 25/10 | 51 | 0 | 0 | 28 |
| 20 GREGARIO | E | E | E | | E | E | E | # | # | - | E | E | | E | E | E | E | | E | E | E | | | E | E | E | | E | E | | 50 | 10 | 10 | 28 |
| 21 LAYOS | E | E | E | E | | E | E | # | # | - | E | E | E | | E | E | E | E | | E | E | # | # | H | - | - | - | - | # | | 51 | 35 | 35 | 28 |
| 22 POLIDO | E | | E | E | E | E | | E | E | E | | E | E | E | | | E | E | E | | E | E | E | | E | E | E | E | | | 50 | 0 | 0 | 28 |
| 23 DALY | D | | D | D | D | | D | D | D | | D | D | D | D | | | D | D | D | D | D | | | D | D | D | | D | D | | 53 | 0 | 0 | 8 |
| 24 THORBECK | DE | | D | D | D | D | D | | | D | D | | E | E | E | E | | D | D | D | D | | | D | D | | E | E | E | 27 | 51 | 0 | 5 | 28 |
| 40 JOHNSON | N | | N | N | N | N | N | | | N | - | - | - | - | # | # | - | N | N | N | N | | | N | N | N | N | N | | | | 6 | 6 | 28 |
| 45 GREEN | DE | D | E | E | | D | D | # | # | B | - | | D | D | D | D | D | | C | C | C | | | E | E | | D | D | D | 25 | 50 | 13 | 13 | 28 |
| 46 GRIESBECK | DR | | D | D | D | | D | D | D | | N | N | N | N | | | D | E | E. | | D | D | D | D | | D | D | D | | 26/10 | 50 | 0 | 0 | 28 |
| 47 SALTZ | DE | D | D | D | | E | E | | D | D | D | D | # | # | # | # | # | D | D | D | D | | | | D | E | E | | D | 24 | 51 | 11 | 11 | 28 |
| 60 MCMILLON | DE | E | | D | D | D | D | | # | D | D | D | | D | D | E | E | | D | D | D | | | D | D | D | | D | D | 23 | 50 | 5 | 6 | 28 |
| 61 SCHMIDT | DE | | D | D | D | D | D | | | E | E | E | E | | D | D | D | D | | D | D | | | # | D | D | D | D | E | 25 | 51 | 5 | 5 | 28 |
| 62 VOKOVICH | E | | E | E | E | E | # | E | E | E | # | E | E | E | | | E | E | E | E | # | E | E | E | # | E | E | E | | | 50 | 5 | 5 | 28 |
| 63 DAVIS | E | E | E | E | | | E | | | | E | | E | E | E | E | E | | | E | E | | | | E | | E | E | E | | 50 | 0 | 0 | 28 |
| 70 CUTLER | E | | | | E | | | E | E | E | | | | | | | | | | | E | E | E | E | | | | | | | 50 | 0 | 0 | 28 |
| 80 DODD | N | N | N | | | | N | N | N | N | | | | N | N | N | N | | | | N | N | N | N | | | | N | N | | | 0 | 0 | 28 |
| 82 STEWARD | N | N | N | N | N | N | | | N | N | N | N | N | | | N | N | N | N | N | | | N | N | N | N | N | | | | | 0 | 0 | 28 |
| 88 STAPLES | N | | | N | N | N | N | N | | | N | N | N | N | N | | | N | N | N | N | N | | | N | N | N | N | N | | | 0 | 0 | 28 |
| 89 HURD | S | | | D | D | D | D | D | | | D | D | D | D | D | | | D | D | D | D | D | | | D | D | D | D | D | | | 0 | 0 | 28 |
| 90 CSICSAY | D | D | D | D | D | D | | | D | D | D | D | D | | | D | D | D | D | D | | | D | D | D | D | D | | | | | 0 | 0 | 28 |
| 91 GLOVER | E | | E | | E | | E | | | E | | E | | E | | | E | | E | | E | | | E | | E | | E | | | | 0 | 0 | 28 |
| 92 WILLIAMS | E | | | E | E | E | E | E | | | E | E | E | E | E | | | E | E | E | E | E | | | E | E | E | E | E | | | 0 | 0 | 28 |
| RNS | NITE | 2 | 2 | 2 | 2 | 2 | 2 | 2 | 2 | 2 | 2 | 2 | 2 | 2 | 2 | 2 | 3 | 2 | 2 | 2 | 2 | 2 | 2 | 2 | 2 | 2 | 2 | 2 | 2 | | | | | |
| | DAY | 3 | 6 | 5 | 6 | 6 | 6 | 4 | 3 | 6 | 5 | 5 | 6 | 6 | 3 | 3 | 6 | 7+ | 6 | 5 | 5 | 4 | 4 | 7+ | 6 | 6 | 6 | 6 | 3 | | | | | |
| | EVEN | 2 | 3 | 3 | 3 | 4 | 3 | 2 | 2 | 3 | 3 | 3 | 3 | 3 | 3 | 3 | ' | 3 | 3 | 3 | 3 | 2 | 2 | 3 | 4 | 3 | 3 | 3 | 2 | | | | | |
| RN+LPN | NITE | 2 | 3 | 3 | 3 | 3 | 3 | 2 | 2 | 3 | 3 | 3 | 3 | 3 | 2 | 2 | 3 | 3 | 3 | 3 | 3 | 2 | 2 | 3 | 3 | 3 | 3 | 3 | 2 | | | | | |
| | DAY | 5 | 9 | 9 | 9 | 9 | 10+ | 5 | 5 | 8 | 7 | 7 | 7 | 8 | 6 | 5 | 9 | 9 | 8 | 8 | 9 | 5 | 5 | 9 | 9 | 9 | 9 | 10+ | 6 | | | | | |
| | EVEN | 4 | 6 | 6 | 5 | 6 | 5 | 4 | 4 | 6 | 5 | 5 | 6 | 5 | 4 | 5 | 6 | 5 | 5 | 5 | 5 | 4 | 4 | 6 | 6 | 5 | 6 | 5 | 4 | | | | | |
| TOTAL | NITE | 4 | 5 | 5 | 5 | 5 | 5 | 4 | 4 | 5 | 5 | 5 | 5 | 5 | 4 | 4 | 5 | 5 | 5 | 5 | 5 | 4 | 4 | 5 | 5 | 5 | 5 | 5 | 4 | | | | | |
| | DAY | 6 | 10 | 11 | 11 | 11 | 11 | 6 | 6 | 9 | 9 | 9 | 9 | 9 | 7 | 6 | 10 | 11 | 10 | 10 | 10 | 6 | 6 | 10 | 11 | 11 | 11 | 11 | 7 | | | | | |
| | EVEN | 4 | 7 | 7 | 7 | 7 | 7 | 5 | 4 | 7 | 6 | 7 | 7 | 7 | 5 | 5 | 7 | 6 | 7 | 6 | 7 | 5 | 4 | 7 | 7 | 7 | 7 | 7 | 5 | | | | | |

# REQUEST; - VACATION; C HOSPITAL BUSINESS; B BIRTHDAY; H HOLIDAY OFF

**FIGURE III.3.1 Cont.**

The first 16 nurses are RNs, the next 9 LPNs, and the last 7 AIDEs. AIDEs work fixed schedules on this unit, by hospital policy.

### Explanation of the "Percentages to Date" Columns

For each scheduling period, certain data are accumulated for each nurse in order to aid in decisions such as the allocation of weekend duty, rotation duty, and the granting of requests.

**RO—Rotation:** Percentage of duty spent on other than a nurse's "home" shift. Calculated as:

$$100 \times \frac{\text{No. of days other than home shift}}{\text{No. of days on all shifts}}$$

(Printed only for those nurses whose rotation is to be equalized.)

**%N—Percentage of Rotation to Night:** Percentage of duty spent on the night shift. Calculated as:

$$100 \times \frac{\text{No. of night shifts worked}}{\text{No. of days on all shifts}}$$

(Printed only for those nurses who are both equalized rotators and who rotate to all three shifts.)

**WE—Weekends:** Percentage of the total number of weekend days a nurse could have worked which she took off. Vacation, holiday, or birthday taken on a weekend day counts as an off day. Calculated as:

$$100 \times \frac{\text{No. of weekend days not on duty}}{\text{No. of weekend days could have been on}}$$

(Not printed for nurses with fixed schedules.)

**RG—Requests Granted:** Ratio of days requested and given off to the total number of days worked, expressed as a percentage. A maximum of two request days a week are accumulated. When on vacation for an entire week, both full and part-time nurses thus accumulate two request days for that week. Calculated as:

$$100 \times \frac{\text{No. of requested days granted}}{\text{No. of days worked}}$$

**RM—Requests Made:** (Same as above, for requests made.)

**#W—Number of Weeks** on which the above data is based.

**FIGURE III.3.2**
Coverage policy

UNIT: Sur

DATE: 4/8/73

| | | S | M | T | W | T | F | S |
|---|---|---|---|---|---|---|---|---|
| MINIMUM RN COVERAGE | N | 2 | 2 | 2 | 2 | 2 | 2 | 2 |
| | D | 3 | 4 | 4 | 4 | 4 | 4 | 3 |
| | E | 2 | 3 | 3 | 3 | 3 | 3 | 2 |

| | | S | M | T | W | T | F | S |
|---|---|---|---|---|---|---|---|---|
| MAXIMUM ADDITIONAL RN COVERAGE | N | 1 | 1 | 1 | 1 | 1 | 1 | 1 |
| | D | 2 | 2 | 2 | 2 | 2 | 2 | 2 |
| | E | 2 | 2 | 2 | 2 | 2 | 2 | 2 |

| | | S | M | T | W | T | F | S |
|---|---|---|---|---|---|---|---|---|
| MINIMUM RN+LPN COVERAGE | N | 2 | 3 | 3 | 3 | 3 | 3 | 2 |
| | D | 5 | 7 | 7 | 7 | 7 | 7 | 5 |
| | E | 4 | 5 | 5 | 5 | 5 | 5 | 4 |

| | | S | M | T | W | T | F | S |
|---|---|---|---|---|---|---|---|---|
| MAXIMUM ADDITIONAL RN+LPN COVERAGE | N | 1 | 1 | 1 | 1 | 1 | 1 | 1 |
| | D | 2 | 2 | 2 | 2 | 2 | 2 | 2 |
| | E | 2 | 2 | 2 | 2 | 2 | 2 | 2 |

| | | S | M | T | W | T | F | S |
|---|---|---|---|---|---|---|---|---|
| MINIMUM TOTAL COVERAGE | N | 4 | 5 | 5 | 5 | 5 | 5 | 4 |
| | D | 6 | 9 | 9 | 9 | 9 | 9 | 6 |
| | E | 4 | 6 | 6 | 6 | 6 | 6 | 4 |

| | | S | M | T | W | T | F | S |
|---|---|---|---|---|---|---|---|---|
| MAXIMUM ADDITIONAL TOTAL COVERAGE | N | 0 | 0 | 0 | 0 | 0 | 0 | 0 |
| | D | 1 | 2 | 2 | 2 | 2 | 2 | 1 |
| | E | 1 | 2 | 2 | 2 | 2 | 2 | 1 |

| | | S | M | T | W | T | F | S |
|---|---|---|---|---|---|---|---|---|
| DAYS/SHIFTS WHICH CAN MOST EASILY SUSTAIN A SHORTAGE OF ONE NURSE (0-5)* | N | | | | | | | |
| | D | | | 4 | 4 | | | |
| | E | 3 | | | | | | |

| | | S | M | T | W | T | F | S |
|---|---|---|---|---|---|---|---|---|
| DAYS/SHIFTS WHERE EXTRA (ABOVE MINIMUM) PERSONNEL ARE DESIRED (0-5)* | N | | | | | | | |
| | D | | 1 | | | 1 | 1 | |
| | E | | | | | | | |

*Rank on a scale of zero to five,
where zero is "least" and five is "most".

NE. Rotators are also identified as "equalized rotators," who in the long run rotate an equal proportion of time to their second shift, or as "special proportion rotators," who in the long run rotate a specified proportion (such as thirty percent or eighty percent) of time to their second shift. Within two-week periods, most rotations are "block" in the sense that, for example, if a nurse rotates to the evening shift for three days, they will be consecutive days. This to minimize the undesirable effect of "jet fatigue," arising from continually adjusting to new time periods.[6]

**Schedule Quality Evaluation** (see figure III.3.3)—Each nurse individually rates certain patterns that may appear in her schedule as to her aversion to working them. Each nurse uses the same total number of rating weights. For example, in figure III.3.3 Nurse Cutler is five times as averse to a stretch of seven days as to a stretch of six days that allows a three-day weekend. These weights, along with certain rotation-related weights made by the head nurse for the unit as a whole (see figure III.3.4), become parameters in the mathematical programming formulation (see appendix).

**FIGURE III.3.3**
Individual aversion to work stretch

NAME Cutler UNIT Sur DATE 4/8/73

Please arrange 50 "aversion points" among the work stretch patterns below to indicate the relative aversion you have to working them. The more points you place on a particular pattern, the higher your aversion to working it.

Single day on 12

| | | ..if allows a 3-day weekend |
|---|---|---|
| Stretch of 5 days | 0 | 0 |
| Stretch of 6 days | 10 | 3 |
| Stretch of 7 days | 15 | 10 |

The second part of the scheduling system is *period-specific input,* which is specified on the Nurse Scheduling Planning Sheet (figure III.3.5). This becomes essentially a "skeleton" of what the final schedule must be including:

**Restrictions**—Special requirements such that, for example, Nurse Griesbeck (see figure III.3.5) cannot work on the night shift on the first Monday, or that Nurse Cheslik will be on vacation the first week. Weekend duty, previously decided by weekend policy, is specified (as modified, if need be) as restrictions in figure III.3.5.

**FIGURE III.3.4**
Unit-wide aversion to certain rotating situations

UNIT Sur DATE 4/8/73

After reviewing the aversion weight distribution on work stretch situations indicated by all nurses on the unit, the following situations that might occur for rotating nurses should be assigned penalties for the "typical" rotating nurse on the unit. The weights assigned should be relative to both (1) one another among the factors below and (2) the average or typical response to the aversions on work stretch. For example, if EWWD is typically "twice as bad" as a six day stretch, the typical (average) weight placed on six day stretches is 10, the EWWD should be assigned 20. If then EV is "110% as bad" as EWWD, it should have a 22, etc. If two situations below are "equal", they should have equal weights. Use as many weights as are appropriate, but keep in mind the balance of the factors below with the work stretch weights.

| | |
|---|---|
| EWWD (to E before weekend off, and D after) | 14 |
| DWWN (to N after weekend off, and D before) | 8 |
| ER (to E before a requested day off) | 15 |
| RN (to N after a requested day off) | 18 |
| EV (to E before a vacation day off) | 20 |
| VN (to N after a vacation day off) | 24 |
| DE (to E without a day off in between) | 1 |
| ND (or NE) (back to D (or E) without a day off) | 2 |
| XX (positive weight for double day off in middle of week for full time) | 3 |

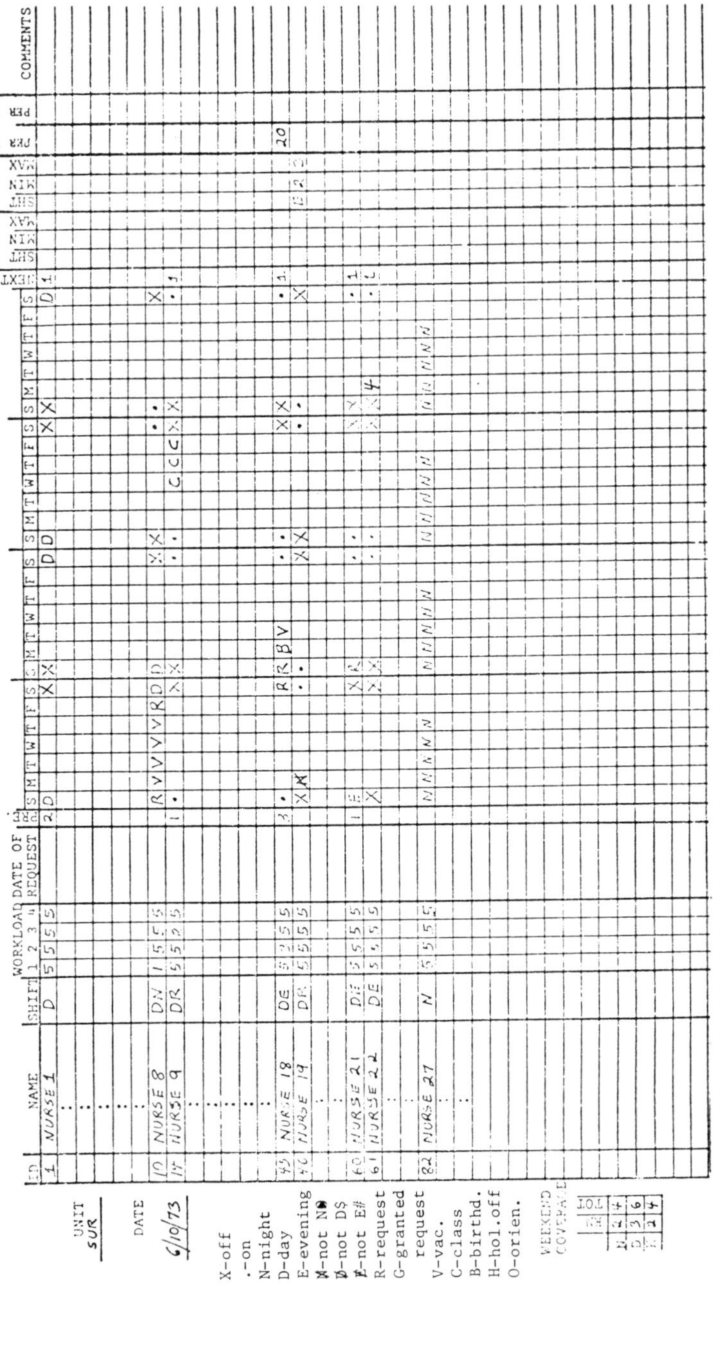


**FIGURE III.3.5**
Nurse scheduling planning sheet

**Requests for days off**—Requests for days off and vacation can be handled in one of three ways:

• The head nurse grants or denies requests according to the nature of the request, other requests, and the nurse making the request. In this case, the requests are specified as days off (or on) in figure III.3.5. (The "R" indicates requested days off.)

• The head nurse quantifies each request in terms of "weights:" the higher the weight, the more likely a nurse will be granted the request. The number of "weights" used for each nurse is accumulated in order to maintain a degree of fairness. The weight associated with a request is balanced against the quantified aversion to poor quality schedules (figures III.3.3 and III.3.4) by the mathematical programming formulation.

• The "weighting" above is done by the nurses themselves. Each month each nurse receives a certain number of weights to place on requested days off (singles, pairs, triplets, etc.). Unhonored weights are refunded. In this way, each nurse is assured of equal influence in the request granting process. In addition, given that coverage must be maintained, the decision of whose request is granted or not granted is entirely in the hands of nursing personnel themselves, reducing any favoritism, inadvertent or not, on the part of the decision maker.

**Rotation**—The shift to which a nurse will rotate each of the two fourteen-day "halfs" of the scheduling period is specified either automatically by the rotation policy or specifically in figure III.3.5. The number of days a nurse will rotate each two weeks is determined in one of two ways:

• A range on the number of days a nurse will rotate is specified in figure III.3.5.

• If no range is specified, the programming model will attempt to equalize the long-run proportion among all nurses for whom no range is specified. Further, for those nurses who rotate to both night and evening, the long-run proportion of duty on the night shift is also equalized.

Using the "penalty" evaluations of figures III.3.3 and III.3.4, the rotation ranges of figure III.3.5 (or the "equalizing" range), and the quantified preferences (if any) and restrictions of figure III.3.5, each possible individual schedule for each nurse is generated and a "value" assigned to it. The value is simply the sum of any applicable penalties, plus the sum of any applicable expressed weights associated with requests. The best fifty of these potential schedules become "valued" variables in the mathematical programming model.

To incorporate fairness the proportion of time each nurse rotates is automatically updated and reported each scheduling period as well as the average amount (sum of the penalty points) of undesirable schedules she has worked in the past (see figure III.3.1). This information is used both as input to the decision and in making postoptimal adjustments in the schedules generated by the computer scheduler.

## Implementation and Evaluation

The system is programmed in FORTRAN IV for interactive use on a terminal. The University of Michigan Hospital has trained payroll secretaries as schedulers, since, except for the head nurse, they are the most familiar with scheduling-type data. The hospital currently uses approximately three-quarters of a full time equivalent secretary, although four secretaries are able to schedule.

First, the scheduler, with the head nurse of the unit, completes the Nurse Scheduling Planning Sheet (figure III.3.5), at the same time noting any changes that need to be made to the unit's permanent data file on the computer (terminations, new staff, a nurse changing from permanent evening duty to rotating status, coverage). Then the scheduler begins interactive conversation on the terminal. The first questions deal with updating the permanent data with the above changes. The scheduler then enters the data from the Nurse Scheduling Planning Sheet in the same format as on the sheet. With these data and the permanent policies, the system formulates and solves a large, nonlinear integer programming problem, and prints out a solution (figure III.3.1). The scheduler then has an opportunity to make changes to this schedule in an interactive mode. Finally, the head nurse may desire to make changes in the schedule before it is posted, and these changes may also be made in an interactive mode (the program saves the "final" schedule for later changes, if necessary).

Typically, the Planning Sheet is completed in half an hour, the interactive scheduling takes forty to ninety minutes (thirty to 120 seconds of IBM 360/67 CPU time is used), and the final review and changes by the head nurse take about half an hour.

The scheduling system was initially implemented on three units of The University of Michigan Hospital in September 1972 and implemented on six other units by September 1973. The system has presently been implemented on eighteen units of several hospitals, involving approximately 600 nurses. Implementation on most of the forty units at the University Hospital is planned, as well as on additional units of several other hospitals in Michigan.

An evaluation of the system on the first three units was made in May 1973, and other units were evaluated in May 1974.[7,8] Generally, the quality of the schedules (in the opinion of the nurses who worked them) was slightly better, and the amount of time devoted to scheduling by the head nurse was reduced by sixty to eighty percent. These findings were later confirmed for other units in a questionnaire to head nurses in Summer 1974, the results of which are summarized in figure III.3.6. (Times in figure III.3.6 represent the complete scheduling process, including gathering and negotiating requests, making last-minute changes, and other "fixed" times.)

**FIGURE III.3.6**
Summary of responses of seven head nurses to questionnaire concerning their experience with computer-aided nurse scheduling

(1) Overall, for my unit the system has taken over 74% of the effort expended to make a schedule. Typically, the decision took about 17 hours a month before the computer-aided system, and now it takes about 4.5 hours.

(The above numbers are averaged; actual responses for the seven units were:

| | | |
|---|---|---|
| Unit A | 75% reduction: | 16→ 4 hours |
| Unit B | 70% reduction: | 14→ 4 hours |
| Unit C | 70% reduction: | 8→ 2.5 hours |
| Unit D | 80% reduction: | 10→ 2 hours |
| Unit E | 50% reduction: | 12→ 6 hours |
| Unit F | 80% reduction: | 40→ 8 hours |
| Unit G | 67% reduction: | 18→ 6 hours) |

(2) The quality of the schedules (after my final adjustment) is

| | |
|---|---|
| Worse | |
| A little worse | X |
| About the same | XX |
| A little better | XXX |
| Better | X |

(3) Overall,

| | |
|---|---|
| The system is a Godsend | XX |
| The system has been very useful | XXX |
| The system has been slightly useful | XX |
| The problems equal the benefits | |
| The problems slightly outweigh the benefits | |
| The problems seriously outweigh the benefits | |
| The system is a failure on my unit | |

## APPENDIX III.3.A

The twenty-eight (or forty-two) day scheduling period is divided into two (or three) fourteen-day periods, which are treated separately except for the work stretch at the end of the previous period. A twenty-eight day problem proved much too large, while solving four seven-day problems introduced serious restrictions for rotating nurses.

**The Variables**—Let i = 1,2, . . . N index the nursing personnel to be scheduled (where i = 1,2, . . . , R, are RNs, i = R + 1, R + 2, . . . , L are LPNs, and i = L + 1, L + 2, . . . N are AIDEs).

Let j index potential fourteen-day schedules for each nurse, where $J_i$ is the number of such schedules for nurse i.

Let $A_{ij}$ be a vector of length 42 (14 days × 3 shifts per day) representing the jth possible schedule for nurse i.

Further, let $A_{ij}$ have a 1 in those positions where nurse i will be on duty and a 0 where she is off duty. For example:

```
       ┌──Sunday               ┌──Sunday               ┌──Sunday
       │┌─Monday               │┌─Monday               │┌─Monday
       ││┌Tuesday              ││┌Tuesday              ││┌Tuesday
       │││   etc.              │││   etc.              │││   etc.
A11 =  11100111010000          00000000001110          00000000000000

          Day                     Evening                 Night
          Shift                    Shift                  Shift
```

would correspond to Nurse i working the following fourteen-day schedule:

(D = day shift; E = evening shift; X = day off.)

| Su | Mo | Tu | We | Th | Fr | Sa | Su | Mo | Tu | We | Th | Fr | Sa |
|---|---|---|---|---|---|---|---|---|---|---|---|---|---|
| D | D | D | X | X | D | D | D | X | D | E | E | E | X |

Finally, the variables are

$$X_{ij} = \begin{cases} 1 & \text{if nurse i is to work schedule } A_{ij} \\ 0 & \text{if not} \end{cases}$$

The computer scheduler generates possible schedules for each nurse, considering both the policy decisions for that nurse and any restrictions on her schedule for this fourteen-day period. Up to 600 such schedules are generated by the program. (From experience with over 3,000 sets of

$A_{ij}$, only two percent of the time will a nurse have over 150 possible schedules, and never has a nurse had 600, although it is certainly possible to construct examples of much more than 600. The average number is about twenty possible schedules). The program selects the "best" fifty for use in the model (the "best" meaning highest $C_{ij}$—see below).

**The Constraints**—Let RN be a vector of length 42 specifying minimum RN coverage (from figure III.3.2), LPN specifying RN + LPN coverage, and TOT specifying total coverage.

Then:

$$\sum_{i=1}^{R} \sum_{j=1}^{J_i} X_{ij} A_{ij} \geq RN$$

$$\sum_{i=1}^{L} \sum_{j=1}^{J_i} X_{ij} A_{ij} \geq LPN$$

$$\sum_{i=1}^{N} \sum_{j=1}^{J_i} X_{ij} A_{ij} \geq TOT$$

Where:

$$\sum_{j=1}^{J_i} X_{ij} = 1 \text{ for each } i=1,2\ldots N,$$

and

$$X_{ij} = (0,1) \text{ for each } i \text{ and } j$$

**The Phase I Objective Function**—Sometimes it is not possible to satisfy the coverage constraints for a particular fourteen-day period, due to reasons like the unit being under budget or nurses being on vacation or in orientation. In this case, the need arises for a mechanism to minimize the seriousness of constraint violation. This is done by specifying a nonlinear phase I objective function which is addressed first in the solution search. If there is no feasible solution, the phase II search begins with the best possible infeasible solution (the one which minimizes the phase I objective), and the phase II search is only among those solutions which do not increase the phase I objective.

Let k index the forty-two day/shift combinations in the scheduling period.

Let $S_k$ be the "sustainability of shortage" from figure III.3.2 for day/shift k, and

Let $U_k$ be the artificial variables associated with the kth minimum RN constraint.

then define:

$$F(U_k) = (10-S_k)^{U_k}$$

Similarly, let $V_k$ be the artificial variables for the RN + LPN minimum constraints, and $W_k$ for the TOT constraints, and define $F(V_k)$ and $f(W_k)$ the same as $f(U_k)$.

The phase I objective becomes

$$\text{Min} \quad b_1 f(U_k) + b_2 f(V_k) + b_3 f(W_k)$$

where the b are relative weights.

**The Phase II Objective**—Let $C_{ij}$ be the relative value of the jth schedule to nurse i. The $C_{ij}$ are obtained by applying:

- The individual aversions (figure III.3.3)
- The unit wide aversions (figure III.3.4)
- "Votes" for requested days off (figure III.3.5)
- A small factor for equalized rotation, calculated by first determining how many days nurse i should rotate (to be equalized), and then decreasing $C_{ij}$ for those $A_{ij}$ where she would rotate more or less than the equalizing amount.

In order to distribute extra (above minimum) personnel optimally among the day/shift combinations in the scheduling period, the slack variables are used as follows:

Let k index the forty-two day/shift combinations in the scheduling period.

Let $E_k$ be the value of having an extra RN on day/shift k (see figure III.3.2).

Let $F_k$ be the maximum additional RN coverage for day/shift k (see figure III.3.2).

Let $s_k$ be the slack variable associated with the kth RN minimum coverage constraint.

Then define:

$$g(s_k) = \begin{cases} 0 & \text{if } s_k = 0 \\ E_k & \text{if } 0 < s_k \leq F_k \\ E_k - (s_k - F_k) & \text{if } s_k > F_k \end{cases}$$

(Also, let $t_k$ be the slack variable associated with the kth minimum RN + LPN constraint and $u_k$ for the TOT constraint, and define $g(t_k)$ and $g(u_k)$ and the same as $g(s_k)$ using the appropriate values from figure III.3.2).

The phase II objective is

$$\text{Maximize} \sum_{i=1}^{N} \sum_{j-1}^{J_i} C_{ij} X_{ij} + \sum_{k=1}^{42} [g(s_k)+g(t_k)+g(u_k)]$$

**Solution of the Programming Problem**—The problem formulated above is a multiple choice programming problem and is solved by a modified version of Balintfy's algorithm.[9 10] A typical problem of 400 variables is solved in five to twenty seconds of CPU time on a 360/67. In agreement with Balintfy's experience, good results are obtained using a maximum block size of two.

## NOTES

[1]R. J. Connor, "A Hospital Inpatient Classification System." Doctoral dissertation, Johns Hopkins University, 1960.

Harvey Wolfe, "A Multiple Assignment Model for Staffing the Nursing Units." Doctoral dissertation, Johns Hopkins University, 1964.

[2]Connor, "Inpatient Classification."

R. C. Jelinek, T. F. Zinn, G. L. Delon, and R. A. Alemon, "A Nurse Allocation and Scheduling System in Operation." Chicago: Medicus Corporation, 1972.

V. Trivedi, "A Management Information System for the Allocation of Nursing Resources." Ann Arbor: Program of Hospital Administration, The University of Michigan, 1973.

D. M. Warner and J. Prawda, "A Mathematical Programming Model for Scheduling Personnel in a Hospital." *Management Science*, December 1972, Vol. 19, No. 4, pp. 411-422.

[3]D. J. Murray, "Computer Makes the Schedules for Nurses." *Modern Hospital*, December 1971, pp. 104-105.

[4]L. L. Schuette, "Development of Criteria for Evaluating Nurse Scheduling." Ann Arbor: Program in Hospital Administration, The University of Michigan, 1973.

[5]M. Melbin, "Curbing Absenteeism and Turnover Among Nursing Personnel." Boston: Massachusetts General Hospital, 1968.

[6]Melbin, "Curbing Absenteeism."

[7]Schuette, "Evaluating Nurse Scheduling."

[8]Curtis Wood, "An Evaluation of the Impact of a Computer-Assisted Scheduling System." Ann Arbor: Program in Hospital Administration, The University of Michigan, 1974.

[9]W. C. Healey, "Multiple Choice Programming." *Operations Research,* Vol. 12, 1964, pp. 122-138.

[10]J. L. Balintfy and C. R. Blackburn, "General Purpose Multiple Choice Programming by Truncated Block Enumeration." Presented at the 36th National Meeting of ORSA, Miami, Florida, November 1969.

# III.4

# Daily Allocation of Nursing Resources

*by Vandankumar M. Trivedi*

## Introduction

This chapter is directed at the last of several steps in nursing staffing problems—the final assignment of nurses and nonprofessional personnel to the various units of the hospital. This assignment occurs at the start of each shift and accommodates to absenteeism, census changes, and special needs of the units. Beginning of the shift allocation can be visualized as a fine tuning to the complete process of scheduling nursing resources to the delivery of inpatient care in a hospital. This process starts with annual budget decisions for a period of a fiscal year. A budget of the expected manpower requirement for all the skill levels in different units of the hospital is prepared. This annual decision is followed by the scheduling decision, when for a period of four to six weeks, days on duty and off duty for the individual nursing personnel are determined. (The budget decision is discussed in section III.2, and the scheduling decision in section III.3). Although in the last two decades a fair amount of research and investigation has been directed towards the allocation problem, comparatively few models for the allocation of nurses have been developed.[1,2]

There is a daily variation in the inpatient demand for nursing care due to the variation in the census as well as patient mix.[3,4] Also, the nursing staff size and mix varies from day to day due to staff absenteeism and the twenty-four hours a day, seven days a week coverage requirement. Considering these important characteristics of inpatient demand and nursing staff, the beginning-of-the-shift allocation decision is a final attempt by nursing management to achieve a balance between the inpatient demand

and the supply of nursing personnel to meet the demand on each nursing unit. The consequences of imbalance can be quite serious. Delays in patient treatments can result in complications or extended hospital stay. Imbalance can augment patient complaints and cause patient and physician dissatisfaction. The daily inequity in workload can result in higher staff absenteeism or a higher staff turnover rate.

There is an added advantage of allocating resources at the beginning of a shift. It has been shown in past research that the patient care loads in different inpatient units of a hospital are independent of each other, which implies that the peak loads in various units do not in general occur simultaneously.[5] This finding suggests a point of view for the beginning of the shift allocation decision. A system called "controlled variable staffing" was introduced by Connor utilizing this point of view.[6] He suggests the operational procedure for controlled variable staffing as follows:

> The hospital wards would be assigned personnel based on their requirements for their lowest loads. The remaining personnel would go into a pool, and be assigned to the inpatient units from the pool. The assignments will be guided by the basic staff assigned and estimated loads.
>
> Inherent advantages in such a system would accrue from the overall staff requirement being reduced and/or the personnel being better utilized. The staff requirement will be reduced by the decrease in the amount of stand-by labor necessary to meet the variation in load. The results of this reduction would be decrease in the payroll and an increase in the efficiency of the staff.[7]

The allocation model presented in this chapter is founded on this concept of controlled variable staffing. The part of the staff Connor refers to above as "basic staff" is termed "core staff" for the purpose of this chapter.

Connor's work was completed over a decade ago; his findings have not been substantially changed by numerous other researchers, and many hospitals have tried to implement controlled variable staffing in one form or another. A variety of difficulties have been encountered, however, and successful practical applications are rare. The size of the variation in demand for nursing care, the difficulty of maintaining the allocation pool, the tendency of unit nurses to upgrade their staffing demands, and the mechanical difficulties involved in collecting the necessary data and analyzing it in a brief time span are among the problems encountered.[8] In this proposal, an effort was made to reduce the data collection needs, speed the analysis, and provide indicators of staffing needs based upon head nurses' perceptions.

The central objective of this research was to devise a nursing allocation system that would be consistent with nursing practice. First, the severity of need for nursing care was measured from head nurses' perception of the need. Second, this perception of need was related to factors that were found to influence it. Finally, an allocation model was developed to make allocation decisions; the objective of the model was to minimize the total severity of need for the hospital while maintaining the difference in severity of need between hospital units below a predetermined level. The major variables found to be significant for measuring severity of need were the staffing hours available in different skill levels. census of the units, and patient classification (found to be significant in only two units). This finding indicates that the variables predominantly influencing the head nurses' perception of severity of need for nursing care in the study hospital are the census and the nursing hours available. The patient classification variables do influence the head nurses' perception, but their influence is not of predominant importance when compared with the former two variables. However, in the past research where severity of need was measured by time study or work sampling methods and not from the head nurses' perception, it was found (or in some instances assumed) that patient classification variables and variables corresponding to nursing procedures performed on the unit have a major influence on severity of need.[9] It should be noted that the findings of the present research are based upon the data from a 296 bed short-term general hospital where the census was stable at ninety-five to ninety-seven percent capacity. Demand for beds was high and an admission scheduling system was successfully operating on three of the five units used in this study. (The admission scheduling system is discussed in section III.2.).

## Measurement of the Nursing Care Need

Figure III.4.1. represents a hypothetical relationship between nursing staff and the severity of need for an additional staff member on an inpatient unit for a fixed demand for nursing care. The severity of need depends upon several factors such as: penalty incurred due to services needed but not provided; penalty due to treatment delays and complications; patient, physician, and employee complaints and dissatisfaction; penalty of not being able to provide a desired quality of nursing care; and problems due to staff absenteeism, turnover, and similar other factors. It is hypothesized (figure III.4.1) that the resultant effect of these penalties (severity of need for an additional staff member) decreases at a progressively decreasing rate with each marginal increment in staff size. In the above discussion, the costs that increase with staff size (employment costs) are not considered. Since the nursing personnel are already scheduled for work when the daily allocation decisions are made, their employment cost is "sunk cost" at that time. Therefore, its effect has not been considered in the discussion on severity of need.

It will be useful to know the nature of the functional relationship shown in figure III.4.1 for every inpatient unit and all skill levels in making daily allocation decisions. Once this curve is known, the person making the allocation decision (usually the house director) will be able to measure the need for additional staff in each skill level in every unit of the hospital before the start of the shift. This may provide an objective and more consistent method for allocation when compared with usual nursing practice. (The usual nursing practice is to allocate the staff based on such factors as the house director's experience, requests from the head nurses, the nature

**FIGURE III.4.1**
Relationship between staff size and severity of need for a fixed inpatient demand for nursing care

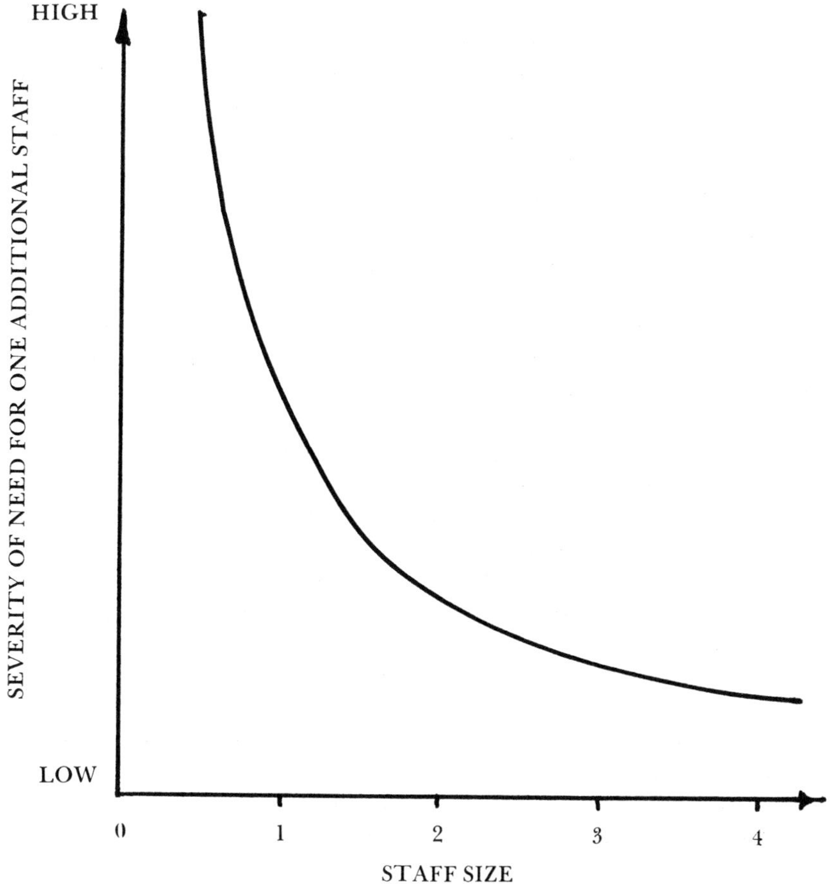

of absenteeism, and the positions' control. Moreover, it will even be possible to utilize these functions (such as figure III.4.1) in a mathematical programming model which will, in turn, make the optimum allocation decisions.

One way to quantify the workload in inpatient units is to use industrial engineering work measurement techniques.[10] Once the workload is computed, the divergence between the available staff size and the workload will provide a scale for severity of need for additional staff. If the workload is far greater than the available staff, the severity of need is high, but when the workload is equal to the staff size, there is no severity of need for an additional person. In past research, similar approaches have been utilized.[11] Some of the drawbacks of such approaches are as follows: work measurement techniques are usually expensive; they measure actual practice at the time of the study, not what ideally should be provided to deliver a predetermined quality of nursing care; and nurses visualize the delivery of patient care as a complete task for the total period of a patient's stay in a hospital.[12] Moreover, a certain number of nursing hours per patient day cannot be considered as standard because of the evidence that exists of a wide variation in this quantity between hospitals. A study by the American Hospital Association showed that the nursing hours per patient day varied between 3.06 and 6.28 hours for fifty-four hospitals under study.[13]

The alternative source of information for determining severity of need is in fact the nursing personnel. The head nurse of an inpatient unit organizes and assigns duties to her staff in a fashion she considers appropriate for providing a predetermined quality of nursing care to the patients in her unit. Her nursing education and experience help her in her judgment. She knows that at times the units are understaffed and overstaffed some other times.

She is aware of the consequences of understaffing and, when the situation arises, orders her staff to cut down on their breaks or some patient care and treatment tasks. She knows when her staff is overworked and when the physicians and patients will be complaining. When the staff is at such a low level that either the patients' welfare will be in danger or the quality of care delivered by the available staff would suffer due to excessive workload, she calls the house director for more help. The decision process, based on all these variables, seems to be part of her professional experience. The evidence that nurses respond to the staffing and patient load environment of an inpatient unit in an orderly and consistent fashion is also found in the literature.[14]

The underlying premise of this research is that the head nurse of an inpatient unit is the best judge of the severity of need for nursing care on her unit.

## Development of Questionnaire

Therefore, in this research, the nature of the severity of need was measured based on head nurses' opinions. In order to extract the head nurses' opinions in a real life situation and not in a hypothetical environment, the data were collected during actual day-to-day operations in the study hospital. Figure III.4.4 shows the questionnaire designed to gather the information for this purpose. (The preamble to the questionnaire is provided in appendix III.4.A)

The first question is designed to measure the severity of need for one person in addition to the staff already existing in the unit. As mentioned earlier, the "need scale" in this question refers to the resultant effect of various tangible and intangible penalties. There were two main reasons for dividing this question into three parts: 1) The nursing staff is usually divided into three major categories—registered nurse, licensed practical nurse, and aide. The need for each skill level could be separately measured since duties are essentially different at each level.[15] 2) Although the major duties for the three skill levels are different, there is some overlap in their duties. Therefore, the severity of need for one skill level can easily affect that of some other skill level. The intent of asking the questions one after another for each skill level is to measure the effect of substitution of duties.

The second question is designed essentially to provide a frame of reference for the head nurse who is answering the questionnaire. The five factors (a-e) included in this question are major factors affecting patient load. These factors were considered from the past research studies and also from consultation with the nursing supervisory staff in the study hospital.[16] The factor "e" (number of highly nursing dependent patients) is based on a patient classification scheme described below.

The third question is for the purpose of measuring the severity of need caused by a unit marginal reduction in the staff. When compared with question one, question three balances the questionnaire. This question is also categorized into three parts similar to question one. Question four provides a frame of reference to the head nurse. The fifth question measures the head nurse's perception of the quality of nursing care delivered during her shift.

The scale used in this questionnaire is a Likert-type five point scale.[17] The head nurses were asked to answer the questionnaire at the end of a shift, when they had the complete picture of the events during the entire shift. It may be observed that the questionnaire does not pertain to any specific organization of nursing care delivery such as team nursing, case nursing, or functional nursing.[18] Therefore, it can be used in any type of inpatient unit setting.

As already mentioned, the objective of the questionnaire is to establish a relationship (as shown in figure III.4.1) between severity of need and staff size, for allocating staff at the beginning of a shift. This suggests that it is not sufficient just to establish the relationship; it is equally essential to be able to predict severity of need even before a shift starts. To achieve this objective, the following information pertaining to the shift was collected along with the questionnaire: nursing hours available; census; number of new admissions; transfers; discharges; number of patients in different care categories; "specialized nursing procedures" performed in the unit; and number of forty-eight hour postoperative patients in the unit. These variables were derived from previous studies and consultation with nursing supervisory staff in the study hospital.[19] The questionnaire was pretested in two other hospitals before it was used for data collection in the study hospital.

## Patient Classification System

One of the variables considered for the measurement of patient load was the number of patients in various levels of care categories. To classify patients in an objective and auditable fashion, it was necessary to use a system. Based on nursing opinion and preliminary statistical analysis, five patient care items were identified for classifying patients according to the time required for their nursing care.

The objective of data collection for this purpose was to derive a patient classification system that would take less time to classify patients than the existing systems. Moreover, the system should maintain unambiguous and precise patient categories based on nursing care time. A summary of the patient classification study follows.[20]

The classification format used was an extension of the Connor format. Fifteen nursing procedures were added to the Connor format after discussion with the nursing supervisory staff. These procedures were added to encompass the complete spectrum of nursing care activities that were either time-consuming or good indicators of the nursing care time consumed by patients. Data were collected on a sixty-eight bed surgical unit of the study hospital for a period of two weeks. For each patient in the unit, all relevant items on the form were checked, and in addition, the head nurse classified patients as low, medium, or high according to the nursing care time required for their care. The data were analyzed to identify the most relevant items for low, medium, or high classifications as perceived by the head nurse.

Analysis of the data revealed that it was possible to identify the most relevant items required for classifying patients based on the head nurses' perception. A workable patient classification system applicable to all hospital units was developed using only five nursing care items. The format is shown in figure III.4.5. These five items are indicators of patients' psychophysiological status. The method for classifying patients in type I (self care), type II (partial care), or type III (total care) categories is described in appendix III.4.B.

## Data Collection

The sample size for collection of the data was determined by statistical sampling methods to be seven weeks.[21] Data were collected simultaneously in five inpatient units of the hospital.[22] The questionnaires were completed by the head nurses of the respective units at the end of their shifts. Since the licensed practical nurses had most familiarity with the patients, they filled out the patient classification forms to save time. The information on new admissions, transfers, discharges, census, forty-eight hour postoperative patients, and staffing for each of the five units was collected from "Daily Report" forms routinely used in the study hospital.[23] In addition, to get a complete picture of the workload on patient units, information on "specialized nursing procedures" performed on every shift for each unit was collected. A list and description of the specialized nursing procedures appear in appendix III.4.C.

## Prediction Equations

The major objective of the data collection was to establish a relationship between severity of need and staff size for each of the three skill levels in the five study units for various levels of inpatient demands.

A "severity index" was developed based on the scales in the questionnaire.[24] The severity index has range of 1.2 through 6.0. A severity index of 1.2 for a skill level indicates a situation of "no need" (see figure III.4.4) for an additional staff member in that skill level *and* "no difficulty" of releasing a person from the same skill level. At the other extreme, a severity index of 6.0 indicates a situation of "very great need" for an additional staff member in a skill level *and* "very great difficulty" of releasing a person from the same skill level. When the severity of need is between these two extreme situations, the severity index has a corresponding value between 1.2 and 6.0.

A multivariate regression analysis was performed on the data. The dependent variable was the severity index, and the independent variables were the various patient load variables hypothesized to affect need and staffing variables. (Only those independent variables were included that were significant at the five percent significance level.) Regression equations for the five study units and three skill levels are given in table III.4.1.

**TABLE III.4.1**
Regression equations for the five study units, day shift

| *Unit* | *Severity index of* | *Constant* | *Independent variables* | *Standard error of estimate* | *Coefficient of determination* | *Significance level (%) of "f" statistic* |
|---|---|---|---|---|---|---|
| | RN | 7.43<br>(p ≅ 0)* | −6.26(RN hrs/census)−0.0023(LPN hrs)$^2$<br>(p ≅ 0) (p ≅ 0.023)<br>(−0.62)** (−0.37) | 0.87 | 0.38 | 0.02 |
| Med-Surg | LPN | 2.74<br>(p ≅ 0) | +9.80(1/(LPN hrs−4.0))<br>(p ≅ 0)<br>(0.42) | 0.62 | 0.41 | 0.00 |
| | Aide | 10.63<br>(p ≅ 0) | −0.082(aide hrs)−4.096(RN hrs/census)$^2$<br>(p ≅ 0) (p ≅ 0.002)<br>(−0.76) (−0.56) | 0.71 | 0.64 | 0.01 |
| | RN | 0.61<br>(p ≅ 0.038) | +8.08(1/(RN hrs−4.0))−0.87 log$_e$(LPN hrs/census)+0.78(# trans)<br>(p ≅ 0) (p ≅ 0.005) (p ≅ 0)<br>(0.66) (−0.44) (0.54) | 0.71 | 0.52 | 0.00 |
| Pediatrics | LPN | 1.39<br>(p ≅ 0.002) | −0.0032(RN hrs)$^2$+0.39(# trans)+0.37(1/((LPN hrs/census)−0.15))+1.67(# type III)<br>(p ≅ 0.007) (p ≅ 0.091) (p ≅ 0) (p ≅ 0.055)<br>(−0.43) (0.28) (0.52) (0.31) | 0.83 | 0.41 | 0.06 |
| | Aide | 1.50<br>(p ≅ 0.002) | +0.12(census)−0.085(LPN hrs)+1.59(1/(LPN hrs−4.0))−0.47(aide hrs/census)<br>(p ≅ 0) (p ≅ 0) (p ≅ 0.003) (p ≅ 0.011)<br>(0.51) (−0.33) (0.26) (−0.23) | 0.95 | 0.43 | 0.00 |
| | RN | 2.21<br>(p ≅ 0) | −1.56 log$_e$(RN hrs/census)−0.66(aide hrs/census)$^2$<br>(p ≅ 0) (p ≅ 0.039)<br>(−0.64) (−0.36) | 0.47 | 0.54 | 0.00 |
| Surgical | LPN | 4.26<br>(p ≅ 0) | −2.29(RN hrs/census)−1.33(aide hrs/census)+12.32(1/(LPN hrs−12.0))<br>(p ≅ 0.024) (p ≅ 0.065) (p ≅ 0.001)<br>(−0.36) (−0.30) (0.52) | 0.66 | 0.35 | 0.08 |
| | Aide | 6.36<br>(p ≅ 0) | −3.33(aide hrs/census)<br>(p ≅ 0)<br>(−0.49) | 0.92 | 0.24 | 0.00 |

| *Unit* | *Severity index of* | *Constant* | *Independent variables* | *Standard error of estimate* | *Coefficient of determination* | *Significance level (%) of "f" statistic* |
|---|---|---|---|---|---|---|
| ICU/CCU | RN | 4.31<br>($p \cong 0$) | $-2.08 \log_e$(RN hrs/census)<br>($p \cong 0$)<br>(−0.54) | 1.03 | 0.29 | 0.01 |
| ICU/CCU | LPN | 7.00<br>($p \cong 0$) | $-1.61 \log_e$(LPN hrs/census) $-1.76$(RN hrs/census)<br>($p \cong 0.008$) ($p \cong 0$)<br>(−0.45) (−0.63) | 1.09 | 0.43 | 0.01 |
| ICU/CCU | Aide | 0.36<br>($p \cong 0.124$) | $+1.45 \log_e$(aide hrs) $-1.67 \log_e$(aide hrs/census)<br>($p \cong 0.002$) ($p \cong 0$)<br>(0.32) (−0.38) | 0.91 | 0.35 | 0.00 |
| Medical | RN | 2.77<br>($p \cong 0.042$) | +7.09(% type II)+0.11(WSec hrs)−8.39(RN hrs/census)$^2$<br>($p \cong 0.013$) ($p \cong 0.052$) ($p \cong 0$)<br>(0.41) (0.33) (−0.57) | 0.91 | 0.52 | 0.00 |
| Medical | LPN | 12.84<br>($p \cong 0.001$) | $-3.22 \log_e$(LPN hrs)+0.004(WSec hrs)$^2$<br>($p \cong 0.005$) ($p \cong 0.018$)<br>(−0.46) (0.39) | 1.00 | 0.33 | 0.72 |
| Medical | Aide | 43.76<br>($p \cong 0$) | +6.78(% type II) $-9.58 \log_e$(aide hrs)<br>($p \cong 0.036$) ($p \cong 0$)<br>(0.43) (−0.75) | 0.72 | 0.68 | 0.00 |

* Numbers in these brackets represent the significance level of the "t" statistic of the coefficients.
** Numbers in these brackets represent the partial correlation coefficients of the independent variables.

The majority of the regression equations (ten out of fifteen) show that the severity index decreases at a progressively decreasing rate with each marginal increment in staffing. This fact concurs with the hypothesis regarding the relationship between severity of need and staff size (figure III.4.1).

The remaining five regression equations represent a linear relationship. Since data were collected only in the region of a marginal increment (or decrement) in staffing and not over the entire staffing range, the linearity in this small range is comprehensible even if the hypothesis is true.

The equations indicate that the factors contributing most to the severity index are staff size and census. Other patient load affecting factors such as patient classification, transfers, discharges, and admissions play a relatively minor role.[25] The equations also represent the presence of the substitution effect between skill levels.

## Allocation Model

The allocation model is designed as an aid to the house director for making the daily allocation decisions at the beginning of each shift. It utilizes the severity index prediction equations to make proper allocation decisions. The following assumptions are made:

**The staff in the hospital is divided into two categories.**

*Core Staff:* The core staff for a unit, as the name indicates, is that part of the staff which is absolutely necessary for keeping the unit open. For example, at least one head nurse, one registered nurse, etc.

*Pool Staff:* The pool staff constitutes that part of the staff that is not assigned to work on any particular unit at the start of a shift. Staff from the pool are allocated to various units at the beginning of a shift. (The model will not pull people from the core staff to allocate elsewhere.)

**The inpatient units over which the allocation decision is made are homogeneous units.** A member from the pool staff could work, if necessary, in any of the units over which the allocation decision is made. This would exclude some specialized units of the hospital where only highly trained staff could work.

The objective of the model is to minimize the total severity index for the hospital (the sum of the severity indices for all units within the hospital), and at the same time maintain the difference in the severity indices between hospital units below a predetermined level.

The model is based on the "branch and bound" principle of mathematical programming.[26] It could be verbally stated in terms of mathematical programming as follows:

**Objective:** Minimize the total severity index for the hospital.

**Subject to the following constraints:**

1. The number of allocations made in each skill level is less than or equal to the total number of pool staff available to that skill level.

2. The allocations are always made in integers (in increments of one whole person only).

3. The difference in severity indices between various units (variance) should be less than or equal to a predetermined constant.

The severity index prediction equations are provided to the model only once. It will theoretically be necessary to change these equations only if there is a major policy change in the hospital's nursing care delivery process; if the quality of nursing care is greatly changed due to new methods, equipment, or change in the staff; if seasonal changes in the number of patients are great enough to require a change in the nursing care delivery process; or due to any other factor of this nature.

To obtain the allocation decision for a shift at the beginning of that shift, it is necessary to provide the following data to the model.

- Up-to-date census for all units
- Up-to-date patient classification (only for those units where required)
- Core staff in different units
- Total pool staff available
- Other information on patient load if required (none in this case)

Figure III.4.2 shows the information flow to and from the model. The model is programmed to be in an interactive mode on a computer terminal so that the house director can "ask" for more solutions if she desires.

## Model Testing and Conclusions

The model was implemented in the study hospital for a period of four weeks to test its validity. Only the five inpatient units in which data were collected were included in the implementation. The implementation took place in two phases. In the first phase, for a period of two weeks, the house director went through the motions required for running the model but did not see the model's solutions. This phase was essentially to orient her to the new system and to adjust the parameters of the model. In the next two weeks, during the second phase of implementation, the model was actually run and the solutions from the model were shown to the house director. The sample output from the model is included in appendix III.4.D. During both of these phases, the head nurses of the five units for which the allocation model was run filled out the questionnaire (figure III.4.4).

Figure III.4.3 compares the model's performance with the actual allocation decisions carried out by the house director for the four-week period. Both the total severity index and the variance for the solutions from the model are less than the house director's solutions in most cases. (The

**FIGURE III.4.2**
Information flow to and from the model

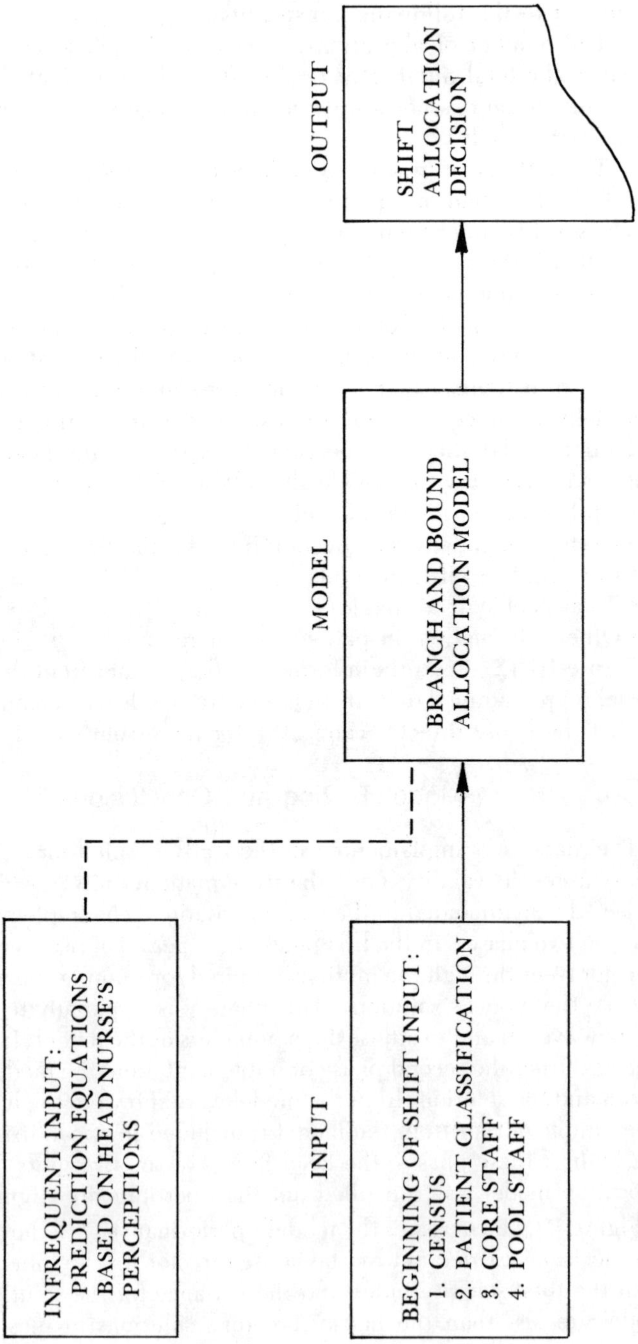

average of the total severity index for the model solutions over the four-week period is 6.42, and for the house director's actual allocation, the average is 6.84). This indicates that the allocation decisions arrived at by the model utilizing the head nurses' opinions follow closely the allocation decisions actually taken by the house director. Moreover, during the testing period there were days when the model solutions had smaller variance between the units and total severity index than the house director's solutions.

Further, responses from the questionnaires filled out by head nurses during the implementation period were compared with the severity indices predicted by the prediction equations. The correlations were found to be significant, thus verifying the reliability of the questionnaire. It was observed during the implementation that the house director and her staff had positive attitudes toward the solutions from the computer. This reaction was essentially due to the fact that those solutions were based on opinions of the head nurses of her staff.

## Applications of The Model

Although the model is primarily designed for the purpose of making daily allocation decisions, there are several other ways it could be used for cost and quality control purposes.

### Nursing Budget Decisions

When budgeting positions for various nursing units, it is essential for the administrator to know if those positions are adequate under average working conditions. It will be possible to input different combinations of core staff and average values of patient load affecting variables into the model. If the values of the severity indices thus obtained are acceptable, the core staff can be considered adequate. It will even be possible to budget positions considering seasonal trends in both patients and staff (for example, when nurses graduate from school in June, they are more readily available for hiring). To accommodate seasonal trends, the average values of the input variables corresponding to that part of the year could be supplied to the model. The decision regarding adequacy of the core staff can be made from the values of the severity indices thus obtained. The resulting cost benefits will be due to reduction in the core staff for different periods in a fiscal year.

### Placement of New Admissions

Since the allocation model is run at the beginning of a shift, it is possible to send the final severity indices to the admissions office, so

**FIGURE III.4.3**
Comparison of model performance and house director's decision

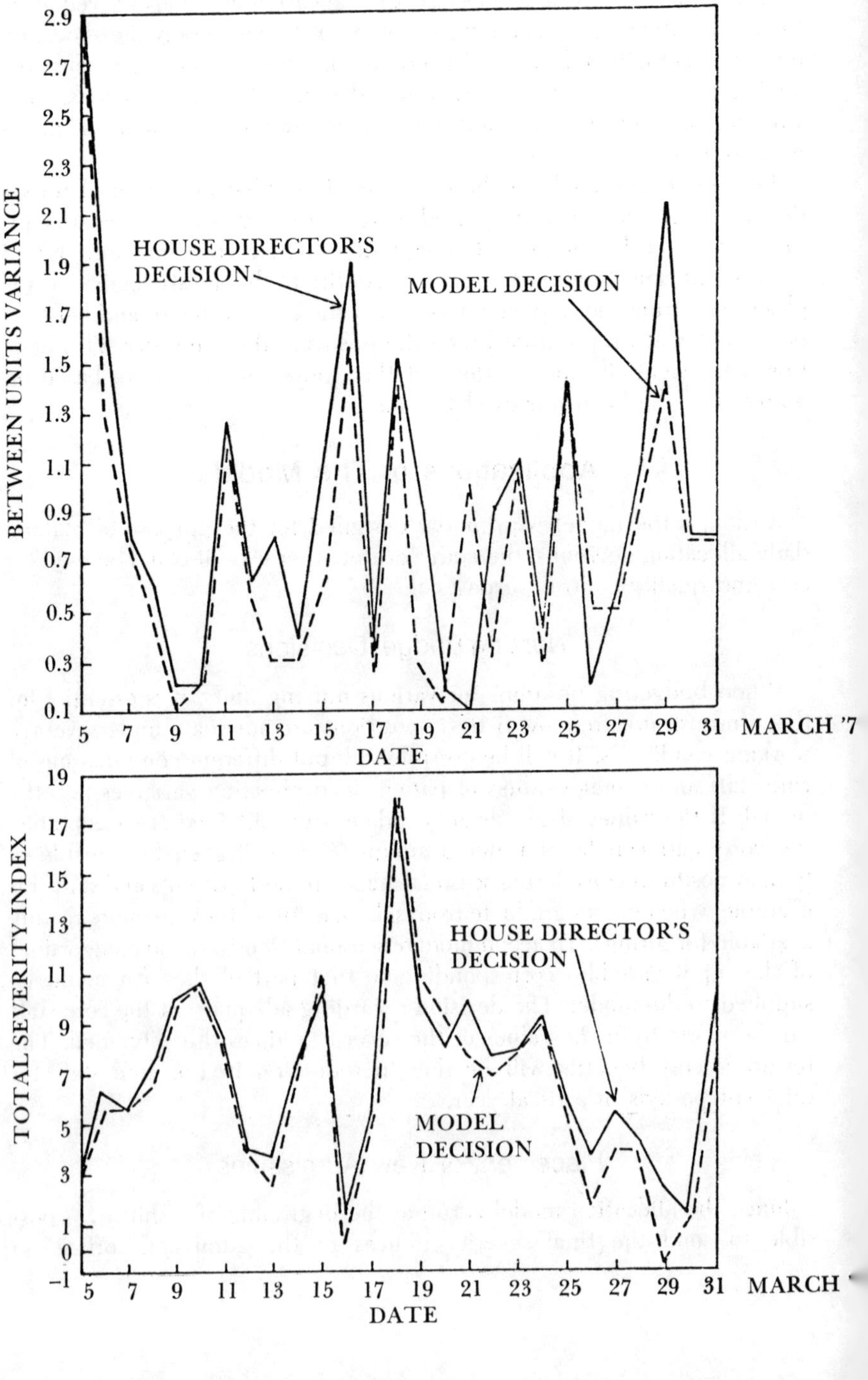

that the admissions officer can place a new admission in a unit where the severity index is low. The result will be to reduce the final variance of the severity indices.

### Use of the System During Staff Shortage

When a severe shortage of staff exists, the normal action by the nursing administrator would be to abandon the float pool and the allocation system. However, it would be beneficial to maintain the system during such times to reduce the variance of severity indices between units.

### Scheduling of Inservice Training

The inservice training schedule for hospital staff is usually prepared without considering the need of staff members for delivery of patient care on a given day. If the allocation model is in operation, it may be possible to schedule inservice training for nurses from units where the severity index is low.

## APPENDIX III.4.A

## Nurses' Estimate of Nursing Needs

You are being asked to answer the attached Nursing Unit Staffing Evaluation to provide information that will help improve the assignment of nursing unit personnel on a day-to-day basis. You have probably experienced many days when you wish there were additional personnel on the unit to help with an unusually heavy workload. On the other hand, you have also experienced days on which you could have managed the workload with less personnel. We are trying to establish a procedure for making the best possible assignment of the nursing staff available in the hospital on any given day (RNs, LPNs, and aides), just prior to the beginning of a shift.

We believe that nursing unit personnel can provide information that can be extremely helpful in assessing the adequacy of staffing on each shift each day. In answering the questionnaire each day, keep the following points in mind:

• Near the end of your shift (during the last half-hour or so), think about the staffing level for the entire shift: Was it adequate? If not, what category of personnel would you have needed most? If it was more than adequate, what category of personnel could you best have gotten along without?

• Please try to consider the shift as a whole. There will probably be times when an hour or two of the shift will be very hectic, and yet you won't need a whole additional person during the entire shift. Try to distinguish between these kinds of situations as you answer the questions.

• While answering the questionnaire, consider only the personnel that actually worked on that shift. For example, if an RN who was supposed to work on the shift was "pulled" from your unit, do not include that RN in your total staff while answering the questionnaire. On the other hand, if you received an additional RN from some other unit, include her in your total staff.

Please feel free to ask any questions or make any suggestions you would like about either the staffing evaluations or the problems of nursing staff allocation. We are interested in your ideas.

APPENDIX III.4.B

## Scheme For Patient Classification[27]

In the patient classification format (figure III.4.5), the columns marked A are weighted 1, the columns marked B are weighted 2, and the columns marked C are weighted 3. For classifying a patient either as type I (self care), type II (partial care), or type III (total care), follow these steps:

1. Count the total number of A columns checked for that patient and multiply that number by one. Let that number be P.

2. Count the total number of B columns checked for that patient and multiply that number by two. Let that number be Q.

3. Count the total number of C columns checked for that patient and multiply that number by three. Let that number be R.

4. Classify the patient as type I (self care) if P is maximum. Classify the patient as type II (partial care) if Q is maximum. Classify the patient as type III (total care) if R is maximum.

Exceptions:

1. In the case of a tie, the patient is classified in a more intense (more time-consuming) category.

2. For classifying a patient as type III (total care), there should be at least two C columns checked. If there is only one C column checked, neglect that column and classify the patient according to the remaining columns, following exactly the scheme described above. (This exception was especially made for those patients who were strictly confined to bed by doctors orders, but were self care patients (type I) in all other respects.)

**FIGURE III.4.4**
Head nurse questionnaire

Name ______________________ Date __________-72 Unit _________ Shift 7:00-3:30 ( ) 3:00-11:30 ( ) 11:00-7:30 ( )

1. If one additional person was available to you on your unit for today's shift:

a) How would you express the need for that person if that person was a RN? (Check one)

| No Need | Little Need | Fair Need | Great Need | Very Great Need |
|---|---|---|---|---|
| ( ) | ( ) | ( ) | ( ) | ( ) |

b) How would you express the need for that person is that person was a LPN? (Check one)

| No Need | Little Need | Fair Need | Great Need | Very Great Need |
|---|---|---|---|---|
| ( ) | ( ) | ( ) | ( ) | ( ) |

c) How would you express the need for that person if that person was an Aide? (Check one)

| No Need | Little Need | Fair Need | Great Need | Very Great Need |
|---|---|---|---|---|
| ( ) | ( ) | ( ) | ( ) | ( ) |

2. Indicate the reasons for your answer to question one (1). (Check only those items which influenced your answer to question one.)

| | Below Average | Average | Above Average |
|---|---|---|---|
| a) New Admissions | ( ) | ( ) | ( ) |
| b) Transfers (into, within, and out of the unit) | ( ) | ( ) | ( ) |
| c) Patients requiring special procedures (e.g., I.V., Catheter, I.O., Suction, Major Dressing Change) | ( ) | ( ) | ( ) |
| d) Postoperative Patients (Today/Yesterday) | ( ) | ( ) | ( ) |
| e) Number of highly nursing dependent patients (based upon ambulation, bathing, feeding, vital signs, and orientation status) | ( ) | ( ) | ( ) |

f) Other (please explain) ______________________________________________

3. If one person had been withdrawn from your unit for staffing elsewhere:

a) With what degree of difficulty could you have released that person (let that person go) if that person was a RN? (Check one)

| Very Great Difficulty | Great Difficulty | Fair Difficulty | Little Difficulty | No Difficulty |
|---|---|---|---|---|
| ( ) | ( ) | ( ) | ( ) | ( ) |

b) With what degree of difficulty could you have released that person if that person was a LPN? (Check one)

| Very Great Difficulty | Great Difficulty | Fair Difficulty | Little Difficulty | No Difficulty |
|---|---|---|---|---|
| ( ) | ( ) | ( ) | ( ) | ( ) |

c) With what degree of difficulty could you have released that person if that person was an Aide? (Check one)

| Very Great Difficulty | Great Difficulty | Fair Difficulty | Little Difficulty | No Difficulty |
|---|---|---|---|---|
| ( ) | ( ) | ( ) | ( ) | ( ) |

4. Indicate the reasons for your answer to question three (3). (Check only those items which influenced your answer to question three.)

| | Below Average | Average | Above Average |
|---|---|---|---|
| a) New Admissions | ( ) | ( ) | ( ) |
| b) Transfers (into, within, and out of the unit) | ( ) | ( ) | ( ) |
| c) Patients requiring special procedures | ( ) | ( ) | ( ) |
| d) Postoperative Patients (Today/Yesterday) | ( ) | ( ) | ( ) |
| e) Number of highly nursing dependent patients | ( ) | ( ) | ( ) |

f) Other (please explain) ______________________________________________

5. How would you rate the overall nursing care provided in today's shift on your unit? (Check one)

| Very Good | Good | Fair | Poor | Very Poor |
|---|---|---|---|---|
| ( ) | ( ) | ( ) | ( ) | ( ) |

**FIGURE III.4.5**
Patient classification format

PATIENT CLASSIFICATION
MEDICAL WEST WING

MIDNIGHT SHIFT

| ROOM | | AMBULATORY | | | B A T H | | | FEEDING | | | TPR/BP | ORIENTATION | | |
|---|---|---|---|---|---|---|---|---|---|---|---|---|---|---|
| | | SELF | WITH ASST | SCB | SELF | PART ASST | COMP ASST | SELF | PART ASST | COMP ASST | Q2H OR OFTEN | ORIENTED | CONFUSED | DISORI |
| | | A | B | C | A | B | C | A | B | C | C | A | B | C |
| 537-A | | | | | | | | | | | | | | |
| 539-A | | | | | | | | | | | | | | |
| 539-B | | | | | | | | | | | | | | |
| 541-A | | | | | | | | | | | | | | |
| 541-B | | | | | | | | | | | | | | |
| 543-A | | | | | | | | | | | | | | |
| 543-B | | | | | | | | | | | | | | |
| 545-A | | | | | | | | | | | | | | |
| 545-B | | | | | | | | | | | | | | |
| 547-A | | | | | | | | | | | | | | |
| 547-B | | | | | | | | | | | | | | |
| 549-A | | | | | | | | | | | | | | |
| 549-B | | | | | | | | | | | | | | |
| 551-A | | | | | | | | | | | | | | |
| 551-B | | | | | | | | | | | | | | |
| 553-A | | | | | | | | | | | | | | |
| 553-B | | | | | | | | | | | | | | |
| 555-A | | | | | | | | | | | | | | |
| 555-B | | | | | | | | | | | | | | |
| 557-A | | | | | | | | | | | | | | |
| 557-B | | | | | | | | | | | | | | |
| 559-A | | | | | | | | | | | | | | |
| 559-B | | | | | | | | | | | | | | |

APPENDIX III.4.C

## Specialized Nursing Procedures

A brief explanation of various specialized procedures follows.

1) I.V.: Setting up equipment and starting I.V. infusion, also maintaining parenteral fluid flow by replacing bottles and/or controlling infusion rate

2) I.O.: Patients on input and output

3) Catheter: Placing and/or maintaining the patency of the urinary catheter

4) Major Dressing Change: Including wound irrigation, observation of drainage, and/or suture removal

5) Suction: (a) Nose, mouth or tracheotomy suction to maintain open air passages and/or (b) Maintaining levine tube for continuous lavage purpose

6) Major Teaching: Patient instruction for self-care. For example: (a) Diabetic care (b) Colostomy care (c) Self-catheterization

7) Surgical Procedures on Unit: Include procedures such as bone marrow, liver biopsy, or C.V.P.

8) Lab, X-Ray, or Surgery Prep: Include glucose tolerance test, enemas, etc.

9) Isolation: Patients in total isolation

10) Incontinent: Patients who are incontinent

11) Special Equipment: Special equipment required by the patients such as: Monitor, Ivac, Traction, Circle Bed, Respirator, Croupett, etc.

APPENDIX III.4.D

## Specimen Output

The specimen output from the teletype terminal (connected to an IBM 360/67 computer) is included in this appendix.

The first page of the output (p. 222) contains the input information provided for day shift on March 30, 1973. The second page (p. 223) contains the severity indices for different units before making any allocations. It provides the total severity index and variance of severity indices between the five units before the allocations are made. It also provides the minimum possible total severity index in the absence of any constraint on the variance. The third page of the output (p. 224) provides the first allocation solution that is obtained by the Min-Max algorithm. The asterisks in the printout represent the units where different skill levels are allocated.

**FIGURE III.4.6**
Specimen output

```
#
 EXECUTION BEGINS


                         GOOD MORNING

   {PLEASE PUT A COMMA AFTER EVERY NUMBER THAT YOU ENTER}

{1}  AVAILABLE CORE STAFF?
              RN,LPN,A/O,
     MED-SURG= 3,2,5,
     PEDS     = 2,1,2,
     SURGICAL= 4,3,7,
     ICU/CCU  = 3,2,1,
     MEDICAL  = 4,3,10,


{2}  AVAILABLE STAFF IN POOL?
     RN       = 0,
     LPN      = 1,
     A/O      = 2,


{3}  CENSUS?
     MED-SURG= 60,
     PEDS     = 15,
     SURGICAL= 66,
     ICU/CCU  = 12,
     MEDICAL  = 81,


{4}  WARD SECS. ON MEDICAL UNIT = 2,

{5}  NO. OF TYPE III PATIENTS IN PEDS = 5,

{6}  NO. OF TYPE II PATIENTS IN MEDICAL = 9,

{7}  NO. OF TRANSFERS IN/OUT OR WITHIN PEDS = 0,


PLEASE CHECK THE ABOVE INFORMATION
IF CORRECT ENTER OK OTHERWISE ENTER REPEAT
ok
```

FIGURE III .4.6 Cont.

DEPARTMENT OF NURSING
BAKER HOSPITAL

STAFFING REPORT 03-30-75 DAY SHIFT
10:10.49

| | AVAILABLE CORE STAFF | | | SEVERITY | INDICES | | |
|---|---|---|---|---|---|---|---|
| | RN | LPN | A/O | RN | LPN | A/O | TOT |
| MED-SURG | 3 | 2 | 5 | 1.3 | 0.6 | 1.3 | 3.2 |
| PEDS | 2 | 1 | 2 | -0.6 | -0.3 | 0.3 | -0.6 |
| SURGICAL | 4 | 3 | 7 | 0.2 | 0.4 | 0.9 | 1.4 |
| ICU/CCU | 3 | 2 | 1 | -0.1 | 0.0 | 0.3 | 0.2 |
| MEDICAL | 4 | 3 | 10 | 0.4 | -0.1 | -1.0 | -0.7 |

TOTAL DAY SHIFT SEVERITY= 3.6 {VARIANCE*= 2.1}

AVAILABLE STAFF IN POOL

| RN | LPN1,2 | A/O |
|---|---|---|
| 0 | 1 | 2 |

LOWEST POSSIBLE TOTAL DAY SHIFT SEVERITY= -0.8**

* This variance represents the variance in the severity indices between the five units.

** This number represents the lowest possible total severity in the absence of any constraint on the variance.

SOLUTION * 1 *

| | SUGGESTED | STAFFING | | SEVERITY | INDICES | | |
|---|---|---|---|---|---|---|---|
| | RN | LPN | A/O | RN | LPN | A/O | TOT |
| MED-SURG | 3 | 3 * | 7 ** | 0.6 | 0.2 | 0.5 | 1.3 |
| PEDS | 2 | 1 | 2 | -0.6 | -0.3 | 0.3 | -0.6 |
| SURGICAL | 4 | 3 | 7 | 0.2 | 0.4 | 0.9 | 1.4 |
| ICU/CCU | 3 | 2 | 1 | -0.1 | 0.0 | 0.3 | 0.2 |
| MEDICAL | 4 | 3 | 10 | 0.4 | -0.1 | -1.0 | -0.7 |

TOTAL DAY SHIFT SEVERITY= 1.7 {VARIANCE= 0.8}

DO YOU WANT MORE SOLUTIONS ?
ENTER YES IF ANSWER IS YES OTHERWISE ENTER NO

yes

ENTER THE CONSTRAINT ON VARIANCE
{E.G. 1.20, 5.50 E.T.C.}
CONSTRAINT= 1.5**

* The first solution is arrived at by "min-max" algorithm and not by "branch and bound" algorithm.

** This represents the constraint on the variance for the next solution as a multiple of the variance for the first solution. For example, in this case the next solution *should not* have a variance greater than $(0.8 \times 1.5) = 1.2$.

**FIGURE III .4.6 Cont.**

SOLUTION # 2

| | SUGGESTED STAFFING | | | SEVERITY INDICES | | | |
|---|---|---|---|---|---|---|---|
| | RN | LPN | A/O | RN | LPN | A/O | TOT |
| MED-SURG | 3 | 3 * | 5 | 0.6 | 0.2 | 1.3 | 2.2 |
| PEDS | 2 | 1 | 2 | -0.6 | -0.3 | 0.3 | -0.6 |
| SURGICAL | 4 | 3 | 9 ** | -0.2 | -0.0 | 0.0 | -0.2 |
| ICU/CCU | 3 | 2 | 1 | -0.1 | 0.0 | 0.3 | 0.2 |
| MEDICAL | 4 | 3 | 10 | 0.4 | -0.1 | -1.0 | -0.7 |

TOTAL DAY SHIFT SEVERITY= 0.9 {VARIANCE= 1.1}

DO YOU WANT MORE SOLUTIONS ?
ENTER YES IF ANSWER IS YES OTHERWISE ENTER NO

yes

ENTER THE CONSTRAINT ON VARIANCE
{E.G. 1.20, 5.50 E.T.C.}
CONSTRAINT= 1.2

SOLUTION # 3

| | SUGGESTED STAFFING | | | SEVERITY INDICES | | | |
|---|---|---|---|---|---|---|---|
| | RN | LPN | A/O | RN | LPN | A/O | TOT |
| MED-SURG | 3 | 3 * | 6 * | 0.6 | 0.2 | 0.9 | 1.7 |
| PEDS | 2 | 1 | 2 | -0.6 | -0.3 | 0.3 | -0.6 |
| SURGICAL | 4 | 3 | 8 * | -0.0 | 0.2 | 0.4 | 0.6 |
| ICU/CCU | 3 | 2 | 1 | -0.1 | 0.0 | 0.3 | 0.2 |
| MEDICAL | 4 | 3 | 10 | 0.4 | -0.1 | -1.0 | -0.7 |

TOTAL DAY SHIFT SEVERITY= 1.3 {VARIANCE= 0.8}

DO YOU WANT MORE SOLUTIONS ?
ENTER YES IF ANSWER IS YES OTHERWISE ENTER NO

no

NO. OF SOLUTIONS CHECKED = 23 NO. OF NODES = 133

HAVE A HAPPY DAY

STOP 0
EXECUTION TERMINATED

At this point, the program also demands a constraint on the variance for the next solution (which is obtained by branch and bound algorithm) as a multiple of the variance for the Min-Max solution (i.e., solution 1).

On the fourth page (p.224), the branch and bound solution is generated. (Notice that the constraint on variance of this solution is provided on the previous page.) On this page, another constraint on variance for the next branch and bound solution is demanded. This constraint is also provided as a multiple of the variance of the Min-Max solution (solution 1). The branch and bound solution with this constraint on the variance is generated on the fifth page of the output. Solution 3 represents the actual staffing made by the house director on that shift.

## NOTES

[1]Two of the issues addressed here, measurement of nursing workload and optimum allocation model, have been elaborated individually in the following publications: V. M. Trivedi and W. M. Hancock, "Measurement of Nursing Work Load Using Head Nurses' Perceptions," *Nursing Research*. V. M. Trivedi and D. M. Warner, "A Branch and Bound Algorithm for Optimum Allocation of Float Nurses," *Management Science*.

The term "model" is used in the sense of mathematical programming or statistical models.

[2]D. M. Warner, "A Two-Phase Model for Scheduling Nursing Personnel in a Hospital." Doctoral dissertation, Tulane University, 1971.

H. Wolfe, "A Multiple Assignment Model for Staffing Nursing Units." Doctoral dissertation, Johns Hopkins University, 1964.

[3]The inpatient demand is defined as explicit requests for nursing care made either by patient, physician, or nursing supervisor and implicit demand from convention or nursing policy.

[4]Robert J. Connor, "A Hospital Inpatient Classification System." Doctoral dissertation, Johns Hopkins University, 1960, p. 66.

[5]*Ibid.*, p. 68.

[6]*Ibid.*, pp. 101-102.

[7]*Ibid.*

[8]David H. Stimson and Ruth H. Stimson, *Operations Research in Hospitals: Diagnosis and Prognosis*. Chicago: Hospital Research and Educational Trust, 1972, pp. 9-14 and chapter 3.

Myrtle K. Aydelotte, *Nurse Staffing Methodology: A Review and Critique of Selected Literature*. DHEW Publication No. (NIH) 73-433, January 1973, pp. 94-95.

[9]Connor, "Hospital Inpatient Classification." A. M. Feyerham, "Measurement of Hospital Patient Care Loads." Kansas State University, 1964.

Richard C. Jelinek, "Nursing: The Development of an Activity Model." Doctoral dissertation, The University of Michigan, 1964. Warner, "Two-Phase Model." Wolfe, "Multiple Assignment Model."

[10]Technique such as time study or work sampling.

Ralph M. Barnes, *Motion and Time Study Design and Measurement of Work.* New York: John Wiley & Sons, 1968.

Commission on Administration Services in Hospitals, *Nursing Procedures Manual.* Los Angeles: The Commission, 1968.

[11]Warner, "Two-Phase Model."

Wolfe, "Multiple Assignment Model."

[12]Dolores E. Little and Doris L. Carnevali, *Nursing Care Planning.* Philadelphia: J. B. Lippincott Company, 1969.

[13]American Hospital Association Nursing Activity Study, "Project Report," p. 2.

[14]Jelinek, "Nursing Activity Model."

Louis E. Freund, "A Model for Measuring the Difficulty of Registered Nurse Assignments." Doctoral dissertation, The University of Michigan, 1969.

[15]In general: medication and supervision for registered nurses; treatments for licensed practical nurses; and patient care for aides.

[16]Connor, "Hospital Inpatient Classification."

Feyerham, "Patient Care Loads."

Freund, "Difficulty of RN Assignments."

Jelinek, "Nursing Activity Model."

[17]Rensis Likert, "A Technique for the Measurement of Attitudes." *Archives of Psychology,* Vol. 22, No. 140, June 1932.

[18]Edythe Alexander, et al., *Nursing Service Administration Principles and Practice.* Saint Louis: C. V. Mosley Co., 1962.

[19]Connor, "Hospital Inpatient Classification."

Feyerham, "Patient Care Loads."

Freund, "Difficulty of RN Assignments."

Jelinek, "Nursing Activity Model."

[20]V. M. Trivedi, "Optimum Allocation of Float Nurses Using Head Nurses' Perceptions." Doctoral dissertation, The University of Michigan, 1974, chapter 3.

[21]*Ibid.*, p. 56.

[22]Medical-surgical, 60 beds; pediatrics, 28 beds; surgical, 68 beds; ICU/CCU, 16 beds, medical, 86 beds.

[23]For each skill level, staff was fivided into two categories: regular staff; and staff in orientation in the unit.

[24]Trivedi, "Allocation of Float Nurses," p. 60.

[25]The census in the study hospital is relatively stable at ninety-five to ninety-seven percent. Therefore, these patient load affecting factors are also relatively stable. Hence, their effect is not predominant in the severity index.

[26]Trivedi, "Allocation of Float Nurses," chapter 5.

[27]Freund, "Difficulty of RN Assignments."

R. K. D. Hausmann, "A Queueing Theory Approach to Measuring Quality of Care: Application in a Burn Unit." Doctoral dissertation, The University of Michigan, 1968.

# III.5

# Resource Allocation and Scheduling for a Radiology Department

*by Ronald F. Perry and Richard F. Baum*

The radiology department is an integral service component of the patient care process, providing the physician with diagnostic assistance in the form of a written report of the radiologist's findings. The major elements of the radiologic process are: patient scheduling and transporting; patient examination, including film processing and quality check for the x-ray; and diagnostic reporting, which includes interpretation of the film by the radiologist, typing a report, and dispatching it from the department. These elements were all included in a simulation model of a radiology department developed for Baker Hospital. Information for the structure and data needed to develop the model were obtained from a data collection study in the department, available department records, and interviews with the chief radiologist and chief technologist.

The purpose of this research was to improve the utility of the information available to decision makers for predicting the impact of radiology department resource allocation and scheduling decisions on the overall patient care process, as well as on the cost of the department operations. The research resulted in forecasting the effect of scheduling and resource allocation decisions for the Baker Hospital radiology department before such decisions were implemented.[1] This research also resulted in developing a pragmatic engineering approach for use in analyzing and improving the overall operations of a radiology department.

Previous works consider only the part of the radiologic process involving patient scheduling, transportation, and examination. Omitted from consideration is diagnostic report preparation, which links the radiology department activities to the physician's diagnostic and treatment process, and hence to the cost of patient care. The measures of performance developed to date reflect only the cost of the resources used to perform radiologic procedures. The level of service provided to the physician, which influences the impact of the radiologic process on total patient care cost, is not considered.

The service view of a radiology department is incorporated in this work through the measures of performance developed to assess the impact of decisions on overall patient care. Specifically, these measures reflect the extent to which diagnostic reports are available to attending physicians when they are needed to aid in diagnosis and treatment, as well as immediate patient related service.

The measure of performance for overall patient care is based on the premise that a diagnostic report should be available to a physician on the visit to the hospital immediately following the one on which the examination was requested, and that any delay beyond this increases patient care cost by potentially increasing a patient's length of stay. The measures of performance which reflect immediate patient service are the average waiting time in the department, and the starting time of the last fluoroscopic examination of the day.

The engineering approach, based on the service function of the radiology department, is to work back through the radiology process. That is, concentrate on the timeliness of report availability as a critical factor in cost and quality for the operations of a radiology department. From this, determine the service measures relating to report dispatch, in the context of the hospital's requirements. Then establish the radiology process time requirements to meet the report service goals. If the process is incapable of meeting these time goals, work backward through the system, starting with report dispatch, to achieve process capability. Identify bottlenecks and delays, and eliminate them as much as possible. Resource and personnel requirements for the system should be planned, as much as possible, to attain reasonable utilization of equipment and personnel. Finally, once the desired process time has been attained, install a monitoring system so that the system performance can be kept in control.

In the following pages the development of service criteria and an objective function for radiology department operations is discussed under the heading "Measuring Radiology Department Performance." The development of the model which takes the form of a computer simulation and its validation are covered under the heading "Model Development." The part headed "Experimental Approach: Problem Decomposition" discusses the role of the model in seeking the optimum value of the objective function, and the use of the model in analyzing a planning decision faced by the study hospital. The hospital has just finished building a new outpatient facility and has expanded the radiology department. Because of construction economies, all of the new examining rooms were built at one time, but it is not necessary to equip all of them immediately. The decisions studied concern the timing of equipment and personnel additions to meet forecast demand without having undue excess capacity. The "Summary and Recommendations" contains a concise description of the radiology department operations model and presents recommendations, based on the experiments conducted with the model, for implementation at Baker Hospital.

In addition to the planning problem, management is faced with the task of monitoring measures of performance on a continuing basis. This requires information to detect and correct deviations of these measures from expected levels. "Performance Monitoring" discusses methods of obtaining this information and its use in the monitoring system.

## Measuring Radiology Department Performance

The demand for diagnostic radiologic services is increasing. The National Advisory Committee on Radiation estimates that the total demand for radiologic services is growing at the rate of 7.2 percent annually, while professional manpower is estimated by Knowles to be increasing at an annual rate of only 5.7 percent.[2,3,4] In addition, inadequacies of space and equipment are claimed to exist. A survey by the American College of Radiology reveals that an average of 1.4 to 3.4 additional exposure rooms are felt to be needed by radiology departments in hospitals of all sizes.[5] Cost is also increasing, according to data collected by Hospital Administrative Services which show that the national median cost per diagnostic procedure increased an average of 8.6 percent per year during the two years ending 1972.[6]

### Service Criteria

The role of diagnostic radiology in the patient care regimen is to provide assistance to the attending physician in diagnosing and treating his patient. In the case of a medium-sized, nonteaching, community general hospital, such as Baker Hospital, this is accomplished in two ways: first, by the written diagnostic report containing the radiologist's interpretation of the patient's radiograph, and second, by consultation of the radiologist with the physician.

The elements of the radiologic process necessary to provide this service to physicians are the following: patient scheduling and transporting, including requisition processing; patient examination, which includes processing and quality check of the x-ray; film filing and retrieval; and diagnostic reporting, which includes interpretation of the film by the radiologist, typing a report, and dispatching it from the department. Figure III.5.1 depicts the flow of requisitions, patients, films, and diagnostic reports through the process.

A complete measure of department performance must include a measure of service provided, as well as the cost of the resources (professional and clerical personnel, equipment, and building space) used to fulfill the demand for radiologic procedures. It is assumed that the professional quality of the diagnostic information is adequate. Therefore, the service measure is concerned with the timeliness of the information, specifically the delay from the time of the examination request by the physician to the time the diagnostic report is available to the physician (subsquently referred to as report delay). Adequate measures of resource costs are available for inclusion in a measure of performance. Also, the resources required for the patient billing process are assumed to be sufficient to provide a system acceptable to the hospital. Hence, the following paragraphs are concerned with the development of a measure of service.

Diagnostic reports which are unavailable when the physician needs them potentially increase patient care cost. In the case of inpatients, the length of stay may be increased by unavailable reports. Gertman and Bucher found that approximately sixteen percent of the inappropriate days of hospital stay were caused by delayed radiology reports.[7] A day was defined as inappropriate if the major reason for that day's stay was not directly related to patient diagnosis or treatment. Further, it is strongly suspected that unavailable reports sometimes cause physicians, thinking that their orders were lost, to reorder a procedure.

In addition to the length of report delay, the timing of report availability is important when the attending physician's presence at the hospital is limited, as is the case for a nonteaching, community general hospital. A study of the pattern of physicians' visits to the study hospital found that eighty-five percent of the doctors visit the hospital once a day, and seventy-five percent of the visits on a given day occur between the hours of 8:00 A.M. and 12:00 noon.

In light of this visiting pattern, the following service criteria are proposed to measure the availability of the diagnostic report to the physician on the visit immediately following the one on which the examination was requested. For the doctors who visit during the morning the criterion is: the fraction of reports produced for examination requests received in the radiology department by 12:00 noon which is available to physicians by 8:00 A.M. on the following day. For the afternoon doctors it is: the fraction of reports produced for examination requests received after 12:00 noon which is available to physicians by 12:00 noon on the following day. These criteria are suitable for both inpatient and outpatient reports since physicians receive outpatient reports in their hospital mailboxes, and since outpatients live in the community and may conveniently obtain x-ray findings on a day subsequent to the examination visit.

Some adjustments for the staffing policies in the hospital are necessary to implement these service criteria. Medical secretaries who type the re-

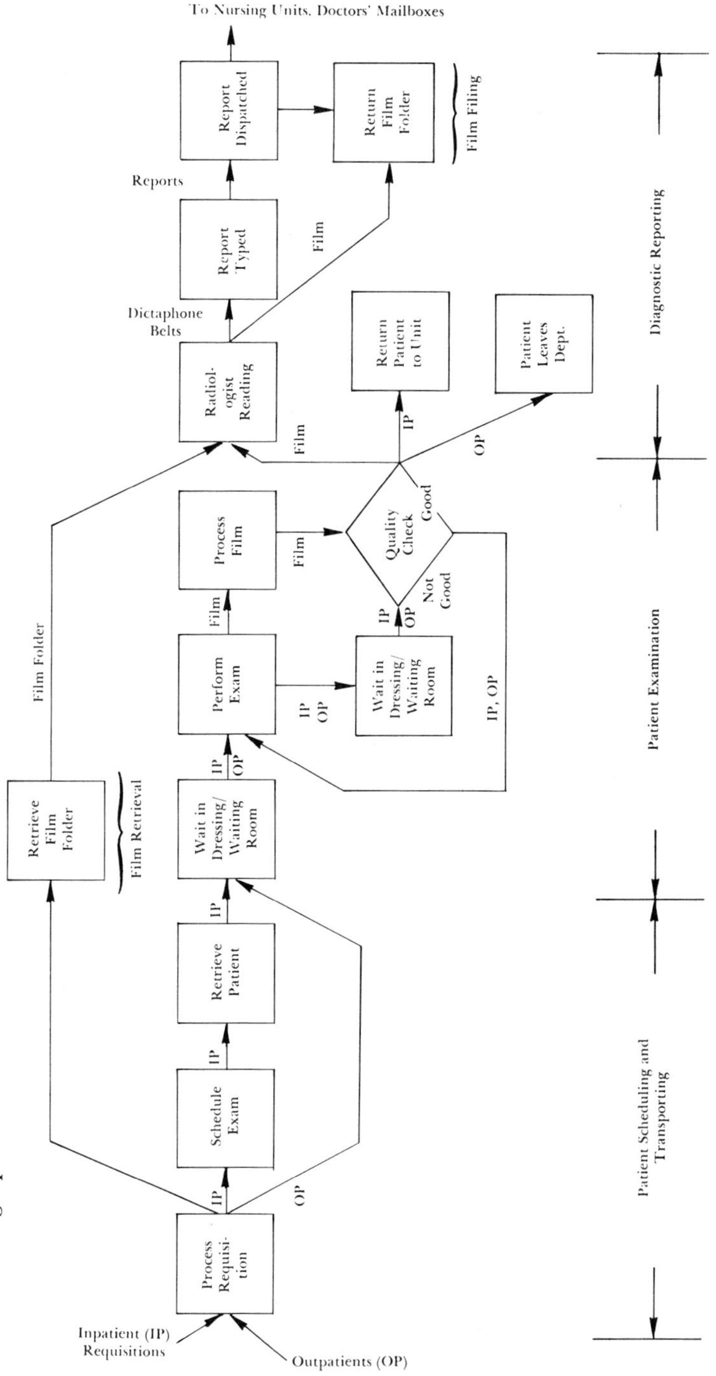


**FIGURE III.5.1**
Radiologic process

ports, and the messenger service which delivers them to the nursing units, are available only during the day shift. Given these constraints, if a report is to be on the nursing unit or in the physician's mailbox by 8:00 A.M., it must leave the radiology department by the end of the previous day shift. For reports to be on the nursing unit by 12:00 noon, allowance must be made for messenger delivery and posting to the patient chart, so that the report should leave the department by 10:00 A.M.[8]

The service criteria for evaluating diagnostic report availability are now defined as follows:

*For morning doctors:* the fraction of reports produced for examination requests received by 12:00 noon which is dispatched from the department by the end of the current day shift.

*For afternoon doctors:* the fraction of reports produced for examination requests received after 12:00 noon which is dispatched from the department by 10:00 A.M. of the following day.

The performance of Baker Hospital relative to these criteria is indicated by data collected in 1972 for model development. For inpatients, reports were dispatched by the end of the current day shift for approximately sixty-five percent of the requests received by 12:00 noon, and by 10:00 A.M. of the following day for approximately fifty percent of the requests received after 12:00 noon. This indicates that about half of the physicians probably did not see a diagnostic report for their hospitalized patients on the day following their examination request. This was further demonstrated by an additional study of diagnostic report turnaround.[9]

The state of the art in modeling and performance measurement of radiology department operations may be summarized as follows. The models developed to date have included only two elements of the radiologic process: patient scheduling and transporting; and patient examination. Measures of performance used are the cost of the resources for these elements, and patient waiting time, which reflects only one aspect of level of service.[10] Operating and design criteria have been concerned almost exclusively with the balancing of patient waiting time against examining room and technologist utilization. The model developed here includes all the elements of the radiologic process necessary to relate department activities to the patient care process, and uses measures of performance which reflect resource costs and level of service. Film filing is not considered since it does not contribute to report delay at medium-sized hospitals such as Baker. The following segment discusses the problem of integrating all of these measures into on objective function.

## Development of an Objective Function

An objective function which expresses the total cost of the measures of performance discussed in the previous section may be defined as follows:[11]

**minimize:** $C_1L_1N_1 + C_2L_2N_2 + C_3W + R$

**subject to:** (1) maximum acceptable values for personnel and equipment utilization

(2) latest start time for examinations requiring the patient to fast

(3) discreteness of resource additions (e.g., the decision variable, examining rooms, must be increased in increments of one unit)

where: $i$ = 1 denotes inpatients, $i = 2$ denotes outpatients

$L_i$ = average fraction of diagnostic reports produced for patient type i requisitions which fail to be dispatched by the service criterion deadline

$N_i$ = number of diagnostic reports produced for patient type i requisitions during a given period

$W$ = average patient waiting time in the department

$C_i$ = cost per unit for patient type i reports failing to meet deadlines, $i = 1, 2$

$C_3$ = cost per unit for patient waiting time

$R$ = costs of resources (personnel salaries, equipment depreciation, etc.)

The first constraint arises from a concern to prevent personnel fatigue and excessive equipment down time, which is caused by prolonged uninterrupted use. The second constraint reflects humane consideration of the patient in attempting to minimize the number of missed meals, and long standing tradition in the radiologist's method of operation. The third constraint prohibits the addition of fractional pieces of equipment, and reflects policy decisions on whether to use part-time employees. Finally, there is an implicit constraint that all demand for radiologic services presented to the department must be met. This is imposed by not allowing any patient demand to be postponed.

The measures $L_1$, $L_2$, and W, and the costs R are functions of the decision variables (patient arrival schedule, number of examining rooms, and personnel staffing patterns) used in defining the scheduling and resource allocation policies. The costs $C_1$, $C_2$, and $C_3$, however, are functions of patient and physician characteristics beyond the control of the radiology department. Because of the difficulty in reliably estimating these costs, their associated measures, $N_1$, $N_2$, and W will be removed from the objective function and constrained to acceptable limits.

The revised objective function is then:

**minimize:** R

**subject to:** constraints (1) through (3) above and:

(4) maximum acceptable value for $L_1$

(5) maximum acceptable value for $L_2$

(6) maximum acceptable value for W

It seems clear that the cost of additional hospital stay necessitated by a late inpatient report ($C_1$) is considerably more than the outpatient cost ($C_2$), and that $C_1$ exceeds the cost of patient waiting time in the department ($C_3$) for either patient type by a still greater margin. Because of the relative magnitude of late inpatient report cost ($C_1$), its impact on the optimum solution is assessed by a sensitivity analysis of constraint (4), the constraint which limits the fraction of late inpatient reports.

## Model Development

Radiology department operations are modeled as a queueing network, (shown in figure III.5.2) of the following elements of the radiologic process: patient scheduling and transporting, patient examination, and diagnostic report generation. Film filing and retrieval is not included in the model because this element does not now, and is not expected to, contribute to report delay. This situation is typical for a medium-sized, non-teaching community hospital.

Since the capability to analytically treat queueing networks as complex as this one is not available, the model takes the form of a computer simulation.[12] For the purposes of this chapter, the definition of simulation provided by Naylor et. al. is appropriate.

> Simulation is a numerical technique for conducting experiments on a digital computer, which involves certain types of mathematical and logical models that describe the behavior of a business or economic system (or some component thereof) over extended periods of real time.[13]

Variables treated as exogenous (i.e., variables specified as input to the model) in the experiments conducted are:

**decision variables**—those which define:

- Number of examining rooms of each type
- Scheduling of certain patient arrivals (e.g., walk-in outpatients)
- Scheduling of films to the radiologist
- Staffing patterns for various categories of personel (technologists, typists, etc.)
- Minimum batch sizes for accumulation between processes

**uncontrollable variables**—those which define:

- Daily demand for examinations, by type
- Arrival pattern for emergency room patients
- Process times:
  - —requisition processing
  - —patient transportation
  - —patient examination
  - —film processing
  - —film interpretation
  - —report typing
  - —report dispatching

Endogenous variables (i.e., output variables) generated by the model are:
**diagnostic report delay**—provided for morning and afternoon service criteria for each patient type
**resource utilization**
- Personnel—by category
- Examination room

**delays between processes**—provided for each patient type:
- Patient waiting time
- Film processing completion to film interpretation start
- Film interpretation completion to report typing start
- Report typing completion to start of report dispatching

The model is constructed in three segments, as indicated in figure III.5.2. The first segment provides the arrival stream of patient requisitions and patients, and their attributes (patient type, examination type). The second segment accomplishes patient scheduling, transporting and examination, and film processing. Segment three consists of diagnostic report generation. Constructing the model in this fashion reduces simulation costs and experimental error in evaluating decisions, since it is possible to feed exactly the same stream of random events from segment 1 into segment 2, or from segment 2 into segment 3, in evaluating different scheduling and resource allocation policies. Additional cost reductions accrue from the decomposition of the problem discussed under "Experiments and Results."

Segments 1 and 2 are relatively easy to adapt for use in other medium-sized hospitals, since the elements of radiologic process which they contain are faily standardized. The report generation process tends to be hospital-specific, and therefore segment 3 would require more adapting to the operating procedures of another hospital.

## Data Collection and Analysis

Information for the structure and data for the exogenous variables in the model were obtained from the Baker Hospital radiology department. This department has three examining rooms and processed approximately 39,000 patients during 1972, the year the information was gathered. Three sources provided inputs to the model: a nine-day data collection study, available department records, and interviews with the chief radiologist and the chief technologist. During the study period, data on 1,000 patients were collected, while information on 4,100 patients was retrieved from department records. The study period data were used to develop the process times, batch sizes for accumulation between processes, and hourly arrival patterns of examination requests and patients to the department. The department data were used to define daily demand for each type of examination.

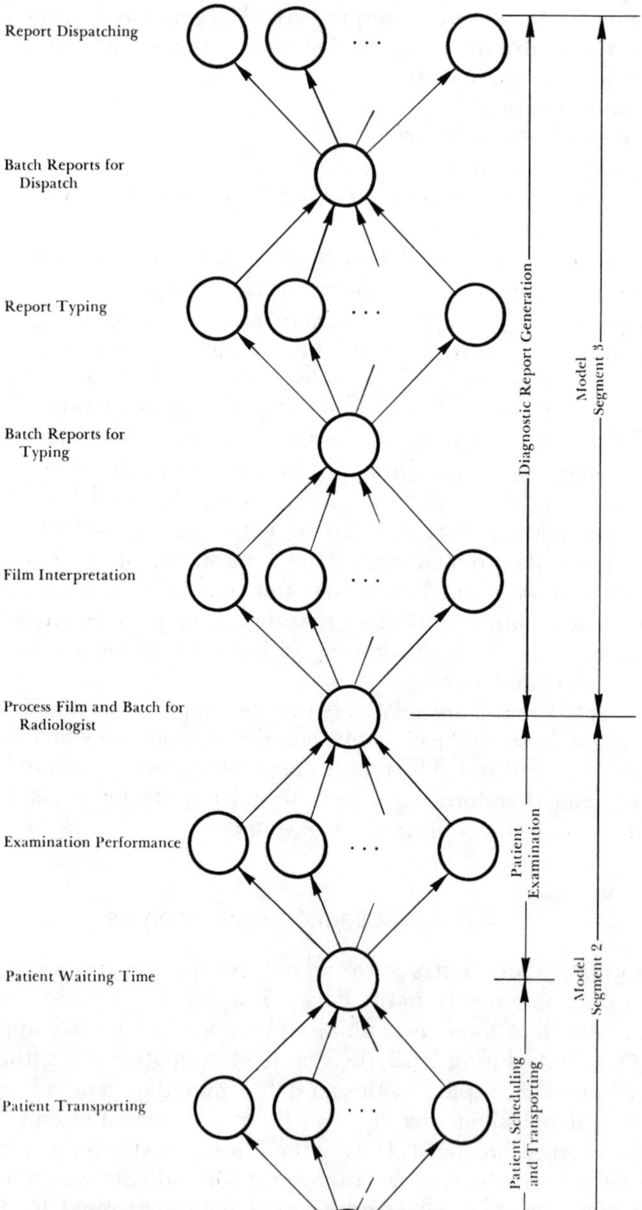


**FIGURE III.5.2**
Queueing network of radiology department operations

In order to minimize the disruption of department operations during data collection, several automatic time stamps were used at selected locations in the department. As the patient passed through these locations, department personnel time stamped a card attached to the patient requisition, thus generating a permanent record of the patient's progress in the department. A sample of the cards used appears in figure III.5.3. The time and date were stamped for the following events: examination request arrival, patient arrival, examination start and finish (for the initial examination and any required repeat films), film processing completion, report typing start and finish, and dispatch finish. The process times and arrival patterns mentioned above were then computed from these data.

Data analysis consisted of the application of statistical methods to: determine differences in mean values for daily examination demand and hourly arrival rates; fit theoretical distributions to the data for these variables; and develop predictor equations for process times. The theoretical distribution fits were helpful in verifying the assumptions of the tests for differences in means. They also permitted simplification of the model where their use (instead of the empirical distribution) was justified by previous findings.

## Model Validation

Model validation is the process of establishing that a model accurately reproduces the system under study. That is, for a given set of inputs, the outputs provided by the model should be the same as those of the system itself, to within a specified degree of tolerance.

In validating the model of Baker Hospital radiology department, a two-week period of time (fourteen days) was simulated. The length of the simulation run was determined by consideration of the cost of computer time and the rate at which the system reached steady state.[14] The cost of a two-week run of all three model segments is approximately $60.00, as opposed to $40.00 for a one-week run. As indicated previously under "Model Development," however, cost savings result from the model segmentation, which requires that additional runs be made only for those segments where decision variable inputs have been changed.

All three model segments were run for a simulated period of two weeks, with interim output being obtained after one week. For all of the patient arrival streams, and almost all of the endogenous (output) variables, there were no significant differences in mean values, and close agreement was observed in the frequency distributions, for a one-week run versus a two-week run. Also, the sample standard deviation decreased by ten percent or less for the two-week run compared to the one-week run. In view of this, it was felt that additional replications beyond two weeks would not produce improvement in the estimate of steady state conditions sufficient to justify

**FIGURE III.5.3**
Sample time stamp card

| | | | | |
|---|---|---|---|---|
| 16 | DAY NO. 65 | 1 | 11.06 Jun5 | Requisition Arrival |
| 15 | PATIENT TYPE: IN | 2 | 11.35 Jun5 | Patient Arrival |
| 14 | | 3 | 11.55 M | Exam Started |
| 13 | EXAM NOS.: 101 | 4 | 11.62 M | Exam Finished |
| 12 | Female Age 23 | 5 | 11.71 Jun5 | Film Processing Finished |
| 11 | NURSING UNIT: OB | 6 | 16.36 Jun5 | Typing Started |
| 10 | | 7 | 16.62 Jun5 | Typing Finished |
| 9 | STRETCHER PAT.? wheel ch. | 8 | 7.36 Jun6 | Report Dispatched |

the computer cost. Further, in view of the consistent values of the output variables for the one- and two-week runs, it was decided that the experiments in the following pages could be conducted using a one-week run, with confidence that the results represented steady state performance.

The validation process consisted of comparing values of output variables for the study data to those of the model, for each segment of the model. Statistical tests were run to detect differences in mean values, and frequency distributions were compared for those variables where a marked departure from the actual distribution could effect or indicate a major anomaly in model operation (daily variation in examination demand and patient waiting time for example). Comparisons of study data to model output indicated no significant differences for any output variable. The detailed results of this analysis are discussed in Perry, Baum, and Warner.[15]

## Experimental Approach: Problem Decomposition

A computer simulation model by itself is a descriptive tool which accepts a set of inputs, including decision variables, and produces outputs, including measures of performance, for the system being modeled. Such a model is used here to provide values for the terms of objective function and constraints formulated previously. The approach to seeking an optimum value for the objective function is experimentation with the simulation model, which requires the use of an appropriate search technique. For the model developed here, the search process would be greatly simplified, and reduced in cost, if each of the latter two major model segments could be searched independently of the other. The following paragraphs divide the problem into two stages, one involving only model segment 2, and one involving only model segment 3. This approach is then used in conducting the experiments described later under "Analysis of a Planning Decision."

The matrix of figure III.5.4 indicates the impact of decision variables on exogenous (output) variables, given that the constraint requiring all demand to be met is satisfied. An asterisk in element (i,j) indicates that decision variable i affects output variable j. It may be observed that decision variables of model segment 3 affect only output variables of segment 3, while decision variables of model segment 2 affect output variables of model segments 2 and 3. If decision variables of segment 2 can be shown to primarily affect only output variables for model segment 2, with little or no effect on segment 3, then the two segments may then be treated separately, to determine the optimum solution. This was the case, as described in the following paragraphs.

The patient schedule, $v_1$, a decision variable of segment 2, can have an affect on late reports ($l_1$, $l_2$), a segment 3 output variable, (for instance,

**FIGURE III.5.4**
Decision variable/output variable matrix

| DECISION VARIABLES | | OUTPUT VARIABLES: MODEL SEGMENT 2 | | | | | | MODEL SEGMENT 3 | | | | |
|---|---|---|---|---|---|---|---|---|---|---|---|---|
| | | $u_2$ = examining room utilization | $u_3$ = technologist utilization | $u_4$ = radiologist utilization, performing exams | $w_1$ = average patient wait, general exams | $w_2$ = average patient wait, prep exams | f = time of last fluoro start | $u_{4a}$=radiologist utilization, reading film | $u_5$=typist utilization | $u_6$=clerk utilization | $l_1$=fraction late inpatient reports | $l_2$=fraction late outpatient reports |
| SEGMENT 2 | $v_1$=patient schedule | | | | * | * | * | | | | * | * |
| | $v_2$=examining rooms | * | | | * | * | * | | | | * | * |
| | $v_3$=technologist hours | | * | | * | * | * | | | | * | * |
| | $v_4$=radiologist hours | | | * | * | * | * | * | | | * | * |
| SEGMENT 3 | $v_5$=typist hours | | | | | | | | * | | * | * |
| | $v_6$=clerk hours | | | | | | | | | * | * | * |
| | $v_7$=interprocess batch sizes | | | | | | | | | | * | * |
| | $v_8$=film reading priority system | | | | | | | | | | * | * |
| | $v_9$=technological improvements in report generation process | | | | | | | * | * | * | * | * |

scheduling all inpatient examinations at the end of the day). However, most hospitals, including Baker Hopsital, have established a policy to examine inpatients as soon as possible after the requisition is received (in the case of examinations requiring patient fasting this may be the following day). Moreover, examination times of other schedulable patients are determined so that waiting time is of reasonable length. Hence the impact of this decision variable ($v_1$) on model segment 3 is inconsequential. That is, $v_1$ may be varied only to satisfy constraints of model segment 2, without having any great impact on model segment 3. This allows the deletion of the asterisks in elements ($v_1$, $l_1$) and ($v_1$, $l_2$) of figure III.5.4.

The number of examining rooms and the technologist staffing pattern, $v_2$ and $v_3$, are decision variables of segment 2 which affect the number of late diagnostic reports ($l_1$,$l_2$). In order to effect a small reduction in late reports, however, an extremely large reduction in patient waiting time would be necessary to materially alter the flow of films in segment 2, and this would be obtained at great expense (for example, by adding at least one half-time technician or radiologist). This insensitivity to changes in waiting time is due to the batching that takes place in the steps subsequent to film processing. Report delay is much more responsive to small changes in the decision variables of segment 3 (such as interprocess batch size, $v_7$, or the film reading priority system, $v_8$). Therefore, $v_2$ and $v_3$ were varied only to meet the constraints of segment 2, where such manipulation is cost-effective. Thus the asterisks in the four elements at the intersections of rows $v_2$ and $v_3$ with columns $l_1$ and $l_2$ may now be deleted.

For the purpose of this model the radiologist performs two tasks: patient examination for certain examinations, and film interpretation. Sufficient radiologist hours must be provided in model segment 2 to meet the constraints on output variables of segment 2. Moreover, if these hours are not sufficient to meet constraints on output variables of segment 3 (specifically $u_{4a}$,$l_1$,$l_2$), additional radiologist hours must be added. However, these hours will not affect examination performance since this additional time is not related to model segment 2 (the examinations having already been completed). Therefore, radiologist hours ($v_4$) can be divided into two variables, $v_4$ and $v_{4a}$, where $v_4$ is the number of radiologists allocated in segment 2 for patient examination, and $v_{4a}$ in segment 3 is the number of radiologists' hours needed for film reading. This permits the deletion of the asterisks in elements ($v_4$,$u_{4a}$), ($v_4$,$l_1$) and ($v_4$,$l_2$). The revised decision variable/output variable matrix is shown in figure III.5.5.

In view of the above arguments, one objective function and constraint set may be written for each of model segments 2 and 3, where the variables, parameters, and functions are defined in figure III.5.6, and an explanation of the formulation is contained in the paragraphs immediately thereafter.

**Model Segment 2 (Patient Scheduling and Examination)**

**minimize:** $\sum_{i=1}^{4} C_i v_i$, where: $C_i$ is a row vector, and $v_i$ is a column vector

**subject to:**
- $u_i = h_i(v_i) \leq U_i,\ i = 2,3$
- $w_k = g_k(v_1,v_2,v_3,v_4) \leq W_k,\ k = 1,2$
- $f = e(v_1,v_2,v_3,v_4) \leq F$
- each element of $v_2$, integer
- each element of $v_3$, $v_4$, multiples of ½ day equivalents
- each element of $v_i = 0,1$; and only one element equals 1

**Model Segment 3 (Diagnostic Report Generation)**

**minimize:** $\sum_{i=4a}^{9} C_i v_i$, where: $C_i$ is a row vector, and $v_i$ is a column vector

**subject to:**
- $u_i = h_i(v_i,v_9) \leq U_i,\ i = 4$ and $4_a$ combined, 5,6
- $l_1 = f_1(v_{4a},v_5,v_6,v_7,v_8,v_9) \leq L_1$
- $l_2 = f_2(v_{4a},v_5,v_6,v_7,v_8,v_9) \leq L_2$
- each element of $v_9$, integer
- each element of $v_{4a},v_5,v_6$, multiples of ½ day equivalents,
- each element of $v_7,v_8 = 0,1$; and only one element equals 1

The objective functions utilize row and column vectors for the $C_i$ and $v_i$, respectively, to conveniently specify costs and hours for the same resource, which vary by shift ($v_3,v_4,v_{4a},v_5,v_6$). In the case of $v_i$, $i=1,7,8$, only one element of $C_i$ and $v_i$ equals one, the remaining elements being equal to zero, since they specify the alternative patient schedule, film priority system, and batch size policies selected respectively, and their associated costs (constraint (6) of each model segment). The cost coefficients ($C_i$) reflect additional costs incurred by the implementation of a particular policy (such as additional clerical time needed to implement a patient scheduling system). In the case of the vector $v_9$, the ith element is associated with a technological improvement which affects only the ith resource decision variable (i.e., $v_i$ for $i=4,4a,5,6$). The elements of $C_9$ are similarly defined.

The constraints on the output variables for each model segment are analogous to those of the combined model. The functions which define the output variables are specified by operating characteristics of the simulation model which, given values of the decision variables and uncontrollable variables, generate values for the output variables. The integer constraints on examining rooms, and technological improvements in the report generating process (constraint (4) of each model segment), reflect the infeasibility of adding a fraction of a piece of equipment. The constraints on personnel (constraint (5) of each model segment) reflect policies on part-time employment.

**FIGURE III.5.5**
Revised decision variable/output variable matrix

| | | OUTPUT VARIABLES | | | | | | | | | | |
|---|---|---|---|---|---|---|---|---|---|---|---|---|
| | | MODEL SEGMENT 2 | | | | | | MODEL SEGMENT 3 | | | | |
| | DECISION VARIABLES | $u_2$ = examining room utilization | $u_3$ = technologist utilization | $u_4$ = radiologist utilization, performing exams | $w_1$ = average patient wait, general exams | $w_2$ = average patient wait, prep exams | f = time of last fluoro start | $u_{4a}$=radiologist utilization, reading film | $u_5$=typist utilization | $u_6$=clerk utilization | $l_1$=fraction late inpatient reports | $l_2$=fraction late outpatient reports |
| SEGMENT 2 | $v_1$=patient schedule | | | | * | * | * | | | | | |
| | $v_2$=examining rooms | * | | | * | * | * | | | | | |
| | $v_3$=technologist hours | | * | | * | * | * | | | | | |
| | $v_4$=radiologist hours | | | * | * | * | * | | | | | |
| SEGMENT 3 | $v_{4a}$=additional radiologist hours for film interpretation | | | | | | | * | | | * | * |
| | $v_5$=typist hours | | | | | | | | * | | * | * |
| | $v_6$=clerk hours | | | | | | | | | * | * | * |
| | $v_7$=interprocess batch sizes | | | | | | | | | | * | * |
| | $v_8$=film reading priority system | | | | | | | | | | * | * |
| | $v_9$=technological improvements in report generation process | | | | | | | * | * | * | * | * |

**FIGURE III.5.6**
Model variables, parameters, and functions

Decision variables ($v_i$ are column vectors):

$v_1$ = patient schedule (integer variable),
$v_2$ = number of examination rooms, by room type (integer variable),
$v_3$ = technologist hours per day, by shift,
$v_4$ = radiologist hours per day (for performing examinations),
$v_{4a}$ = additional radiologist hours per day (for interpreting films),
$v_5$ = typist hours per day, by shift,
$v_6$ = clerk hours per day, by shift,
$v_7$ = batch size policy for interprocess accumulation (integer variable),
$v_8$ = priority system for film reading by the radiologist (integer variable),
$v_9$ = technological improvements in report generation (e.g., automated film viewing devices, automatic typewriters), (integer variable).

Output variables:

$u_i$ = average utilization of resources; i = 2, 3, 4, 4a, 5, 6; i is defined as indicated above for decision variables,

$w_k$ = average patient waiting time; k = 1 denotes routine examinations, k = 2 denotes examinations requiring patient preparation (preparation examinations),

$\ell_j$ = average fraction of diagnostic reports produced for patient type j requisitions which fail to meet the service measure deadlines; j = 1 denotes inpatients, j = 2 denotes outpatients,

f = average starting time of the last fluoroscopic examination of the day.

Parameters and policy variables:

$C_i$ = cost per hour of resource i, by shift, or cost per day, i = 2, 3, 4, 4a, 5, 6, 9; cost of implementing the policy associated with $v_i$, i = 1, 7, 8; i is defined as above ($C_i$ are row vectors),

$W_k$ = maximum allowable average patient wait; k = 1 denotes routine examinations, k = 2 denotes preparation examinations,

$U_i$ = maximum allowable average utilization of resources for a given shift; i = 2, 3, 4, 4a, 5, 6; i is defined as above,

F = maximum allowable average start time for the last fluoroscopic examination of the day,

$L_j$ = maximum allowable average fraction of diagnostic reports produced for patient type j requisitions permitted to fail the service measure deadlines; j = 1 denotes inpatients, j = 2 denotes outpatients.

Functions:

$h_i(v_i)$ = operating characteristics of the model which determine $u_i$; i = 2, 3, 4, 4a, 5, 6; i is defined as above,

$g_k(v_1,v_2,v_3,v_4)$ = operating characteristics of the model which determine $w_k$; k = 1 denotes routine examinations, k = 2 denotes preparation examinations,

$e(v_1,v_2,v_3,v_4)$ = operating characteristics of the model which determine f,

$f_j(v_{4a},v_5,v_6,v_7,v_8,v_9)$ = operating characteristics of the model which determine $l_j$; j = 1 denotes inpatients, j = 2 denotes outpatients.

## Optimizing the Objective Function

Two common search techniques used in determining the optimum solution through experimentation with a simulation model are: (1) a predetermined experimental design, and (2) a predetermined search pattern.[16] These approaches may be very costly in higher dimensional problems when the sensitivity of the objective function to changes in decision variables is not known, and when each run in the experimental design or search pattern is relatively expensive in computer time. This is the case for the model of this paper, as was discussed previously. A third approach which greatly reduces the impact of these problems is a sequential search in which the values of the decision variables for each run are determined by the results of the previous run. A number of formal techniques, sometimes called optimum seeking methods or response surface techniques, have been developed.[17] The optimum seeking technique used here is a variant of the so-called "one-at-a-time" method. Briefly, resources are added sequentially, maintaining minimum cost, and the process is terminated when all of the constraints are satisfied. The procedure is described in detail in the following paragraphs, and applied to model segments 2 and 3 in following pages under the heading "Analysis of a Planning Decision."

We begin by listing all reasonable combinations of values of decision variables in order of increasing cost. For model segment 2, the unit cost of decision variables may be ranked from the most expensive to the least expensive as follows: radiologist hours, examining rooms, technologist hours, and patient schedules. For each decision variable there is a range of values from a minimum cost value to a maximum cost value. Minimum values are those necessary for the department to perform its function (one examining room, one technologist, etc.), or those which cannot be reduced (the number of existing examining rooms or radiologists under contract), and maximum values are those for which it is certain that all constraints will be met. The desired rank-ordered list for model segment 2 is represented by the tree diagram of figure III.5.7. For model segment 3, the unit cost of decision variables may be ranked from the most expensive to the least expensive as follows: radiologist hours, typist hours, clerk hours, automated film viewing device, and film priority system and interprocess batch sizes. The rank-ordered list could be represented by a tree similar to that of figure III.5.7.

The optimum seeking technique now proceeds as indicated in the flow chart of figure III.5.8. In blocks (1) through (14) we employ a "forward search" to find an initial feasible solution with "low" cost, and in blocks (15) to (23) we employ a "backward search" to refine the initial feasible solution to obtain an optimal solution. Let us first consider the forward search.

**FIGURE III.5.7**
Rank-ordered list of decision variable combinations

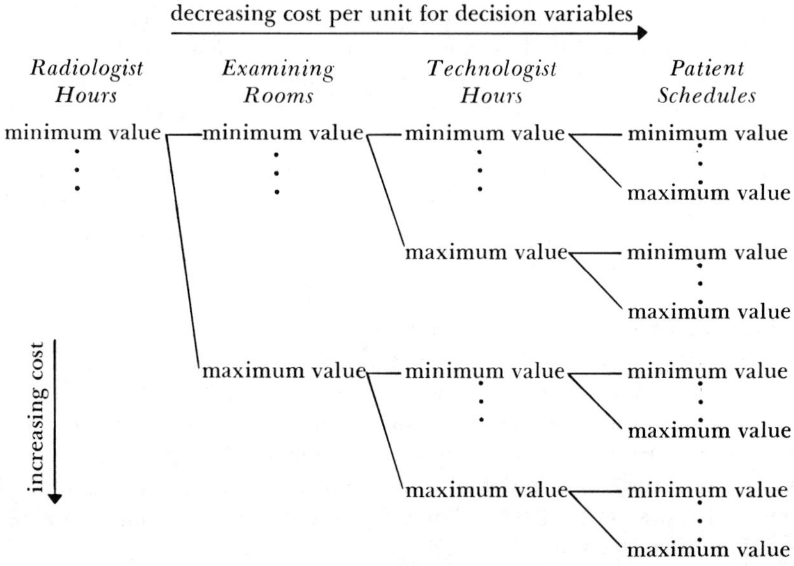


In blocks (1) through (4), values of the resource decision variables, and their associated technological improvement decision variables, are found which just satisfy the resource utilization constraints (constraint (1) of model segments 2 and 3).[18] In block (1), the resource decision variables for which we lack any previous operating experience (or prior model output) are set at their minimum values. For certain resource decision variables, however, data on current operations or prior model output may indicate that minimum values are not sufficient. Any information from these sources is used to reduce the number of runs required, by setting these variables at levels determined by operating experience or model output. The remaining decision variables (those relating to operating policies) are set at their minimum values. The model is then run in block (2), and in block (3) it is determined if all the resource utilization constraints are satisfied. If all of these constraints are not satisfied, we proceed to block (4) and select the next largest value in the rank-ordered list for each resource decision variable (or its associated technological improvement decision variable) in an unsatisfied constraint. The rationale for the action taken in block (4) is explained in the following paragraph.

In every resource constraint, each resource decision variable, or its associated technological improvement decision variable, but not both, is advanced to its next value in the rank-ordered list for a given run (as op-

**FIGURE III.5.8**
Optimum seeking procedure

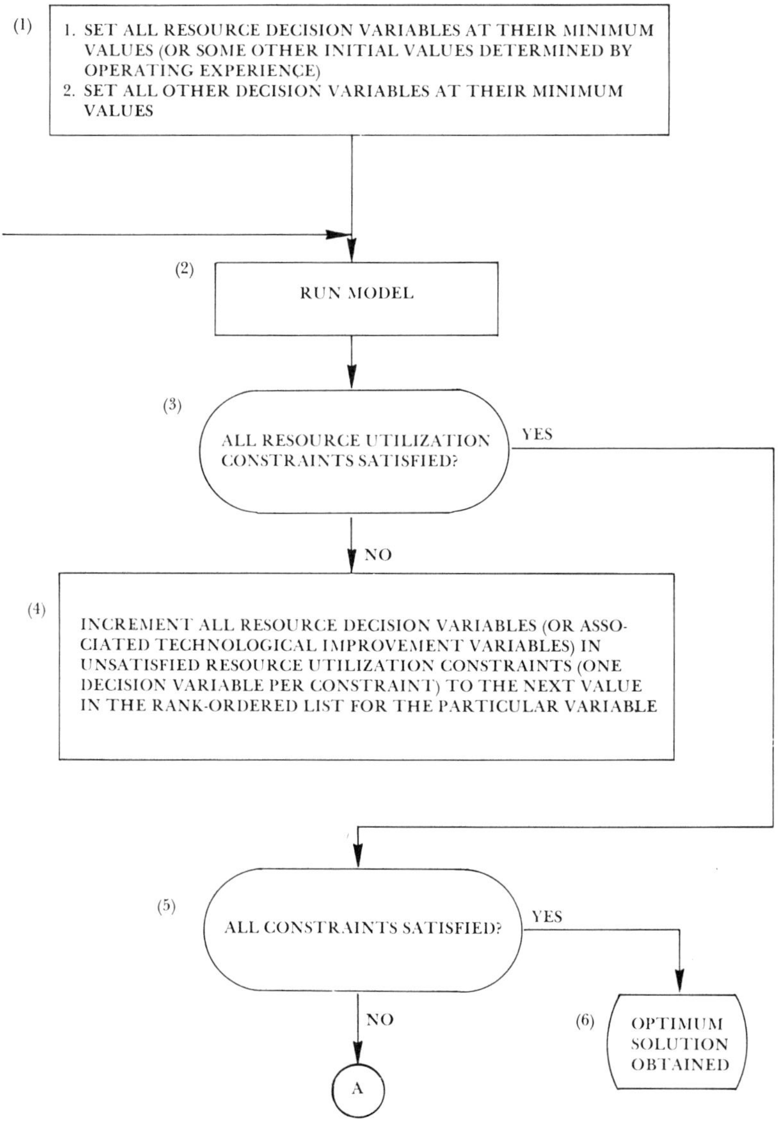

**FIGURE III.5.8 Cont.**

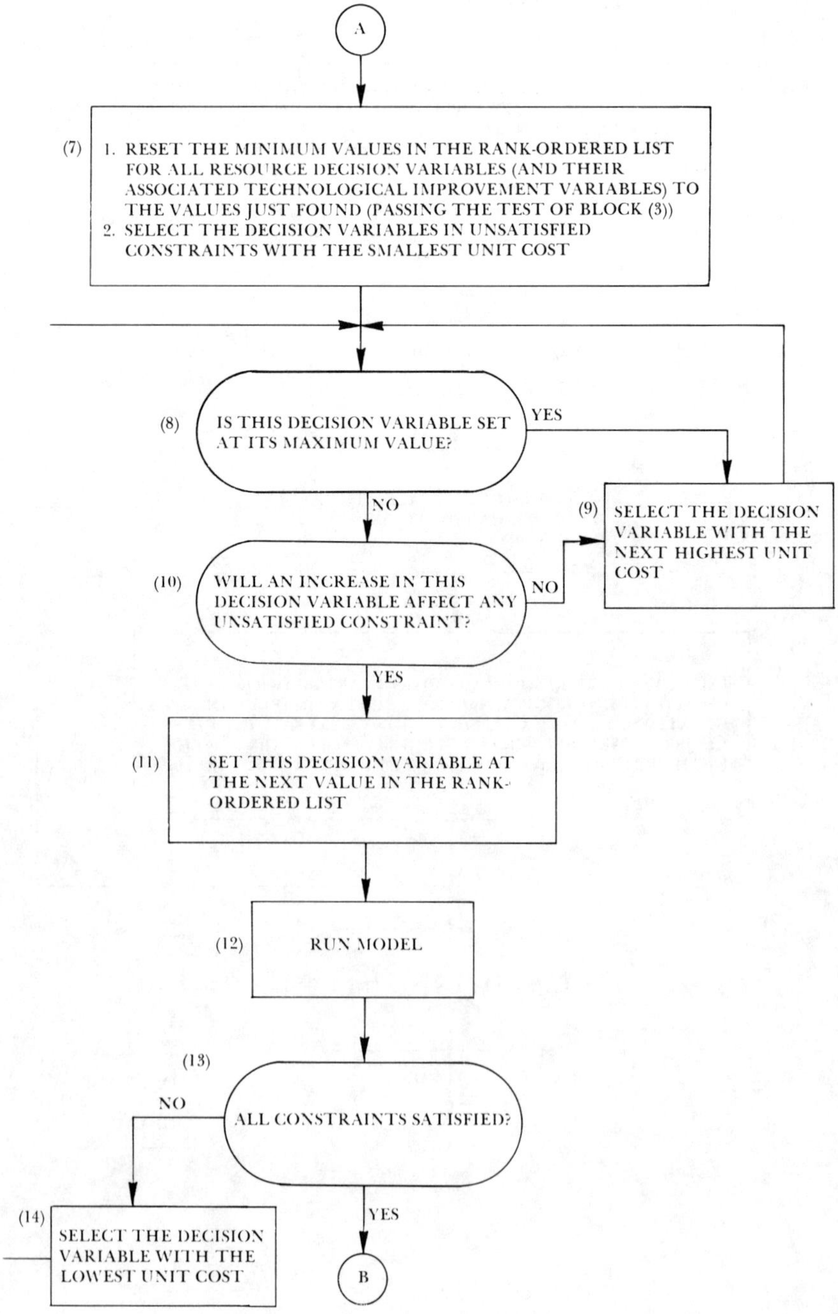

**FIGURE III.5.8 Cont.**

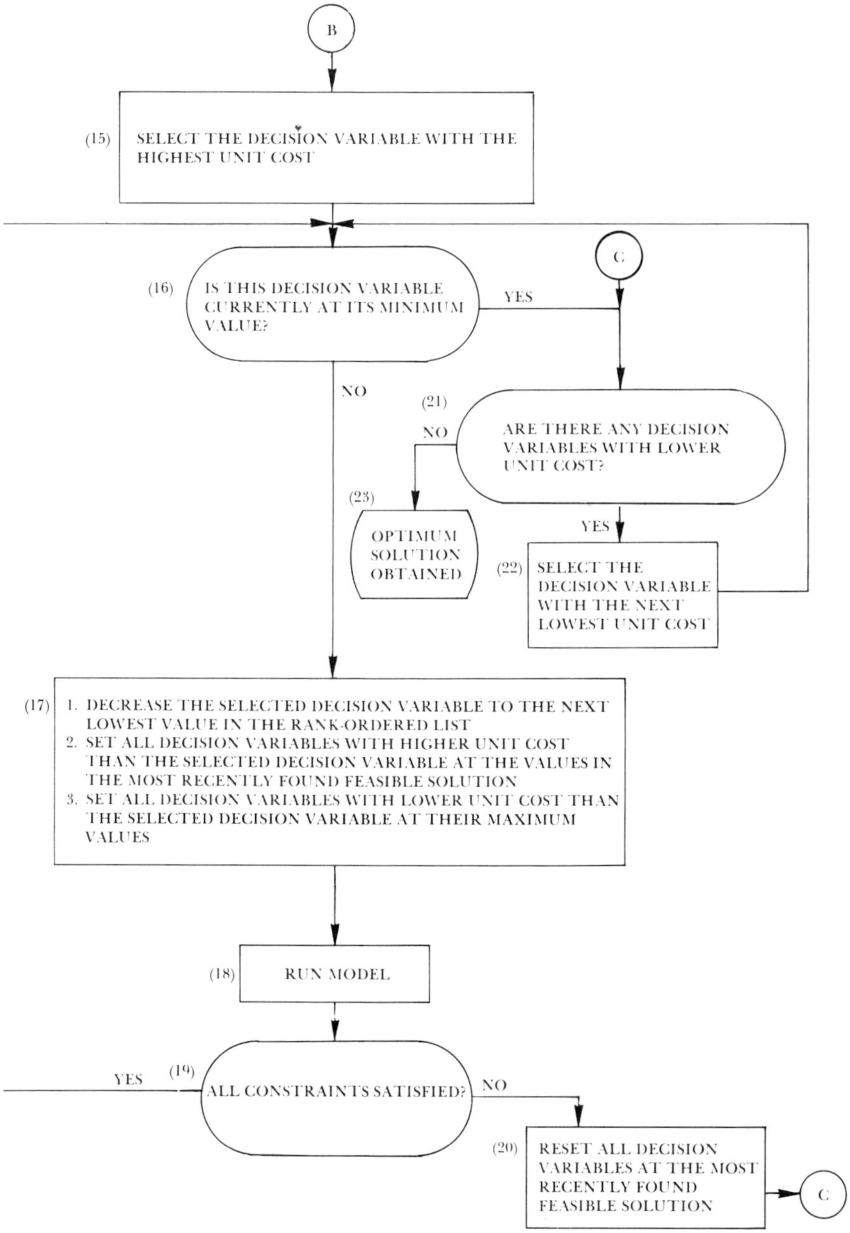

posed to advancing the decision variables one at a time). However, we never vary more than one decision variable in any one constraint. If we did, it would be difficult to assess the individual impact of each decision variable on the constraint. For example, the resource utilization constraints of model segment 2 each involve only the one resource decision variable. The resource utilization constraints of model segment 3 each involve a resource decision variable, and an associated technological improvement decision variable (an automated viewing device for radiologists). Both of these decision variables are means of adding resource hours, but at different costs. However, either one or the other (but not both) is altered for a given run.

Proceed as described above (moving sequentially through blocks (2), (3), and (4)) until all of the resource utilization constraints are satisfied, as determined in block (3). In block (5) we determine if the remaining constraints are satisfied. If all of the constraints of the model are satisfied using the set of decision variable values thus found, the solution is optimal, and the algorithm stops at block (6).

If all the constraints are not satisfied, proceed to block (7) and reset the minimum values of all resource decision variables (and their associated technological improvement variables) in the rank-ordered list to the values just obtained which satisfy the utilization constraints (as tested in block (3)); also select the decision variable in the unsatisfied constraints with the smallest unit cost. In block (10) it is determined if an increase in this decision variable will aid in satisfying the unsatisfied constraints. If a change in this decision variable will aid in meeting any unsatisfied constraint (as determined from knowledge of the actual department operating characteristics, and previous model runs), and if the variable is not already set at its maximum vlaue (which is tested in block (8)), then proceed to block (11) and set the decision variable to the next value in the rank-ordered list of figure III.5.7. The model is then run in block (12), and the satisfaction of all constraints is tested in block (13). If any constraint is still unsatisfied, proceed to block (14), where the decision variable with the lowest unit cost is selected. This permits a reassessment, at each new level of decision variable settings, of the impact of all decision variables on the unsatisfied constraints (as tested in block (10)). Return to block (8) and continue altering decision variables, one at a time, until all constraints are satisfied. Note that if either of the conditions in blocks (8) or (10) is met (that is, the unsatisfied constraints will not be aided by this variable, or the variable is already set at its maximum value), proceed to block (9), select the decision variable with the next highest unit cost, and return to block (8) and proceed as described above.

When an initial solution is found which satisfies all the constraints (as tested in block (13)), a backward search of the tree diagram of figure

III.5.7 is conducted to determine if substitutable properties of the decision variables will permit a reduction in the value of the objective function, while maintaining feasibility (blocks (15) through (23)). The search is begun with the current set of decision variable values, which are decreased one at a time, beginning with the decision variable with the highest unit cost. This procedure is continued until changes in the decision variable with the lowest unit cost have been explored. The set of decision variable values thus found, which satisfies all the constraints, then determines the optimal value of the objective function.

Specifically, the decision variable with the highest unit cost is selected in block (15), and if it is not at its minimum value (as determined in block (16)), then it is decreased in block (17) to its next lowest value in the rank-ordered list. Also in block (17), the decision variables with higher unit costs (than the selected decision variable) are set at the values in the most recent feasible solution. Those decision variables with lower unit costs (than the selected decision variable) are set at their maximum values. The model is then run in block (18) and the satisfaction of all constraints is tested in block (19). If all constraints are still satisfied, then an attempt is made to reduce the current decision variable (the decision variable just reduced) by another increment by going to block (16) again.

Alternatively, if block (19) determines that feasibility was lost by the reduction of the current decision variable, reset the decision variables to their previous values in block (20) (so that feasibility is attained). Then, in block (21), it is determined if any decision variable, with lower unit cost than the one previously considered (and decreased in block (16)) exists. If there are none, then all possible feasible decision variable reductions have been tested, and hence we are at an optimal solution in block (23). If there are decision variables with lower unit costs than the one previously considered, pass to block (22) and determine the decision variable whose unit cost is the next lowest, as compared to the unit cost of the previous decision variable. Then, attempt to reduce this variable by again going to block (16). Again, this procedure will terminate in a finite number of steps and will have implicitly examined the feasible reduction of all the decision variables of the initial feasible solution determined in block (13). Thus, the resulting decision variable values provide a least-cost feasible solution, that is, an optimal solution.

The procedure described above is not as lengthy as it might seem. For the forward search, all branches of the tree of figure III.5.7 need not be explored in obtaining an initial feasible solution. Some branches are excluded due to the lower bound placed on resource decision variables by constraints on utilization. Some branches will be known a priori, from previous model runs, to be ineffective in meeting certain constraints. For example, if the average starting time of the last fluoroscopic examination of the day is to be decreased, and the fluoroscopic rooms are utilized to near capacity during the period when these examinations are conducted, it would be ineffective to increase technologist hours, even though they are less expensive than additional examining rooms.

For the backward search, it turned out that it was not necessary to explicitly use it in the model segment 2 optimization procedure for any of the years in the planning horizon, due to the following reasons. Both radiologist hours and the number of examination rooms were in the initial feasible solution at their minimum values, and therefore could not be reduced. Technologist hours were set at a minimum operating level as part of the forward search, and patient waiting time constraints were violated; hence the technologist hours could not be reduced. Finally, the patient scheduling policy could have been eliminated, but the cost reduction is minimal, and the validation run for the model indicated that it is likely that a waiting time constraint would be violated.

Similarly, the backward search of the optimum seeking procedure was not required for model segment 3 either, for the following reasons. Radiologist hours, typist hours, and clerk hours were in the initial feasible solution at their minimum values, and therefore could not be reduced. The automated viewing device could have been eliminated. However, this device was added during the forward search, as an alternative to the more expensive radiologist hours, to satisfy the radiologist utilization constraint. Hence its deletion would cause the solution to have a higher cost (since radiologists are more "expensive" than automated viewing devices). Finally, the film priority and batching policies could have been replaced by the original policies, while retaining the automated viewing device. However the fraction of late reports was found to be so sensitive to changes in these policies that the late report constraint would surely have been violated, and also, the cost savings accruing would be minimal.

## Analysis of a Planning Decision

Although the model developed is capable of addressing a wide variety of scheduling and resource allocation problems, the decision selected for analysis is based on the particular circumstances of the radiology department in the demonstration hospital. The hospital had just finished building a new outpatient facility and had expanded the radiology department. Because of construction economies, all six of the new examining rooms were built at one time, but they did not need to be equipped at once. The planning decision studied concerns the timing of equipment and personnel additions to meet an increasing demand over a planning horizon without having undue excess capacity in either category.

The planning horizon was taken as five years. A forecast for each patient type over this period was generated using linear regression analysis, and adjusting for seasonality with the "ratio-to-trend" method. The seasonally high month of October was selected for model input in order to provide conservative indications of department performance. Table III.5.1 shows the average weekly forecasts for the planning horizon by patient type.

Due to the growing concern about malpractice suits, many physicians are utilizing more laboratory tests and x-ray procedures in arriving at a diagnosis. In incorporating the impact of this phenomenon into the radiology model, both the number of patients receiving the x-ray examinations and the number of multiple x-ray procedures performed could potentially increase. The former effect would be reflected in the forecast of patient volume, while the later would alter the mix of procedures performed. In order to accurately include these effects in the model, it would first be necessary to ascertain the extent to which the number of x-ray procedures is being inflated. This could be accomplished by a carefully designed survey of physician practices.

Segment 1 of the model uses these forecasts to generate patients to be processed. Then, using the optimum seeking method described in the previous section and the generated patients, the minimum cost solution to the objective functions for model segments 2 and 3 which satisfies all the constraints, is determined for each year in the planning horizon. These results determine the acquisition plan for equipment and personnel. This plan will have minimum total cost over the planning horizon, as measured by the present value method, unless multiple purchases of machines provide discounts, or inflation causes price increases, sufficient to justify earlier equipment purchase. This contingency may be evaluated by computing present values for all acquistion plans where equipment is added sooner than the model indicates is necessary, and comparing them to the present value of the model-determined plan.

The constraint values used in the experiments appear in figure III.5.9. Patient waiting time and room utilization constraints are based on

**TABLE III.5.1**
Weekly x-ray patient forecast 1974–1978

| | YEAR | | | | |
|---|---|---|---|---|---|
| *Patient Type* | *1974* | *1975* | *1976* | *1977* | *1978* |
| Inpatient | 393 | 403 | 413 | 422 | 432 |
| Outpatient | 194 | 206 | 218 | 230 | 242 |
| Emergency Room | 276 | 293 | 310 | 327 | 344 |
| Total Patients | 863 | 902 | 941 | 979 | 1,018 |

**FIGURE III.5.9**
Constraint values used in the model

MODEL SEGMENT 2:

$W_1$ = maximum allowable average patient wait; general examinations = 25 minutes
$W_2$ = maximum allowable average patient wait; prep examinations = 30 minutes
$U_2$ = maximum allowable average utilization; examining rooms = 65 percent
$U_3$ = maximum allowable average utilization; technologists = 88 percent
F = maximum allowable average start time for last fluoroscopic examination of the day = 11:45 A.M.

MODEL SEGMENT 3:

$U_{4,4a}$ = maximum allowable average utilization of radiologist hours for examination performance and film interpretation = 80 percent
$U_5$ = maximum allowable average utilization; typists = 88 percent
$U_6$ = maximum allowable average utilization; clerks = 88 percent
$L_1$ = maximum allowable average fraction of reports produced for inpatient requisitions permitted to fail the service criterion deadlines = 10 percent
$L_2$ = maximum allowable average fraction of reports produced for outpatient requisitions permitted to fail the service criterion deadlines = 40 percent

recommendations in Nuffield, *Towards a Clearer View.*[19] Constraints on utilization of technologists, typists and clerks, are based on values suggested by Barnes for these jobs or similar ones.[20] It should be noted that the upper limits set for utilization of examining rooms and the three personnel categories are about one and one-half to two times those typically observed in studies.[21] The value for the latest starting time of the last fluoroscopic examination of the day is prompted by a desire to have the patient back in his room as close to the normal meal times as possible. A study by Drui suggested values for the constraint on radiologist hours.[22] The constraints on the late diagnostic reports were deemed reasonable initial goals for the department in light of present performance (reports dispatched by the end of the day for sixty-five percent of the requests received by 12:00 noon, and by 10:00 A.M. of the following day for fifty percent of the requests received after noon).

The results of runs of model segment 2, including the validation run, are summarized in table III.5.2. Based on experience with the model during the validation process, each run was of one week in length. This also was the case for segment 3 runs. Following the procedure for optimizing the objective function previously described, the decision variables specifying the number of examination rooms and personnel staffing for run 1 were set at values which appear to just satisfy utilization constraints.

Patient scheduling for outpatients was also included in this intial run, since it is assumed to add minimal operating cost to the objective function. It should be noted, however, that some administrative costs will be incurred in initiating such a system. The patient schedule used was one which was thought to have a reasonably good chance of implementation, and therefore it demands little of patients or referring physicians. Specifically, outpatients requiring prep examinations arrive randomly between the hours of 8:30 A.M. and 10:00 A.M., instead of between 7:30 A.M. and 10:00 A.M., as is the current practice. Examinations for these patients commence at 9:00 A.M. Outpatients requiring general examinations arrive randomly between the hours of 1:00 P.M. and 6:00 P.M., instead of between 7:30 A.M. and 6:00 P.M., as is the current practice.

For run 1, technologist staffing is set at three for the first half of the day shift and one for the balance of the shift. The results indicate that a single technologist during the second half of the day shift is not sufficient to keep waiting time within its constraint.[23] Therefore, a half-time technologist was added to this shift in run 2, to provide two technologists during the afternoon hours when all the outpatients requiring general examinations arrive. During the years 1975, 1976, and 1977 the decision variable settings of run 2 provide acceptable values for all of the output variables. In 1978 (run 6) the average starting time for the last fluoroscopic examination was statistically different from its constraint value. Since the existing fluoroscopic rooms are devoted exclusively to this type of examination during the fluoroscopic period, and since they were already heavily utilized, it was necessary to add a fourth room to satisfy the constraint. This was done in run 7.

For all of the runs, technologist utilization is much greater than examination room utilization. This is so for two reasons. First, technologists perform tasks between examinations, such as fetching patients from the dressing rooms or waiting room and delivering processed film to the darkroom. The time required to accomplish these tasks is included in their utilization measure, while the room utilization measure includes only the time during which the examination is being performed. Second, the current configuration of three rooms cannot be reduced because a room is needed to perform general examinations in the morning, when the other two rooms are totally dedicated to fluoroscopic examinations.

The model segment 3 run results are summarized in table III.5.3. For run 1, 1974, the trial values of the decision variables used to just satisfy the utilization constraints were the values in use during the data collection study period. This choice was based on the results of the validation run, which indicated that any reduction would lead to constraint violations. Also, the film priority system and interprocess batch sizes were changed as follows, since it is assumed that these changes can be effected with essen-

**TABLE III.5.2**

Summary of the runs for model segment 2

| Run | Year | Decision variables | | | | | | | | Output variables[c] | | | | |
|---|---|---|---|---|---|---|---|---|---|---|---|---|---|---|
| | | Patient schedule ($v_1$) | Number of exam rooms ($v_2$)[a] | Personnel by shift[b] (Monday-Friday) | | | | | | Average patient waiting time (minutes) | | Average resource utilization--day shift (%) | | Average starting time of last fluoroscopic exam of the day (f) |
| | | | | Technologists ($v_3$) | | | Radiologists ($v_4$) | | | | | | | |
| | | | | Day | Evening | Night | Day | Evening | Night | Routine exams ($w_1$) (25) | Prep exams ($w_2$) (30) | Exam rooms ($u_2$) (65) | Technologists ($u_3$) (88) | (11:45 AM) |
| Validation | 1972 | No patient scheduling | 3 | 3 | 2 | 1 | 1.5 | - | - | 11 | 32 | 30 | 49 | 11:15 AM |
| 1 | 1974 | Outpatients scheduled | 3 | 2 | 1 | 1 | 1.5 | - | - | 55*c | 34 | 31[d] | 68[d] | 11:15 AM |
| 2 | 1974 | Outpatients scheduled | 3 | 2.5 | 1 | 1 | 1.5 | - | - | 20 | 28 | 33[d] | 63[d] | 11:23 AM |
| 3 | 1975 | Outpatients scheduled | 3 | 2.5 | 1 | 1 | 1.5 | - | - | 19 | 28 | 34 | 57 | 11:26 AM |
| 4 | 1976 | Outpatients scheduled | 3 | 2.5 | 1 | 1 | 1.5 | - | - | 20 | 29 | 34 | 67 | 11:43 AM |
| 5 | 1977 | Outpatients scheduled | 3 | 2.5 | 1 | 1 | 1.5 | - | - | 20 | 30 | 36 | 71 | 12:03 PM |
| 6 | 1978 | Outpatients scheduled | 3 | 2.5 | 1 | 1 | 1.5 | - | - | 24 | 27 | 36 | 73 | 12:23 PM* |
| 7 | 1978 | Outpatients scheduled | 4 | 3 | 1 | 1 | 1.5 | - | - | 24 | 23 | 28 | 60 | 11:37 AM |

[a] Two of the three examination rooms, and three of the four rooms can perform fluoroscopic examinations.

[b] Part-time technologists and radiologists are on the first half of the day shift.

[c] Maximum allowable values appear in parentheses at the head of each column. An asterisk beside an output variable entry indicates that the value of this variable is significantly greater than the upper limit at the 0.05 level or lower.

[d] Lower utilizations occur for the same demands in run 1 versus run 2 because fewer patients are examined on the evening shift for run 2.

**TABLE III.5.3**
Summary of the runs for model segment 3

| Run | Year | Decision variables[a]: Personnel by shift[b] (Monday-Friday): Typists ($v_5$): Day | Typists ($v_5$): Evening | Typists ($v_5$): Night | Clerks ($v_6$): Day | Clerks ($v_6$): Evening | Clerks ($v_6$): Night | Techno-logical improve-ments ($v_9$) | Output variables[d]: Per cent of reports[e] which are late: Inpatient ($\ell_1$): AM deadline (10) | Inpatient ($\ell_1$): PM deadline (10) | Outpatient ($\ell_2$): AM deadline (40) | Outpatient ($\ell_2$): PM deadline (40) | Average resource utilization--day shift (%): Radiologists ($u_4+u_{4a}$) (80) | Typists ($u_5$) (88) | Clerks[g] ($u_6$) (88) |
|---|---|---|---|---|---|---|---|---|---|---|---|---|---|---|---|
| Validation | 1972 | 2 | - | - | 1 | - | - | | 34*d | 53*d | 32*d | 82*d | 75 | 37 | 21 |
| 1 | 1974 | 2 | - | - | 1 | - | - | | 0 | 14 | 0 | 33 | 81 | 47 | 31 |
| 2 | 1975 | 2 | - | - | 1 | - | - | Automated film viewing device | 0 | 12 | 0 | 25 | 64 | 48 | 34 |
| 3 | 1976 | 2 | - | - | 1 | - | - | Automated film viewing device | 0 | 13[f] | 0 | 18[g] | 65 | 51 | 33 |
| 4 | 1977 | 2 | - | - | 1 | - | - | Automated film viewing device | 0 | 10 | 0 | 16 | 66 | 52 | 34 |
| 5 | 1978 | 2[c] | - | - | 1 | - | - | Automated film viewing device | 0 | 11 | 0 | 38 | 70 | 53 | 32 |

[a] Reduced interprocess batch sizes ($v_7$), and inpatient-first film reading priority system ($v_8$) used for all runs beginning with run 1 in 1974.

[b] No additional radiologist hours ($v_{4a}$) were required for any of the runs.

[c] An average of 20 minutes per day of typist overtime is required for this run.

[d] Maximum allowable values appear in parentheses at the head of each column. An asterisk beside an output variable entry indicates that the value of this variable is significantly greater than the upper limit at the 0.05 level or lower.

[e] Deadlines apply only to requisitions received Monday through Friday.

[f] Closer coordination of typists finishing a batch and clerks beginning dispatch, during the hours of 7 AM to 10 AM, began in 1976.

[g] Clerks have other duties besides report dispatching, hence the low utilization.

tially no additional personnel costs being added to the objective function: (1) inpatient films were assigned priority over outpatient and emergency room patient films for interpretation by the radiologist; and (2) interprocess batch sizes were reduced between film processing and the radiologist, the radiologist and the typist, and the typist and the dispatching clerk. The details of these changes are discussed in the following paragraph.

The film priority system is implemented by separating processed films brought to the radiologist for interpretation into three groups: inpatients, outpatients, and emergency room patients. The films are then read in the above order on a first-come-first-served basis within groups. Emergency room patients are given the lowest priority, since the radiologist communicates an immediate oral report of findings, and hence the written report is for the patient record, not for diagnosis. Interprocess batch sizes are reduced by requiring processed film, dictation belts, and typed reports to be delivered to the next operation in the radiologic process at more frequent intervals.

Run 1 yields acceptable values for all of the output variables, but it is apparent that the radiologist utilization is about to exceed its constraint. A considerably less expensive alternative to more radiologist hours is an automated viewing device to allow the radiologist to work more efficiently. At least one study has shown reductions in reading time of fifty percent or more due to this device.[24] In runs 2 through 5 the use of this device was reflected by a conservative reduction in radiologist reading time of forty percent. This saving in radiologists' time requires some additional, but comparatively inexpensive, clerical time. However, there should be sufficient slack in the model-determined clerical staffing to accomplish this task. This change provided acceptable values of output variables for the years 1975 through 1977. In 1978, it was necessary to introduce some typing overtime in order to meet the constraints on late diagnostic reports.

Although hospital policy precluded the reduction of typing personnel, due to the difficulty in obtaining qualified people, the low utilization of forty-seven percent in 1974 suggests that such a reduction might still provide a feasible solution. A run using only one typist (instead of the two currently used) was made, and the utilization for typing personnel rose to seventy-six percent, but the service criterion for inpatient reports was not met. The results indicated that the second typist had the greater impact on reports for afternoon doctors. In light of this, a possible means of reducing typing staff is the following: use two typists during the hours of 7:00 A.M. to 12:00 noon to promptly process reports on examinations of the previous day for afternoon doctors, which must be dispatched by 10:00 A.M., and use one typist (with the necessary overtime) from 12:00 noon until all reports of morning doctors, which must be dispatched by the end of the current day shift, are completed. The difficulty in obtaining well-trained personnel even on a full time basis, however, may prevent the hospital from changing its policy to adopt this solution.

As indicated previously, it is desirable to know the sensitivity of the output variable, fraction of late diagnostic reports, to the decision variables which affect it. The relative sensitivity and cost of these decision variables would assist in determining the marginal cost of improving service. The results in table III.5.3 indicate that the fraction of late reports is extremely sensitive to the decision variables $v_7$ and $v_8$ (interprocess batch size and priority for film reading by the radiologist). Dramatic improvement occurred in report lateness in 1974 versus 1972, the study year, by changing only these two variables. Inpatient report lateness decreased from thirty-four to zero percent for the morning doctors and from fifty-three to fourteen percent for the afternoon doctors. These improvements occurred even though the demand increased by twelve percent.

It is doubtful that the same improvement could have been obtained using staffing changes and the old policies for $v_7$ and $v_8$. Even if it could, the cost would have greatly exceeded the minimal cost associated with the new policies for $v_7$ and $v_8$. This finding is not even considered in a speculative fashion in previous research, and yet it is seen here to be of major impact in establishing policies for radiology department operations.

The following segment summarizes the radiology department model and its application, and specifies recommendations for implementation in the study hospital.

## Summary and Recommendations

The previous sections of this chapter have described the development, validation, and experimentation for a simulation model for radiology department operations at Baker Hospital. The purpose of the model is to assist decision makers in minimizing the cost of resources (personnel, equipment, etc.) needed to meet the demand for radiologic procedures, while maintaining specified levels of service to patients and referring physicians. Service is measured in terms of delay in performing examinations and delay in making diagnostic reports available to physicians. The elements of the radiologic process included in the model are: patient scheduling and transporting; patient examination, including film processing and quality check of the x-ray; and diagnostic reporting, which includes interpretation of the film by the radiologist, typing a report, and dispatching it from the department. Information for the structure and data needed to develop the model were obtained from a data collection study in the department, available department records, and interviews with the chief radiologist and chief technologist.

The measures of performance which reflect patient service are the average waiting time in the department, and the starting time of the last fluoroscopic examination of the day. The measure which reflects service to the physicians is based on the premise that a diagnostic report should be available to a physician on the visit to the hospital immediately following the one on which the examination was requested, and that any delay beyond this increases patient care cost by potentially increasing a patient's length of stay. A study of the physicians' visiting pattern at Baker Hospital found that eighty-five percent of the doctors visit the hospital once a day, and seventy-five percent of the visits on a given day occur between the hours of 8:00 A.M., and 12:00 noon.

In light of this visiting pattern, and unavoidable delays in the report delivery and posting processes, the following criteria were developed for evaluating diagnostic report availability.[25]

*For morning doctors:* the fraction of reports produced for examination requests received by 12:00 noon which are dispatched from the department by the end of the current day shift.

*For afternoon doctors:* the fraction of reports produced for examination requests received after 12:00 noon which are dispatched from the department by 10:00 A.M. of the following day.

Adherence to the first criterion permits reports to be delivered to the nursing unit by the beginning of the evening shift, posted on patient charts during this shift, and available to physicians for their morning visits. The second criterion allows two hours (10:00 A.M. to 12:00 noon) for delivery to the unit and posting on patient charts, so that reports will be available to physicians for afternoon visits.

The radiology department expansion decision, to which the model is applied, concerns the timing of equipment and personnel additions to meet forecast demand, while maintaining a specified service level, and without having undue excess capacity. In analyzing this decision a five-year planning horizon was used. Table III.5.1 shows average weekly forecasts over the planning horizon by patient type.

Table III.5.4 summarizes the operating decisions determined by the simulation model and optimization technique. The resource allocations indicated for each year minimize the cost of resources for the year, while providing acceptable values for all measures of performance. The maximum allowable values for the measures of performance (which appear in parentheses at the head of each column), and upper limits for equipment and personnel utilization (which also appear in parentheses and were set to control equipment down time and personnel fatigue), were obtained from the literature and numerous interviews with personnel in the radiology field.[26] Acceptable values for these utilizations were achieved for each year in the planning horizon.[27]

**TABLE III.5.4**
Summary of experiments and recommendations

| YEAR | AVE.PAT./MONTH | RESOURCE ALLOCATION: NO.EXAM RMS.[1] | PERSONNEL BY SHIFT (MON-FRI): RAD.[2] DAY | RAD.[2] EVE | RAD.[2] NITE | TECH.[3] DAY | TECH.[3] EVE | TECH.[3] NITE | MED.SEC. DAY | MED.SEC. EVE | MED.SEC. NITE | CLERK DAY | CLERK EVE | CLERK NITE | MEASURES OF PERFORMANCE AND UTILIZATION[5]: PERCENT OF LATE REPORTS, DEADLINES[4]: INPAT. AM (10) | INPAT. PM (10) | OUTPAT. AM (40) | OUTPAT. PM (40) | RESOURCE UTILIZATION % DAY SHIFT: EXAM ROOMS (65) | TECH. (88) | RAD. (80) | MED.SEC. (88) | CLERK[6] (88) | AVE PAT WAIT (MIN): GEN EXAMS (25) | PREP EXAMS (30) | AVE. START LAST FLUORO. (11:45) | REMARKS |
|---|---|---|---|---|---|---|---|---|---|---|---|---|---|---|---|---|---|---|---|---|---|---|---|---|---|---|---|
| 72 | 3050 | 3 | 1.5 | - | - | 3 | 2 | 1 | 2 | - | - | 1 | - | - | 34 | 53 | 32 | 82 | 30 | 49 | 75 | 37 | 21 | 11 | 32 | 11:15 | Year of data collection for model development. |
| 74 | 3420 | 3 | 1.5 | - | - | 2.5 | 1 | 1 | 2 | - | - | 1 | - | - | 0 | 14 | 0 | 33 | 33 | 63 | 81 | 47 | 31 | 20 | 28 | 11:23 | New patient scheduling, film priority, and batch size policies begin. |
| 75 | 3580 | 3 | 1.5 | - | - | 2.5 | 1 | 1 | 2 | - | - | 1 | - | - | 0 | 12 | 0 | 25 | 34 | 67 | 64 | 48 | 34 | 19 | 28 | 11:26 | Automated viewing device added. |
| 76 | 3730 | 3 | 1.5 | - | - | 2.5 | 1 | 1 | 2 | - | - | 1 | - | - | 0 | 13 | 0 | 18 | 34 | 67 | 65 | 51 | 33 | 20 | 29 | 11:43 | |
| 77 | 3890 | 3 | 1.5 | - | - | 2.5 | 1 | 1 | 2 | - | - | 1 | - | - | 0 | 10 | 0 | 16 | 36 | 71 | 66 | 52 | 34 | 20 | 30 | 12:03 | Med. sec. overtime required. |
| 78 | 4040 | 4 | 1.5 | - | - | 3 | 1 | 1 | 2 | - | - | 1 | - | - | 0 | 11 | 0 | 38 | 28 | 60 | 70 | 53 | 32 | 24 | 23 | 11:37 | Med. sec. overtime required. |
| 78a | 4040 | 3 | 1.5 | - | - | 2.5 | 1 | 1 | 2 | - | - | 1 | - | - | 0 | 11 | 0 | 38 | 36 | 73 | 70 | 53 | 32 | 24 | 27 | 12:23 | Med. sec. overtime required, and latest start time for last fluoro relaxed. |

NOTES:
[1]Two of the three exam rooms for 72, 74-77, 78a, and three of the four rooms for 78, are capable of performing fluoroscopic exams.
[2]One part-time radiologist on first half of day shift.
[3]Part-time personnel are on the first half of the day shift; tech. assignments do not include students.
[4]These deadlines apply only to requisitions received Monday through Friday.
[5]Maximum allowable values for measures of performance and utilizations appear in parentheses for each measure of performance and utilization.
[6]Clerk has other duties besides report dispatching, which accounts for low utilization figures.

In addition to the resource allocations indicated in table III.5.4, labor saving equipment was added, and certain policies were implemented for some or all years in the planning horizon (as indicated in the "Remarks" column) to achieve acceptable values of measures of performance, and equipment and personnel utilization. First, for 1974-1978, outpatients requiring general examinations begin arriving at 1:00 P.M., rather than as walk-ins during the entire day shift; and outpatients requiring prep examinations begin arriving one half-hour before the start of the fluoroscopic period rather than one and one-half hours before the period. Second, for 1974-1978, priorities for films to be read by the radiologist were changed from a first-come-first-served basis to inpatients first, outpatients second, and emergency room patients last. (Emergency room patients are given the lowest priority because the radiologist communicates an immediate oral report of findings for these patients.) Third, for 1974-1978, the size of batches of films accumulating between film processing and the radiologist, batches of dictated reports between the radiologist and the medical secretary, and batches of typed reports between the medical secretary, and batches of typed reports between the medical secretary and the dispatching clerk, was reduced. Fourth, in 1975, an automatic viewing device was added to keep radiologist utilization below its upper limit (approximate cost: $10,000). And fifth, in 1978, it was necessary to use some medical secretary overtime to keep late diagnostic reports within their upper limits.

## Recommendations to Baker Hospital: January 1974

The recommendations, stemming from the simulation model experiments, for implementation at the study hospital are to implement the resource allocations indicated in table III.5.4 for the years 1974-1977 and 1978a, and the policies detailed in the previous paragraph. The fourth room indicated for year 1978 is not recommended due to the very low room utilization (twenty-eight percent) which would result. In lieu of adding this room, it is recommended that the limit on latest start time for the last fluoroscopic examination be relaxed, and that these examinations be conducted until noon and then resumed after a lunch break.

An indication of the potential improvement in service to be derived from the recommended resource allocations and policy changes is provided by comparing the actual late diagnostic report fraction for 1972 to the fraction predicted by the model for 1974. As indicated in table III.5.4 inpatient late reports decreased from thirty-four to zero percent for the morning service criterion, and from fifty-three to fourteen percent for the afternoon criterion. If it is conservatively assumed that only five percent of late diagnostic reports cause an increase in length of stay of one day, and that all other late reports have no impact on length of stay, then twenty-seven patient days per month of unnecessary hospital stay were incurred for 1972, as compared to only two patient days per month for 1974. It should be noted that this reduction in unnecessary days of hospital stay occurs in spite of a twelve percent increase in demand.

In order to assure that the criteria for report availability continue to be met, an ongoing monitoring system is recommended. Suggestions for collecting and processing the required data for such a system are contained in the following part of the chapter.

## Performance Monitoring

The model developed here aids the decision maker in selecting a particular policy, but an ongoing information system is needed to detect deviations from the level of performance predicted by the model for that policy.

This section considers how to collect the data needed to monitor and control the two most important measures of performance for radiology department operations: the number of late diagnostic reports, and resource utilization. A performance monitoring system for late reports will be discussed first. Two methods will be described for collecting the necessary data for this system: one using notations in the department's daily log, and another using a time stamp technique similar to that discussed previously. A method for monitoring resource utilization using data from existing department records is also described at the end of this part of the chapter.

The daily log method for report delays is as follows. When examination requisitions are received, the patient's name and radiology department file number are recorded in a daily log (along with the examination to be performed, physician's name, and other information). An additional notation of whether the requisition is received before or after 12:00 noon will be made in the log. When the diagnostic report is ready to be dispatched, reference will be made to the log, and the date and time will be recorded beside the patient's name. If it is determined that the report is late (a report for which the requisition was received before 12:00 noon is not dispatched by the end of that day), this will be noted on the log sheet. To aid in this determination, notations of arrival times for requisitions received before noon could be made in one color, and those received after 12:00 noon in another.

In the second method, which uses an automatic time stamp, a copy of the exam requistion travels with the patient or film through the enitre radiologic process. This requisition has the patient's hospital identification number, and would be stamped with the date and time when the requisition arrives in the department and when the diagnostic report is dispatched. The information would then be available to determine the number of reports which failed to meet service criteria. To facilitate manual processing of this data, arrival times for requisitions received before noon could be stamped in one color, and those received after noon in another.

The daily log method is suitable for gross control of report lateness. By performing a manual tally of the information in the daily log, the fraction of reports which failed to meet the service criteria could be computed. In searching for the cause of deviations, however, it would be necessary to refer back to the log sheets for information such as patient type and the number of hours the reports were late. Also, no information is provided on how late a report is relative to others of the same patient type or different patient types, except by futher extensive search of the daily log.

The time stamp method of collecting data on report delays minimizes the clerical time required, and permits much more sensitive control. It provides the same data as the daily log method, but in a more convenient format for analysis. The data for each patient is on a separate sheet (as opposed to a handwritten entry on a line of the daily log), which allows easier extraction of desired items, such as patient type, time and date of requisition arrival, and time and date of report dispatch. This also permits patient types not of concern (emergency room patients) to be readily separated from the others. This data format makes it feasible to compute relatively easily, not only the fraction of reports failing the service criteria, but also the frequency distribution (by patient type) of the number of hours by which they fail (or exceed) the service criteria. The kind of information contained on the patient requisition (and outlined above) permits one to begin searching for the cause of deviations without reference to the data source (the long record in the daily log method described above). To provide this type of information on a timely and regular basis, it might be preferable to use a computer to process the data collected on the patient requisitions. Computerized processing would be more desirable if it could be combined with the billing process. However, this method could be easily operated without computerization. Moreover, either method of data collection would require a total of no more than thirty minutes per day.

Given that either of the data collection methods described above determines the average fraction of late reports to be greater than the desired value, the question is then, whether the difference is "large enough" to require action. Statistical quality control techniques provide a probabilistic answer to this question.[28] A form of the fraction defective control chart may be used to indicate when the deviation from the desired average fraction of late reports is sufficiently large that the given lower probability (specified by the user) of it occurring has been exceeded, and that one should search for an assignable cause. The process of establishing such a chart is described in the following paragraphs.

Since the purpose of the fraction defective chart is to maintain an operating system at a desired level, the decision variable values which are believed will achieve this level must first be determined. The decision variable settings in this case come from the experimental results and recommendations reported previously. Once these recommendations are implemented and the system is stabilized, one can begin to collect the late report data to calculate a trial upper control limit. The upper control limit is based on the binomial probability distribution, and depends on the estimate of the average fraction defective for the process and the size of the samples used in computing the fraction defective for the individual points on the chart.[29] The probability of experiencing a fraction of late reports greater than this value is usually set at .05. The upper control limit allows determination of a deficient service level (too large a fraction of late reports). However, the use of upper and lower control limits would permit determination of improvement as well as degradation in service, and hence might be more valuable.

Sample size is often determined by consideration of the cost of inspection versus the cost of defectives not being found. For late reports, the cost of inspection is minimal. A pilot test indicated that approximately one to two hours of clerical time per week would be quite adequate for the forecast demand levels. Therefore, all of the available late report data should be used, that is, 100 percent inspection. One advantage of 100 percent inspection is that a random sampling system, which could be confusing to the clerical personnel, is not needed. The statistical assumptions for this control chart require that each point on the chart be calculated from a homogeneous population. To achieve this, the five-day week, Monday through Friday, is taken as the population.

Given the trial values for either upper, or both upper and lower control limits (usually calcuated from about twenty-five sample points), the limits and the individual points are plotted on the chart to determine if the process is "in control," that is, if all the points fall within the limits. Revised control limits are then computed by discarding any points which fall beyond the trial limits, which upon investigation are shown to have acceptable assignable causes, and then recomputing the control limits. A monitoring system using this control chart requires a minimal amount of time to operate (one to two hours per week at most, as indicated above), and will permit corrective effort to be concentrated where it can be most effective, namely, on statistically significant degradations in service.

Detailed measurement of resource utilizations can only be obtained by direct observation of their use, using a technique such as work sampling. This approach is expensive, however, and not conducive to routine monitoring. For purposes of detecting resource utilizations which are different from desired values and in need of adjustment, a measure such as the number of manhours per examination performed could be used as a proxy for utilization. The information for calculating this ratio, such as monthly summaries of the number of examinations performed, and the number of hours worked for various personnel categories, is available and readily accessible in existing department records at Baker Hospital.

## NOTES

[1]Only decisions of an administrative nature are considered; those involving medical judgment are taken as given.

[2]National Advisory Committee on Radiation, *Report of the Surgeon General: Protecting and Improving Health Through Radiological Sciences.* Washington: U.S. Public Health Service, 1966.

[3]John H. Knowles, "Radiology: Case Study in Technology and Manpower." *The New England Journal of Medicine*, June 5, 1969.

[4]There are recent indications, however, that the latter rate has accelerated somewhat.

[5]Wendell Scott, ed., *Planning Guide for Radiologic Installations, Second Edition.* Baltimore: Williams and Wilkins, 1966.

[6]American Hospital Association, *Hospital Administrative Services National Group Medians for Three Months Ending December 1969.* Chicago: The Association, 1970.

American Hospital Association, *Hospital Administrative Services National Group Medians for the Three Months Ending January 1972.* Chicago: The Association, 1972.

[7]P. M. Gertman and B. M. Bucher, "Inappropriate Hospital Bed Stays and Their Relationship to Length of Stay Parameters." Paper presented at the annual meeting of the American Public Health Association, October 1971.

[8]Experimentation with the model is used to evaluate the effect of removing the constraints under the control of the radiology department (for example, the typist staffing pattern).

[9]Richard F. Baum, et al., "The Diagnostic Test Cycle." Unpublished University of Michigan MIS report, December 1972.

[10]"Computer Simulation Program for a Diagnostic Radiology Department." Final report of U.S. Public Health Grant HS00179, Health Systems Research Center, Georgia Institute of Technology, October 1971.

Covert, R. P., et al., "Simulation Program for a Diagnostic Radiology Department." USPHS Grant HM00427, The University of Missouri, 1968.

J. J. Kenny, et al., "Diagnostic Radiology" in *Clinical Teaching and Health Care Systems: Models and Evaluation.* New York: The Commonwealth Fund, 1969.

B. Lev, et al., "Patient Flow and Utilization of Resources in a Diagnostic Radiology Department." *Investigative Radiology*, November-December 1972.

R. Lindheim, *Uncoupling the Radiology System.* Chicago: Hospital Research and Educational Trust, 1971.

George Revesz, et al., "Patient Flow and Utilization of Resources in a Diagnostic Radiology Department." *Radiology*, July 1972.

W. G. Sullivan, et al., "Cost Sensitivity for Radiology Department Planning." *Health Services Research*, Winter 1971.

Nuffield Provincial Hospitals Trust, *Towards a Clearer View: The Organization of Diagnostic X-Ray Departments*. London: The Trust, 1962.

J. Vora, "Long Range Facility Planning System for Ancillary Departments in Hospitals." Doctoral dissertation, Rennselaer Polytechnic Institute, 1970.

[11]A following part of the chapter under the heading "Model Development" contains a list of the variables used in the model. Under "Experiments and Results" is a more detailed statement of the objective function and performance measures are shown as a function of the decision variables.

[12]The model is written in GPSS/360 and implemented on the University of Michigan Terminal System. For further information about the simulation write the Bureau of Hospital Administration, The University of Michigan.

[13]George H. Naylor, et al., *Computer Simulation Techniques*. New York: John Wiley & Sons, 1966, p. 3.

[14]When a system has achieved steady state, the probability distribution of the output variables obtained from the simulation run provide approximations of the limiting, time independent probability distributions of those variables.

[15]Ronald Perry, Richard Baum, and Michael Warner, "A Scheduling and Resource Allocation Model for a Radiology Department." Technical Report No. 74-3, Industrial and Operations Engineering Department, The University of Michigan, 1974.

[16]R. Meier, et al., *Simulation in Business and Economics*. Englewood Cliffs, NJ: Prentice Hall, Inc., 1969.

[17]George M. Nemhauser, *Introduction to Dynamic Programming*. New York: John Wiley & Sons, 1966.

D. J. Wilde, *Optimum Seeking Methods*. Englewood Cliffs, NJ: Prentice Hall, Inc., 1964.

[18]A constraint is satisfied if the value of the decision variable, or function of decision variables, does not differ from the constraint value by a statistically significant amount. The $t$ test for differences in means is used for all constraints except constraints (2) and (3) of model segment 3, which utilize a normal test for differences in proportions.

[19]Nuffield, *Towards a Clearer View*.

[20]R. Barnes, *Motion and Time Study, Fourth Edition*. New York: John Wiley & Sons, 1958.

[21]B. Lev, "Patient Flow."

R. Lindheim, *Uncoupling the Radiology System*.

George Revesz, "Patient Flow."

Nuffield, "*Towards a Clearer View*."

[22]A. Drui, "Work Measurement and the Radiologist." *Operations Research*, November-December 1970.

[23]Output variables are compared to constraint values of model segments 2 and 3 using the statistical tests specified in note 18.

[24]J. R. Thombury, "A Comparative Study of Radiologists' Time Utilization in Various Reporting Systems," *The American Journal of Roentgenology, Radium Therapy, and Nuclear Medicine*, March 1971.

[25]Baum, et al., "The Diagnostic Test Cycle."

[26]Nuffield, *Towards a Clearer View.*

[27]An acceptable value for a measure of performance or utilization is one which does not exceed its maximum allowable value by a statistically significant amount.

[28]A. J. Duncan, *Quality Control and Industrial Statistics, Third Edition.* Homewood, IL.: Richard D. Irwin, Inc., 1965.

[29]*Ibid.*

# III.6

# Criteria and Procedures for Establishing Accounting Based Control Systems[1]

*by John R. Griffith*

Systems for the control of routine expenditures exist in any enterprise, but their complexity and effectiveness are a function in part of the severity of the economic environment. The economic climate of hospitals has become markedly more demanding in recent years, and the trend is likely to continue. Management's adjustment to this change, therefore, should include improvements in these control systems.

Effective cost controls consist of three elements: a budget system for preparing and distributing the financial plan, a reporting system for assessing actual performance and identifying variation from plan, and a set of incentives and sanctions to encourage acceptable performance. The last component is the least developed in most community hospitals. The whole of the hospital should be included in cost control systems, and there are a variety of sometimes conflicting criteria and constraints governing system design.

This chapter is based on four years' experience assisting Baker Hospital in upgrading these systems. It includes a review of the goals for their construction and the constraints which derive from these goals. It also suggests a systematic approach to the process of reviewing and upgrading these systems. The following chapter reviews the revisions to accounting systems which were found to be necessary (section III.7).

## Goals For A Cost Control System

### Controlling Costs

The objective is to devise systems which will aid and encourage supervisors to set expenditure standards—budgets—which are as low as quality considerations permit, and then to hold actual expenditures within the narrowest possible tolerances of those standards. (Clearly these tolerances are in both directions. If a budget is set so that there is no impairment of quality or service when actual expenditures are substantially lower than the budget, then it is too high.) Both the budget systems and the reporting systems relate to complex managerial activities involving the operating discipline (the set of quality considerations, technology, and policies governing the work and how it is done) and human factors (the interaction of individuals in small work groups and more formal organizational hierarchies).

Successful cost control systems require strong motivation at all levels of supervision, sufficient professional skills to recognize and subjectively assess the many aspects of quality, a provision for the ongoing review and adoption of new technology and procedures, and an organization robust enough to handle both the stresses of differing individual and professional viewpoints and those imposed by change in policies and procedures. In setting the appropriate nursing manpower budget, for example, all of the following are likely to be important to the administration and to nursing supervision:

- An appreciation of quality and the impact of changes in staffing upon quality.
- A knowledge of new methods and procedures which will change the operating discipline, such as changes in nursing care patterns, changes in organization, and changes in scheduling systems.
- A knowledge of the past performance of the department. (This would include information from the reporting system, but also general knowledge of departmental strengths and weaknesses.)
- An understanding that both viewpoints and values differ and that the best solution requires the most constructive adjustment of these differences.
- A recognition that improvement rather than maintenance of past performance is desirable; in other words that lower costs of nursing care at continued levels of quality is the goal.
- The existence of incentives to both parties to seek the best solution.

A similar set of requirements can be developed for an effective reporting system, which in addition requires a prompt, efficient, well coordinated data return plan, rather than simply the haphazard dumping of all available facts.

The mechanical and procedural components of budgeting and control systems are clearly only a part of the totality. One way to restate the central objective is that the design of these systems is an ongoing exercise to maintain and improve mechanical and procedural components of the budgeting and control systems in a manner which facilitates the effective interaction of individuals in the organization and changes in the operating disciplines to bring about continued improvement in performance.

## Strengthening the Existing Management Structure

The manpower, material, and capital resources of hospitals are actually converted to services by small work groups at or below the departmental level. These teams provide services from intensive nursing care to bookkeeping, which are frequently of a personal and vital character and often require direct professional supervision with a high degree of autonomy. Thus, the hospital is by virtue of its multiple and complex technologies a highly decentralized organization with substantial authority assigned to first line managers. These managers frequently negotiate or influence the quantity of resources used for their work team, its supplies and equipment. Often, they also have routine intercourse with physicians and can influence the demand for their services in a variety of ways. A large fraction of the budget of any hospital is the direct result of aggregating the resource requirements of these teams. We have identified these work teams as responsibility centers (RCs), and their supervisors as responsibility center managers (RCMs). (Head nurses and small department managers are examples of RCMs.)

It is clear that a systematic approach to cost containment must parallel the formal delegation of authority to responsibility center managers. It should incorporate them in budget development and cost control in a manner which recognizes the character of their work and their traditional influence and autonomy, while still directing their efforts toward an overall financial and expenditure position established by top management.

## Emphasizing Major Cost Components

At Baker Hospital, eighty percent of the budget is allocated in decisions which are usually influenced by and executed by RCMs. Eighty percent of this component, by far the largest proportion of RCM expenditures, is in salaries. Only six areas handle concentrated volumes of supplies expenditures. Other nonmanpower expenditures are dispersed in a wide variety of small sums of money (often less than $1,000 a year). The remaining twenty percent of all annual expenditures is the result of decisions made and executed at the trustee and top management level. Such items as depreciation, capital costs, executive salaries, consultation fees, and general insurance protection fall into this category. A well planned system will direct managers' attention to important cost elements, which at Baker, and probably at most hospitals, means a heavy concentration on payroll cost.

## Encouraging Supervisory Participation

At the start of work at Baker Hospital, budgets and cost standards were developed almost entirely by top management with minimal participation or even consultation from lower levels. No data were systematically or promptly reported to lower management on cost performance. In 1971, twenty managers of the largest departments were given an opportunity to state their impressions of the goals and standards for the operation of their departments. Not one of these people mentioned cost control, efficiency, or economy in their responses.

We believe that active involvement of the RCMs in the decision areas where they are expert is a necessary first step to a sound budget procedure. Thus, in the Baker manpower budget, RCMs propose the basic staffing of their centers for discussion and negotiation with administration. This is in no sense an argument for increasing the independence of cost-center heads to decide for themselves what they need. Rather, it is an argument for a much closer linkage of the administrator and department heads in the initial determination of required expenditure levels.

Increased participation of RCMs in budget development, as well as increased willingness to be responsible for cost control are both consistent with Likert's "System 4" management. Likert gives three basic concepts for participative management (which he calls the System 4 approach):

(1) The use by the manager of the principle of supportive relationships,

(2) His use of group decision making and group methods of supervision, and

(3) His high performance goals for the organization.[2]

In Baker, and perhaps in most hospitals, the initial emphasis is appropriately on high performance goals for cost control. Joint decision making on standards, including cost targets, is necessary to achieve such goals. Also necessary is the provision of help to RCMs in achieving the goals, the most basic help being the provision of performance and planning information to the RCMs. It is known that the feedback of information can be used to support a highly authoritarian system of management, that the techniques of participation are sometimes used to make autocratic decisions palatable, and that high performance goals are a characteristic of all management systems. The emphasis is therefore not on the techniques, which may serve a variety of purposes, but on the purposes themselves. There are no management methods which can enforce RCM initiative, only methods which facilitate it. The accounting based cost control systems proposed here accept the importance of such initiative, and are designed to help in its development.

The approach we outline is only a step in the direction of System 4 management and gives initial emphasis to explicit objectives. It is in this sense somewhat closer to "management by objectives" and to the underlying concept of exception reporting in hierarchical control systems.

The major elements of management by objectives are:

1. The manager assumes responsibility for identifying the common goals which all his subordinates share with him, and toward whose achievements he must converge their combined talents.
2. Each person is able to state, in advance of the attempt, *areas of responsibility* and *measures of acceptable results* for his position.
3. Each person has knowledge of the goals he is to achieve, has worked out a plan for achieving them, and is measured by his results, insofar as these can be attributed to conditions under his own effective control.[3]

Restated in the terms of the general performance control system described by Hancock (section III.1), a given manager must have: a set of objectives, developed in concert with his organization superior; the ability in an exception reporting system to measure results; and the ability to modify results as the situation may require.

Relating this budgeting and cost control approach to more conventional hospital practices shows that points of difference include more explicit attention to specifying measurable objectives in advance, developing these jointly between the RCM and administrator, and providing adequate information return. The points of difference between this approach and System 4 are the emphasis on joint (superior-subordinate) rather than group (superior-subordinates) decision making, and on only one aspect of supportive relationships, that involving the development of standards (or goals) and the use of performance information.

## Simplifying Calculations and Improving RCM Understanding

Closely related to the goal of encouraging supervisory participation is the problem of an efficient, comprehensible format for standard setting information, discussion, and performance information. This suggests that data be presented, discussed, and dealt with in forms close to those routinely used by the RCM, and that calculations be minimized. Many approaches to budgeting and reporting appear to be oriented more to forms convenient to upper levels of management; early work on the Baker budget process suffered from this defect. Gross statistics such as manhours per patient day are a case in point. "What does 'hours per patient day' mean," the director of nurses asked us, "when I have three shifts with no rotation and strict area nursing assignments on the day shift?" How, she implied, could such a concept be used for budget development or control? The points she identifies call for preparation of budgets and control reports on a shift basis and for recognition of the need for certain fixed staffing in an RC to cover specialized tasks or geographic areas. Even in a large nursing unit there are different ranges of variability for each shift, and certain minimum staff which are best described not in hours per patient per shift but in terms of numbers of head nurses, medication nurses, and staff nurses which are set by policy rather than according to the activity level. Negotiations of budgets in the most common reference frames—total dollars, manhours, or FTEs, or manhours per patient day—do not illuminate this problem. Although they permit quick comparisons and are therefore desirable, the more central problem of providing information relevant to RCM decisions which determine these outcomes is ignored. Attention should be directed to how specific decisions are made and problems are encountered, and other information should be summarized. We believe, therefore, that budget forms should stress actual decisions about real resources (principally manpower scheduling) and report forms should stress the existence of deviation and give useful detail in determining its cause.

The problem of calculations is simpler. RCMs are neither motivated nor competent as accountants or arithmeticians. Using them as such erodes their enthusiasm for budgeting and control, wastes their time and reduces accuracy. Worst of all, it diverts their attention from their central budgeting responsibility, that of identifying the minimum amount of resources necessary to provide service of appropriate quality.

For these reasons, the Baker budget process approaches the manpower decision from the viewpoint of the RCMs' normal staffing decision: the number of people necessary to cover a standard work week for each work shift. Variability may be incorporated by providing staffing for both high and low volume weeks. Forecasts of activity are tentatively prepared by the budget director or a member of the controller's staff, for review and adjustment by the RCM and line management. All calculations of total manhours and dollars costs are computerized after the hours worked per week for each class of employee are summed manually from the approved work schedules.

Interviews with Baker RCMs and administration indicate these steps were well received. To them the budget was easy to understand, easy to negotiate, and freed of needless drudgery. After its completion, it appeared that RCMs were more aware of its meaning, and its implication for cost control.

## Dealing with Variability in Hospital Activity

Hospital activity levels can change during a budget cycle, and theoretically there should be adjustments in the resource expenditures to meet these changes. The concept of variable budgeting has frequently been advocated as a way to encourage RCM response to activity fluctuation. In variable budgeting, resource requirements are expressed as standards of manhours per unit of activity, and RCMs are encouraged to vary manpower and other resources according to actual activity or short-range forecasts. The investigations at Baker indicate, however, that this concept is a serious oversimplification of the problem. While supplies expenses are generally variable, most other nonmanpower expenses are fixed. The manpower expense, in addition to having important fixed components as noted above, is difficult to vary over short horizons (day-to-day) and difficult to forecast accurately over longer horizons (weekly or monthly). A useable forecast must be sensitive enough to predict changes, and the changes must be of sufficient magnitude to permit adjustments in expenditures. Much of the application of variable budgeting founders upon this rock: there is no useful forecast because there is no measure of activity, no substantial changes to forecast, or no way to predict changes. Whenever these conditions occur, the expected manpower must be treated as a constant. Even where these conditions are met, variable budgets are more expensive to develop and to administer. Frequent adjustments of the work force often have hidden costs in morale, training level of employees, and supervisory time. In many cases, it is actually preferable to eliminate activity level changes rather than to build variable budgets. Thus nursing RCs for adult medical-surgical floors become constant budget centers when admission scheduling reduces occupancy variation below the ability of the department to vary work force.

When these factors were understood at Baker, it appeared that of the total of forty-four RCs:

- Twenty-nine had either no convenient activity measure or no variation in activity substantial enough to adjust staffing. They accounted for thirty-eight percent of the payroll. (Most of these were small. The largest was housekeeping, which Baker treats as a constant staff.)
- Three had measures and were forecastable, but variation dropped below work force change capability when the admission scheduling system was installed. These accounted for twenty-four percent of payroll expenditures (the three medical-surgical nursing floors).

• Twelve had measures and substantial variations. They accounted for thirty-eight percent of the payroll. (Laboratory, linen supply, dietary, cafeteria, intensive-coronary care, obstetrics, operating room, anesthesia, x-ray, physical therapy, and pediatrics).

In a theoretical sense, only the last category of RCs are candidates for variable budgeting at Baker. In a practical sense, even these have not yet been established as such. The practical problems include activity measure difficulties, forecasting difficulties, difficulties in relating work force requirements to activity forecasts, and the priority of other goals than direct cost reduction (specifically, in reducing service times in laboratory and x-ray). (See section IV.5.).

While variable budgets remain a goal for part of the hospital, two general conclusions from our work with Baker Hospital should be noted. The first is that where variability exists it is better to explore ways of reducing the variability in demand, such as the admission scheduling and occupancy control system, before attempting to construct variable budgets and establish variable manpower control systems. Second is that any variable system can be budgeted as a constant or seasonal system, and that an effective fixed or seasonal budget is a preliminary step to establishing a variable budget. The effective operation of a fixed budget is likely to be superior to the poor operation of a variable one, even in the limited number of responsibility centers where variation is required.

There are two additional considerations relating to the variability of activity. First, even when adjustments to day-to-day changes in activity levels are impossible or undesirable, seasonal variation can often be forecast, and changes in work force can be accommodated for a few periods. A well designed budget will encourage consideration of economies possible because of summer or Christmas lulls, for example. Second, the budget preparation process should be efficient enough to permit rebudgeting for major revisions during the cycle. These elements are frequently omitted because of the cost and difficulty of incorporating the calculations. If the input forms are simplified, forecasts provided, and the calculations automated, both seasonal budgeting and rebudgeting to accommodate change become feasible. They are desirable for all departments and are a sound interim step toward variable budgeting for applicable departments.

One possibility which has been uncovered as a result of the Baker studies (and others) is the possibility of contingency reserves to handle unexpected variation. The budget should be developed for the most likely output expectations, including seasonal variations where these are likely to occur. Expenses should be firmly negotiated to the minimum acceptable levels of quality for each responsibility center for these expectations. It is clear that not all of these expectations will come true; some departments will be unable to recruit the agreed manpower and others may have volume variation either above or below expectations. If these variations are allowed to accumulate in the responsibility center accounts, there is a tendency to balance out activities by the year's end, spending more in later months to consume surpluses, or less to absorb shortages. Such a pattern is obviously fallacious. Patients who were treated in the shortage months received below minimum care, by definition. Giving more to other patients at another time simply wastes resources. Another solution, which also appears to be common, is simply to raise the minimum to allow for variation from expectations. While this reduces the probability of low quality, it builds in a permanent waste.

If the problem is viewed over several departments or the whole hospital, however, two elements change. First, the odds of having several estimates in error in the same direction are at least slightly diminished. (The activities of hospitals are not "independent events" in a statistical sense, yet neither are they all perfectly correlated. Among the major activities, it is unlikely that obstetrics, pediatrics, and other inpatient and outpatient activities will all move unexpectedly in one direction.) Second, it is possible to establish a reserve upon which RCMs can draw to meet unexpectedly large demands. Such a reserve would permit closer negotiation of the resource requirements. It goes without saying that drawing upon the reserve would call for the same approvals as the negotiated budget itself, yet the criteria for judging the requests could be agreed upon in advance. Also, the reserve should be dispensed equitably and in good faith, in order to preserve a participative management style. Any actual expenditures below budget, regardless of cause, would be automatically credited to the reserve.

This innovation has not been tried at Baker, nor does the author know of its use elsewhere. (There are two aspects to be included: the establishment of a reserve expense and its use to meet revised conditions on appeal from the RCM.) It appears to have theoretical merit, and may be of considerable practical value as part of an incentive reimbursement system, both to provide flexibility for the hospital as a whole and to aid in transferring incentives to the RCM level.

## Building Upon Existing Data Systems

There are numerous important advantages to using existing data systems. Accuracy is improved, cost is reduced, and multiple uses of data justify larger investments in the systems themselves. There are drawbacks as well, however. Conflicts with original uses must be resolved, and changes must be carefully preplanned to avoid disrupting important activities. These inevitably mean longer planning and implementation schedules. On balance, however, the data requirements of a sound budget and control process are so large that it must rely on an existing payroll and general accounting system.

A manpower control system requires measures of activity from the revenue accounting system or other sources, and data on manhours and expenditures from the payroll system. Three important constraints may require substantial revision of these systems, particularly the payroll system:

• *The budget and reporting periods must be the same, and must be of equal length.* (A thirteen-period four-week system is incorporated in the Baker budget.)

• *The end points of the periods must be simultaneous for each budget group.* That is, the entire payroll must end on the same date, or separate budget periods and report periods must be established so that they are uniform for reasonable groups of RCs. (Nursing RCs could be budgeted on periods ending in even numbered weeks, for example. This appears to be less satisfactory than having all RCs on simultaneous periods, which Baker plans to implement.)

• *The payroll must be accurately assigned to RCs and frequently to shifts within RCs.* (Nurses who are reassigned to different RCs during single tours of duty must have that reassignment reflected in payroll accounting. Manhours and dollars for float or unassigned personnel must be distributed to the cost centers where those persons actually worked.)

The reason for these constraints is that they are necessary to provide accurate control data. In each case where one of these constraints—equal periods, uniform period end points, and accurate direct cost accounting—is violated, potential errors are larger than the control tolerances which can be expected of competent RCMs. The inevitable discovery of these errors causes RCMs to lose confidence in the system and to become frustrated over their ability to control. Errors introduced by using calendar month periods can exceed ten percent in departments working mainly on a Monday to Friday basis. Differing end points require adjustments similar to end-of-month accrual entries which estimate, rather than measure, actual expenses. While these adjustments are generally acceptable for financial accounting purposes, they violate the requirements of sound managerial accounting. Faulty direct accounting encourages the misuse of transferred and pooled personnel.

The shift to thirteen-period accounting provided little difficulty at Baker and was carried through in both general accounting and revenue accounting, so that even reports to the board of trustees are prepared on a four-week cycle. The shift to simultaneous pay periods has proven substantially more troublesome, and is not yet a reality. Revisions of duties of payroll clerks and a change in the supplier of computer services have been the main causes of delay.

We believe the kinds of delays encountered in Baker are to be expected in undertaking a project of this kind. Frustrating as they may be, it is better to work with them patiently than to take expensive or inaccurate shortcuts. As a result, limited short-range goals carefully ordered to be consistent with larger objectives are necessary, and some priority of elements is in order. We believe there should be two criteria for selecting these short-range goals:

1. *Attention should be devoted first to the larger dollar volume routine expenses.* In most situations, this implies an initial concentration on manpower.
2. *The system should build upon the stronger elements of existing data systems.*

## Stimulating Continued Improvement

The preceding seven goals, taken as a whole, strongly suggest the view that budgeting and control systems are an ongoing process of management rather than static systems. As performance improves, standards should improve and tolerances should diminish. Parallel to this process, the budget and control systems themselves should be refined by increasing the quality, quantity and specificity of data which they supply the RCMs and upper management. Such problems as extension to non-payroll costs, improving measures of activity, and better handling of variability are handled gradually, upon a base of full understanding and proven system capability. This suggests that there are three measures of management performance which should be monitored:

1. *Ability to attain actual performance consistent with the budget.*
2. *Ability to improve standard setting and budget development.* That is, ability to refine and reduce budget requests consistent with quality needs.
3. *Ability to improve the data systems and the process of budgeting and controlling.* That is, ability to improve and extend the process itself.

Each of these is important, and none should be overlooked in applying the rewards and sanctions available to the organization. These should include both the intangible and informal incentives—thanks, praise, training, verbal encouragement, technical and professional assistance—and tangible ones—salary increases, bonuses, and promotions. The effective use of these incentives depends on having clear objectives and measures of performance such as those which a sound budget and control system provides. With the development of prospective reimbursement for hospitals, the need for such systems is increased. The institutional incentives which frequently accompany prospective reimbursement open new opportunities for tangible rewards.

## Process of Developing Budgeting and Control System

Figure III.6.1 shows a flowchart of the activities necessary to develop a budgeting and control system like the Baker Hospital system in a community hospital. While it is impossible to identify which of these elements will be most critical or time-consuming in a specific institution, those elements on the main horizontal row are the core activities which must be taken in the sequence listed and which, in many cases, are repeated annually. In a few instances the Baker demonstration failed to follow this order. In each case the result was lost time and backtracking to correct oversights. The following discussion amplifies the activities shown in figure III.6.1

### Introduction and Goal Setting

It is important to start with a consensus at all levels of management that the purpose of the budgeting and cost reporting activity is the provision of data to assist management in containing costs. The responsibilities of RCMs in development and cost control must be introduced and explained. The endorsement and support of the trustees and the implications in terms of requests of third parties, such as prospective reimbursement programs, should be explained. The interrelation of the development of budgets and cost control systems with other accounting purposes should be noted and placed in perspective for both accounting managers and line management. The interrelation of this program to other programs which may be going on must also be noted.

If a satisfactory set of budget procedures and policies is already in existence, these should be reviewed and the responsibility of different groups and individuals in the hospital for various steps should be delineated. If not, it should be made clear in the introduction that considerable attention will be devoted to step 5, a review of the budget policies, and the timetable and responsibilities for this review should be identified.

### Responsibility Accounting System

A thorough review of the expense side of the chart of accounts, its parallelism with the revenue chart and with the formal organization of the institution is necessary. This review is normally the function of the controller or the accounting department, in consultation with appropriate line managers.

**FIGURE III.6.1**
Installation of accounting based cost control systems

Flowchart of Activities

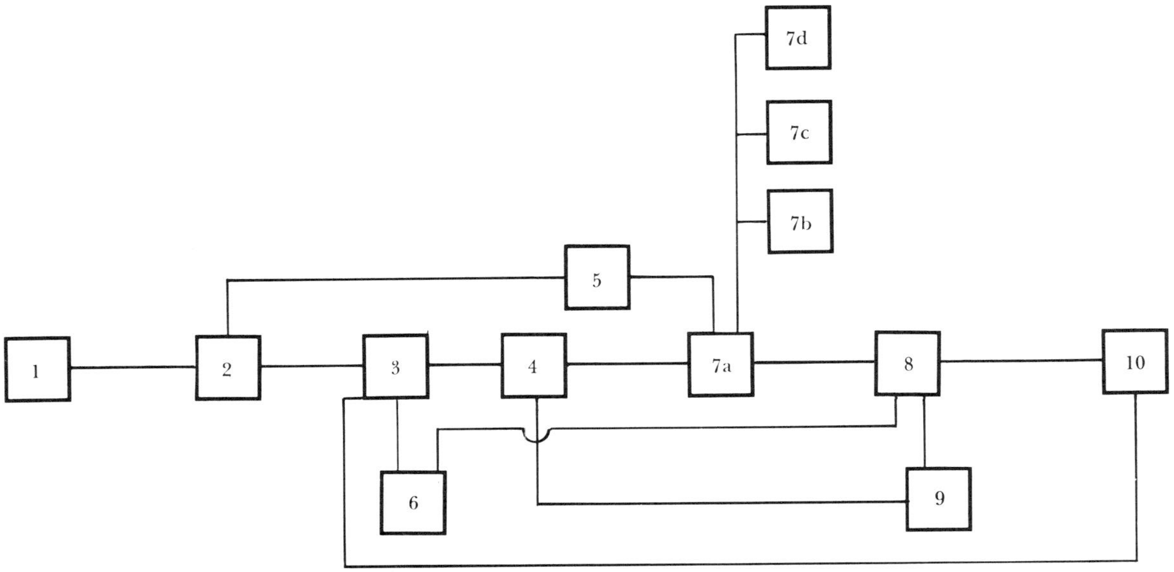


A. Introduction
- (1) Introduction and Goal Setting

B. Accounting and Information Systems
- (2) Responsibility Accounting System
- (3) Data Processing Policies
- (6) Data Processing Mechanics

C. Budget Process and Policies
- (4) Forecasting
- (5) Budget Policies
- (7a) Budgeting
- (7b) Revenue and Cash Budgeting
- (7c) Manpower Planning
- (7d) Related Planning Activities

D. Reporting Systems
- (8) Manpower Cost Reporting
- (9) Short-Term Output Forecasting
- (10) Noncost Reporting Systems

## Data Processing Policies

It is necessary to bring at least the payroll accounting system, the systems for measuring productivity (that is, collecting departmental statistics), and the categories of the budget into congruence with regard to responsibility centers, period ending dates, and account identification.

## Forecasting

Several elements need to be forecast over the budget period. The detail and sophistication of these forecasts depends on whether variable budgets are to be used. In general, all major measures of activity such as patient days, outpatient visits, meals, tests, and so forth should be forecast, at least to the extent of identifying expected trends and seasonal variations. While much of this work can be done statistically by members of the accounting staff, line management review is highly desirable. It is also necessary to forecast the prices of labor and supplies. These functions are presumably best assigned to the experts in these areas.

Finally, it may be desirable to forecast some upper limit on feasible cost increases. This is essentially a financial matter reflecting the environment in which the hospital is working. There are pros and cons to such a forecast, however. If it is provided, it will reduce the amount of time necessary to renegotiate and adjust the budget, and it may reduce thoughtless or irresponsible requests for increases. On the other hand, an overall estimate, such as 105 percent of last year's costs, if handled arbitrarily, may lead some members of the organization to overlook opportunities for growth and quality improvement which they should carefully evaluate.

It should be noted that two of the elements which comprise the total budget are explicitly not forecast in the sense of being projected forward from last year's or the current year's experience. These are the quantities of manpower required to meet output expectations and the prices the hospital will charge. The former are suggested directly by the responsibility center managers and negotiated with their superiors in step 7a of the flowchart. The latter are not directly relevant to a cost containment budget and are taken up in step 7c by the controller's office with appropriate consultation.

## Budget Policies

It is necessary to have a clear and consistent set of policies for both the negotiation of the budget and its administration. Many of the details of these policies are unique to individual institutions.

## Data Processing Mechanics

A second output from step 3 is a set of specifications for either manual or automated data processing. While it may be possible to operate a budget and cost control system in a purely manual system, it is doubtful that this is any longer desirable. At least the payroll system must be automated to produce the proper control reports in a timely fashion. On-line capability is not required, and it appears feasible for the necessary data processing to be done by contractual arrangement if turnaround time and the format and content of reports are carefully specified. The extension of the system to other accounts may depend on the automation of other accounting functions as well. Although figure III.6.1 does not show the relationship, provisions should be made for processing the budget documents themselves in the components of step 7.

## Budget and Related Activities

The central activity 7a of figure III.6.1 is the negotiation of the manpower requirement or expectation. It is completed by line management, using standard work schedules as described in Stephen H. Lipson and Mary D. Hensel, *Hospital Manpower Budget Preparation Manual.*[4] The results are coupled mechanically with labor price expectations and volume forecasts from step 4 to generate a manpower expense budget. Either line management or the controller's office is responsible for step 7b, provisions of expectations in nonlabor cost areas to develop the complete cost budget, analyses of unit costs (including indirect cost allocation) and rate changes for the services sold by the hospital, and the development of cash flow budgets and recommendations as to the fiscal soundness of the proposals. It is frequently necessary to cycle through these steps which are shown as 7a and 7b one or more times. Once agreement has been reached, the ancillary uses of the budget for manpower planning and other planning activities as shown in steps 7c and 7d can be activated. These would, of course, include the review of consistency with prior long-range plans and revision of those plans and the capital budget.

## Manpower Cost Reporting

Data on actual volumes of output and hours and dollars expended by the responsibility centers, together with costs on other parts of the budget as these are developed, should be reported promptly and frequently.

## Short-Term Output Forecasting

In areas where variable budgets are used, it is probably desirable to develop short-term forecasts of one or two periods in advance to aid responsibility center managers and their supervisors in making short-run manpower and other decisions.

## Noncost Reporting Systems

The complete operation of the hospital is not described in accounting systems, yet these systems contain data of potential value in measuring other objectives. Certain framing of productivity measures such as nursing hours per patient day can be used in quality surveillance. For example, minimum coverage requirements can be specified, and the payroll data base can show the number of times these minimums were violated. Turnover, absenteeism, and tardiness data are indicators of employee satisfaction and can be reported for this purpose.

## NOTES

[1]A revised version of this paper entitled "Budgeting Process Integral to Effective Cost Control System" was published in *Hospital Financial Management*, July 1974.

[2]Rensis Likert, *The Human Organization: Its Management and Value*. New York: McGraw-Hill Book Co., 1967, p. 47.

[3]George S. Odiorne, *Management by Objectives*. New York: Pitman Publishing Corp., 1965, p. 61.

[4]Stephen H. Lipson and Mary D. Hensel, *Hospital Manpower Budget Preparation Manual*. Ann Arbor: Health Administration Press, 1975.

# III.7

# Improving Accounting Information Systems

*by Stephen H. Lipson*

This chapter describes the prerequisites of accounting based control systems—responsibility center accounting and measurement of output in hospital activities—and the problems which must be resolved before using the payroll system for managerial data. A brief review of concepts and definitions relevant to responsibility center accounting[1] is followed by a discussion of the problems encountered in the application of this concept at Baker Hospital and the solutions or proposed solutions to those problems. The practical problems of output measurement and use of the payroll systems are presented with the solutions which proved satisfactory at Baker Hospital.

## Responsibility Center Accounting

Responsibility center accounting is a concept of accounting in which costs, revenues, and other accounting data, both financial and nonfinancial, are codified for, collected, and reported to an organizational unit headed by a responsible person, its manager. The goals of responsibility center accounting include performance measurement, identification of problem areas, and development of management attitudes through a cost control system. While revenue control can be incorporated in a responsibility center system, the focus of the Baker Hospital work was cost control. Therefore, revenue data were not reported to the centers. In addition, manpower costs received almost the total available consideration.

In establishing responsibility centers, the aim is to identify each small, homogeneous work group under a single supervisor, and to provide that supervisor with routine data on the group's performance, similar in concept to the data each group would have if they were operating as small, independent enterprises. Nursing stations and laboratory sections such as bacteriology, hematology, and blood bank are examples. The groups should not be trivially small, and should be distinct from other groups. Thus, one would not be likely to segregate inpatient physical therapy from outpatient, except in very large hospitals and where work areas and personnel are separated. Neither should the centers cover work groups that are too big or too broad in function. For example, the food service operations of a hospital, while under the responsibility of a single director, should be subdivided in the accounting system according to its actual managerial divisions, perhaps "food preparation," "inpatient food service," and "cafeteria service." These centers can then be aggregated as necessary to present data on the parent department, or for sections of the hospital under each assistant administrator.

The possibility of aggregation implies that a hierarchic grouping of responsibility centers exists in a hospital at levels such as shift supervisor, department head, assistant administrator, and administrator. In each case, the responsible person is held accountable for all responsibility centers below his point in the hierarchy. An organization chart and a clear understanding of supervisors' scope of responsibilities are required to develop a successful responsibility center accounting system.

Whenever the delegation of responsibility is unclear, as in many circumstances involving nonemployee physicians, the design of a responsibility center accounting system will be difficult. An unusual distribution of responsibilities in an organization is justification neither to abort the responsibility center accounting system nor to arbitrarily change the shape of the organization. However, during the design and implementation of the accounting system, many policies influencing the organizational shape and the assignment of responsibilities can be reviewed, and either confirmed as appropriate or redesigned.

A responsibility center accounting system is wholly compatible with the principles of participative management. Through direct reporting and careful use of incentives and sanctions, lower level managers can be fully informed about activities within their responsibility centers, given the first chance to correct deficiencies, and encouraged to participate in the planning of standards and goals. The result of a well designed system is more clearly defined areas of authority and responsibility for the individual responsibility center managers, and greater authority and responsibility within those defined areas. While the system does not automatically decentralize management, it provides the information base by which management can be decentralized without sacrificing top management participation in goal setting and control.

In performing its functions, each responsibility center consumes resources, or *inputs*. Inputs include manpower, supplies, equipment, and services. The costs of these inputs are assigned to each responsibility center by the payroll and general accounting systems. The costs assigned to responsibility centers are measures of the value of the inputs consumed within a specified period of time. The development and management of well audited basic data systems to account for these inputs are a primary function of the controller's office.

In addition to costs, responsibility center accounting should include measures of *output*, which can be either product, such as sterile packs in the central supply room, or service, such as nursing care, or x-ray diagnosis. Accounting for output is usually accomplished through accounts receivable posting, but many categories of output are not used for revenue. Special accounting for these categories, such as inpatient meals, becomes necessary. Thus responsibility center accounting calls for an expansion of normal data collection.

In holding responsibility center managers accountable for costs, a distinction must be made between controllable and noncontrollable costs for each of the specific centers. While direct costs such as depreciation can be *assigned* to specific responsibility centers, these costs are fixed for the short run. Even in the longer run when new capital is invested and increases the depreciation expense, the decision involves others than the responsibility center manager. Indirect costs are also substantially out of the control of the managers to whose centers such costs are assigned, but they are always direct costs of other responsibility centers. Control over direct costs is primarily the responsibility of the manager. The system of responsibility accounting should focus on direct costs only and need not include capital costs. Extensive study and revision of accounting systems may be necessary to establish responsiblity accounting in some hospitals. Others, however, are better prepared. In those, a brief review at the time of the annual budget cycle is recommended.

## Application at Baker Hospital

At Baker Hospital when the study began, the hospital's accounting system was a limited adaptation of the American Hospital Association's Standard Chart of Accounts. The actual asset, equity, expense, and revenue account titles and their uses were satisfactory, but the entities for which these items were accounted did not conform to the principles of responsibility center accounting. Most of the problems related to the increase in the number of cost and responsibility centers which led to smaller units of management.

Specific criteria were established for the redesign of the accounting system to responsibility center accounting:

• The accounting system should reflect the organizational realities and practicalities, but should not group unrelated activities.

• No responsibility center should be so large that the span of control is unmanageable, nor include more than one specific supervisor for the activities of each center.

• If secondary purposes of a center represent significant costs of the center, a new center should be created. (The same person may be responsible for both centers.)

• Activities not related to existing centers should be assigned to other centers or to new centers if necessary.

An example of unrelated activities appeared in the emergency room, which included nursing service activities, patient registration activities, and general outpatient registration activities. Although the accounting system aggregated all of these activities as one cost center, the director of nursing was responsible for the nursing service activities and the business manager was responsible for all of the patient registration activities. Data for manpower use and costs were aggregated in the existing accounts, so that planning and reporting could not be identified with a responsible individual. The proper handling of this situation called for the provision of three separate responsibility centers, one for the nursing activities, identified with the director of nursing and her subordinates; one each for emergency room patient registration and outpatient registration, both identified with the business manager.

The nursing department, at the start of the study, was one large cost center, with all activities aggregated for accounting purposes. This amounted to more than forty percent of all hospital costs, and approximately one-half of all hospital employees. This size (approximately $350,000 per month and 400 employees) is simply too large. The response to this was to establish each patient care area within nursing as a separate responsibility accounting center. Nursing administration, central supply, and nursing education also became cost centers.

The problem of too many individuals being identified with responsibility for the same center came up in nursing and in those departments that had a physician and a nonphysician head, such as pathology and radiology. The nursing problem was particularly complex. Essentially, overlapping supervisors for each patient care area were assigned according to shift of work and day of the week leaving no one with total responsibility for all activities in any given center, except the director of nursing. The most sensitive issue in the establishment of responsibility center accounting in nursing was whether to categorize each of the geographic patient care areas as centers or to categorize each of the three shifts of work (day shift, afternoon shift, night shift) as centers, crossing patient care areas within each shift. The organization was not static even at the shift level, with different supervisors on different days. Management's choice was to specify the geographic centers of activity as responsibility centers, emphasizing that the activities relating to patients encompass all shifts and that the focus should remain on the patient care units. Considerable internal disagreement with this decision existed, but the lack of clarity of shift responsibilities made that choice even less attractive.

The problem in departments that have nonemployee physician heads, such as pathology and radiology, was in identifying the responsible individual and the costs over which he had control rather than in defining the scope of the responsibility center. This was resolved by defining the nonmedical department head as the responsibility center manager since he routinely made those resource allocation decisions comprising the bulk of the operating expenses. There are several potentially conflicting objectives in these departments, including minimizing expenditures, speeding return of information to the medical staff, and maximizing the physician-specialist's income. In such a situation, considerable tolerance and restraint is necessary, but the principle of cost responsibility remains important. So far, this solution has been easily accepted within the organization.

In some departments the Bureau staff found secondary purposes which were substantial in terms of manpower and costs and were uniquely different from the primary purpose. The most notable was a nursing service education program which supported the clincial experience of licensed practical nursing students as well as the usual inservice education functions. The students, who received token compensation from the hospital in support of their education, and the instructors, full time paid employees of the hospital, were originally treated as a part of the nursing administration. This activity was separated from other nursing activities for accounting purposes, and a separate cost center was established.

A similar situation was the accounting for physician services for the emergency room and coverage for all hospital patients around the clock. These costs had been accounted for as part of the cost of the emergency room. Since these physicians were not the responsibility of either the director of nursing or the business manager, this situation clearly violated the concept of responsibility center management. Furthermore, the requirement that unrelated activities should not be grouped was violated since the house physicians were routinely concerned with some medical needs of inpatients. Therefore, a new responsibility center was established to segregate these costs and other reporting data. The administrator, who coordinated this program directly, became the responsibility center manager.

The new alignment assigned all costs to those responsibility centers where the responsibility lay for their control. Associated costs, such as fringe benefits could also be identified more directly with the appropriate activities and allocated accordingly. The review of centers generally led to an increase in number—from about thirty to forty-four—which called for some revisions in basic accounting practices. Labor costs, for example, were much more accurately accounted. Transfers of personnel among centers required more reporting, particularly in nursing, where they are common, and several new responsibility centers were created. It turned out, however, that the nursing department was already recording these transfers. All that was required was a transfer of information to the time cards.

When the realignment in centers was complete, the chart of accounts had to be recoded to reflect the hierarchy of the organization by which the individual centers were grouped. This also provided for future groupings of responsibility centers for management reporting.

Several additional elements of activity are necessary to reap the benefits of the revision of the accounting system. These include the development of convenient, participative budget policies and procedures, revisions of other parts of the accounting and information systems (especially payroll), and revision of the accounting cycle to provide timely and accurate information.

## Output Data Systems

Each department in a hospital is responsible for some *output*, whether it be services to patients or to other departments, dealing with insurance companies or other outside agencies, or fabricating products for use by patients or employees. Each activity requires a process in which various resources are used. Outputs are a cause of growing concern in terms of quality, quantity, availability, and cost. Naming and counting, or *measuring*, outputs is an inescapable result of this concern, and all systems using these measurements are limited by their success at this basic level.

In the control of costs, measuring both inputs and outputs is important, for the relative efficiency of a production process over time is the ratio of inputs over outputs. The measures used for inputs are fairly easy to identify. The resources themselves, supplies, manhours worked, plant and equipment, and so forth, are measured by long established accounting systems. Dollars, as calculated by accountants consistent with generally accepted accounting principles, are used as the common denominator.[2] Measurement of outputs in hospitals is far more complex. All departments have multiple processes, many of which are personal services individualized for each patient. This problem has received much less attention.

It is possible to control inputs alone, without a measure of output. Such a decision is common in two situations: (1) *Where measurement of output is very difficult or costly, such as medical records or social service.* Despite the size or importance of these activities, it is common to discuss only their inputs, or to relate inputs to a nonspecific output, such as discharges. (2) *Where the value of individual outputs is small, or difficult to use in adjusting inputs, such as telephone switchboards or information desks.* These activities too are frequently budgeted and measured by inputs alone. The general rule is that outputs should be measured, and exceptions should be made only in cases where the value, or utility, of output and efficiency measures is unlikely to exceed the cost of obtaining the measu. s. The situations described above are simply two different conditions of this rule. The rule can be extended to evaluate approximations and substitute measures of output. A proxy measure is useful if its value exceeds the cost of obtaining it, yet it should not be used if the added value of a better measure exceeds the added cost of obtaining the improvement. "Value" can be interpreted in terms of contribution to quality or cost control.

Apparently many hospitals have not systematically explored the value of added information. Certainly this was true of Baker Hospital, where the outputs of the dietary department and central supply were never counted despite the obvious control implications and the relative simplicity of maintaining the counts.

The general criterion can be expanded to a set of indicators regarding the need to measure specific outputs. These indicators are based on presumptions about whether or not use of measurements can be helpful to hospital management in controlling costs. They are:

**Quantity**—The value and quantity of output must be great enough to impact materially on cost control. (That is, trivial outputs have a low priority.)

**Variation**—The volume of output from time period to time period should be nonstationary. (Highly stable outputs have a low priority, at least for cost control purposes.)

**Consistency**—The output from time period to time period should be comparable. (If counts or measures cannot distinguish between varying outputs, they have a low priority.)

**Predictablity**—Management must plan production activities before they occur in order to have the necessary quantity and variety of resources available when needed. (Therefore, unpredictable output has a low priority.)

Examples of situations where these criteria are *not* met would be:

**Quantity**—Almost any department of a hospital has several byproducts or sidelines, such as answering questionnaires and inquiries. Completing questionnaires would generally be a trivial part of a department's production and would not routinely be counted as output.

**Variation**—The accounting department may be responsible for preparing the hospital's monthly financial statement. Precisely one such statement would be prepared each month. Therefore, tallying "monthly statements prepared" per month would not contribute to cost control.

**Consistency**—In the administration responsibility center of a hospital, the output is always changing as management directs its efforts to the issues that arise. Since the nature of the output is different in each month, tallies of specific tasks would not be useful for controlling the departmental costs.

**Predictability**—Delivery rooms of hospitals generally experience unpredictable levels of demand during short time periods such as days or weeks. Their activity is important for uses other than cost control and is always counted. The same kind of unpredictability occurs in the security department. Counting of its activity is difficult and is probably not useful for cost control of short-run expenses.

In these situations and others like them, inputs alone tend to be used for cost control purposes.

Once the input/output approach has been selected for cost control, the examination of measurement alternatives comes to the fore. The choice is often clouded by the multiplicity of processes in each department, and the specific purposes of the measurements, as well as the technical ability to measure and quantify.

The criteria for the selection of output measures for purposes of cost control are:

- *The measures should be valid. That is, they should represent the result of the activity of the responsibility center, and should bear a relationship to input consumption.* Measures should quantify the outputs whose production consumes the majority of the responsibility center's inputs.
- *The measures and the measurement system must be reliable.* That is, the same level of activity should yield those same measurements when measured repeatedly over time, or by different personnel.
- *The measure should be practical to quantify and use.* That is, it should be feasible for data collection, inexpensive to obtain, auditable, and understandable to management at all levels.

The purpose of measuring in this case is cost control. If quality control or revenue control were the goal, particularly the first criterion and its application might be very different.

These criteria tend to be conflicting; greater validity and reliability are obtained at the expense of practicality. For instance, in nursing it is known that patient days are not uniform measures of patient care requirements. A number of other factors have been identified in the literature, and in fact, are incorporated in daily nurse assignment models reported in section

III.4. The addition of sickness classification of patients and of time consuming tasks such as interfloor transfers and special treatments improves the reliablity and validity of the output measure, but at the cost of increased data collection expense, auditability, and clarity of the measure. Patient days alone are routinely double counted, by nursing and the business office, to verify the statistic. Such a procedure is impossible with more complex measures, until an automated data system extracts and processes a considerably larger volume of statistics from business office records (such as transfers and special treatments) than is currently the practice at Baker.

The development of output measures should be evolutionary, following rather than being a precondition to systems for budgeting, cost control, personnel and patient scheduling, and automated data processing. That is, where there is no output measure, budgets and controls should be based on inputs alone. Where imperfect measures, such as patient days, exist, they should be used to the extent that they are acceptable to line management in terms of validity and reliability, and to accounting in terms of practicality. As automated systems evolve, they should incorporate improvements in output measures where these can be justified as improvements in the control function.

The actual output measures initially used at Baker Hospital were:

| | |
|---|---|
| All Nursing Units | — patient days |
| Emergency Room | — patients seen |
| Operating Room | — relative value units[3] |
| Delivery Room | — live births |
| Radiology | — examinations |
| Pathology | — relative value units[4] |
| Physical Therapy | — treatments |
| Respiratory Therapy | — relative value units[5] |
| EKG-EEG | — procedures |
| Anesthesia | — procedures |
| Pharmacy | — prescriptions |

The responsibility centers in which these units were used accounted for a large part of total hospital expenses, and although some of the criteria are crude, they did help management begin to focus on output and results, efficiency measures of input to output, and management by objectives.

Problems existed with the above measures, most notably in operating room, pathology, and respiratory therapy. Despite the weighting of the operating room scale, it did not meet the reliability criterion because of high variation in the length and mix of procedures. In pathology, the practicality of the scale used must be questioned. It was costly to collect, unaudited, and misunderstood by some people called upon to use it. Finally, in respiratory therapy, the scale failed on two counts, reliability and practicality. It was originally adopted as a trial, not tested, but never abandoned. It simply did not produce reliable results, was not understood by most of its users, and was not subject to audit. These experiences confirmed the importance of following the criteria detailed above and the importance of routinely examining the validity of the measures selected in a dynamic system.

## NOTES

[1]American Hospital Association, *Budgeting Procedures for Hospitals.* Chicago: The Association, 1971, pp. 7-9.

Robert N. Anthony, *Management Accounting: Text and Cases.* Homewood, IL: Richard D. Irwin, Inc., 1970, pp. 378-381.

Arthur Battauer, "Responsibility Accounting Provides Controls." *Hospitals,* Vol. 45, August 1, 1972, Part 1, pp. 67-70.

Charles T. Horngren, *Accounting for Management Control.* Englewood Cliffs, NJ: Prentice-Hall, Inc., 1970, chapter 11 and p. 579.

Thomas R. Prince, *Information Systems for Management Planning and Control.* Homewood, IL: Richard D. Irwin, Inc., 1970, chapter 5.

[2]Paul Grady, *Inventory of Generally Accepted Accounting Principles for Business Enterprises, Accounting Research Study No. 6.* New York: American Institute of Certified Public Accountants, Inc., 1965.

[3]Howard J. Berman and Lewis E. Weeks, *The Financial Management of Hospitals, Second Edition.* Ann Arbor: The Health Administration Press, 1974.

[4]College of American Pathologists Relative Value Unit Scale. Published periodically by the College of American Pathologists, 230 N. Michigan Avenue, Chicago, Illinois 60601.

[5]Berman and Weeks, *Financial Management.*

# Section IV

# The Human Problems of Implementation

Control systems do not implement themselves, regardless of how well they are designed. As Aesop pointed out in his fable, once the warning system of alerting the mice by putting a bell on the cat was determined, there remained the problem of implementing it. The focus of this study is control systems, but in this section we consider some of the issues which arise when implementing these systems in hospitals. The first chapter deals directly with the problem of implementing new systems, and proposes several guides for successful implementation. The second chapter considers the reasons for long-term deterioration in control systems, and identifies the system characteristics necessary to avoid such deterioration. The three following chapters report the experience of the Bureau research team as it was working in two study hospitals; the final chapter draws some conclusions from the Bureau team's experience in implementing change.

# IV.1

# Implementation of Hospital Control Systems[1]

*by Fred C. Munson and Walton M. Hancock*

Organizational requirements for the successful introduction of control systems are outlined here. It is easy to state a requirement, more difficult to know how to meet it. Therefore we will also outline the mechanisms we found useful in implementing our control systems in the study hospitals.

Successful organization change usually happens only when a good idea is well implemented. These normative criteria, excellence of idea and application, often cause attention to focus on one or the other of two distinct bodies of knowledge. Assuring the merit of the innovation requires technical experts in whatever discipline or profession is relevant; assuring the success of the implementation process requires the use of behavioral experts in the unique, dynamic, and richly complex sociotechnical system in which the innovation will be introduced.

From the technical and behavioral orientations come separate streams of scholars (industrial engineers versus organization psychologists), scholarly literature (*Operations Research* versus *Human Relations*), and indeed conceptions of purpose. The behavioral group defines success within a homeostatic model, the technical group in an optimization model. Thus a fertile ground for conflict is provided. Behavioral specialists ridicule the management scientist who designs a cost saving innovation that is never accepted; technical specialists ridicule the change agent who labors mightily for participation in the design of a system that a beginning student in plant layout could improve. Although the title of our chapter suggests the behavioral point of view as a starting point, our purpose is to consider the necessary interfacing between the two approaches.

Implementation is a process, a set of events which occur in sequence. The underlying framework is one of unfreezing, moving, and refreezing the task behavior of individuals, and our purpose is to operationalize certain concepts when this framework is applied to the introduction of control systems.[2]

In changing control systems, many persons may be involved. Figure IV.1.1 shows the major linkages in the admitting process for adult, nonemergency, surgical patients. The content and order of communications is not shown. For other admissions, minor differences would appear, and for the associated discharge process, a separate diagram with additional boxes would be needed.

A change in the admitting/discharge process would not only involve persons linked in these networks, but one or more persons in central administration, the same in nursing administration, the medical staff (as an organization) and its executive committee, plus the external group if the source of the innovation is outside the hospital. The importance of mere numbers arises from the complex nature of the change process. To unfreeze, move, and refreeze the conception of task in a large number of individuals is not a trivial problem.

We are satisfied that success in implementing a change in a control system has three basic requirements:

- The innovation be well devised in a technical sense, so that it clearly achieves the objective that gave rise to it.
- The attitude of critical actors be favorable, or at least neutral, toward the innovation.
- Those who must perform new tasks learn to perform the required actions correctly.

We understand each of these to be necessary and, taken together, sufficient conditions for the successful implementation of change. Excluded here is an important precondition for change, that goals of powerful members be consistent with the purposes of the innovation. We specify this as a precondition because the basis of power for such members often arises outside of the organization, and is therefore likely to be impervious to internal modifications of structure. We cannot ask the change process to do well on something it cannot affect. Therefore we treat goal congruence among powerful members as a precondition, rather than as a variable within the control of the innovators. The balance of this chapter will spell out the significance of the three criteria and will identify a process of negotiating and renegotiating the substance of the innovation. The final paragraphs will discuss some typical problems of handling the negotiating process.

## The Innovation Be Well Devised in a Technical Sense

Technical requirements for an innovation require an explicit statement of the objective, so that the technical requirements can be continuously reviewed against it. Examples of objectives that exist in the hospital field are as follows:

**a.** To minimize the cost of community health care.

**b.** To minimize the cost of operating a hospital where the quality of care is maintained at stated levels.

**c.** To provide a radiology service that will minimize the total cost of care per patient.

**d.** To provide a radiology service at minimum cost with respect to the radiology department's budget.

Each of the above objectives is sufficiently different that the technical requirements of designing an innovation would be affected. For example, **objective a** would require a detailed examination of duplicating services between hospital facilities within a community; **objective b** would not contain such a requirement. **Objective c** and **objective d** are different because **objective d** would require an examination of the use of resources used to meet a predicted demand where the radiology department would be considered a separate entity. **Objective c** would require that not only the operation of the department itself be examined, but the interaction of the department with the physicians and nurses be examined regarding the timeliness of the information. It is quite conceivable that the implementation of **objective d** would result in a nonoptimum solution with regard to **objective c.**

Once an objective is stated, the role of the technical expert in the innovation process is to provide an explicit statement of the best method with respect to contemporary technology. The technical requirements must be stated without consideration of the local environment under which the innovation might occur. The reason for the emphasis on a technical solution independent of local conditions is that the technical expert's initial function is to provide the most complete solution possible to accomplish the objective. The explicit statement of the solution then forms a basis for evaluating the cost of the compromises that may have to be made during any particular implementation of the system. Knowing this cost, in terms of what is being considered versus what is technically possible, decision makers will be in a better position to evaluate whether or not the compromise should be made. Once we permit the technical expert to take into account local conditions, it is very difficult to evaluate whether or not his recommended solution is consistent with contemporary technology.

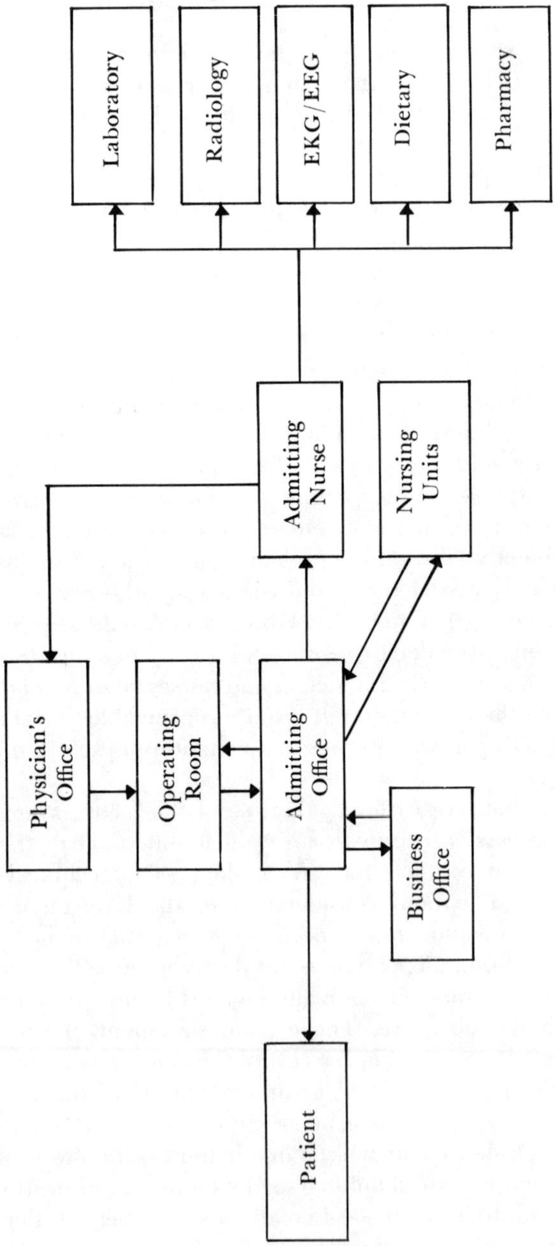


**FIGURE IV.1.1**
Admitting process for adult, nonemergency, surgical cases

As an example of the role of the technical expert, let us consider **objective b**—that we desire to minimize the cost of operating a hospital with quality levels maintained. This, in terms of operation research methodologies, is an optimization problem with quality constraints. If there is sufficient legitimate demand (demand that excludes unnecessary admissions or excessive lengths of stay), one of the ways to minimize the cost is to maximize throughput. The correct technical solution to this problem should contain the following elements:

• An analysis of the demand placed upon the hospital with respect to the patient inflows for the day of the week, between weeks, and between seasons. Specific applications would include separate analyses for inpatient and outpatient services, medical, surgical, psychiatric, or other subclasses of patients within the hospital.

• Any constraints imposed by the physical structure should be examined. Where actual physical constraints exist, then patient waiting lines will also exist. The significance of the constraints in many cases can be measured by the length and rate of turnover of the waiting line. Characteristic of typical constraints are the number of beds or the number of operating rooms.

• The operating procedures which affect the allocation of resources should be examined. For example, since the admissions department in many hospitals commits the resources of the hospital to the patient upon admission for a period of time in the future, the role of admissions, the interaction of admissions and the service departments and the knowledge of the state of use of resources at any given time have to be determined. A minimum cost solution requires that the resources available are sufficient to meet all quality needs, but not in excess.

Sufficient resources must be available at the time the service is needed for it to be rendered. Resources here clearly include personnel, and the training and qualifications of people necessary to give the service have to be examined.

In brief, a technically feasible model to minimize the cost of operating a hospital requires that we allocate resources as a function of the input demand, subject to the constraints that all of the resources will be consumed and that no physical or quality constraints are violated. For example, in Able Hospital the analysis of demand indicated that the hospital physical facility would not be fully utilized over a ten-year horizon. In addition, there were wide variations in the census in the hospital which reflected an admissions policy of admitting patients immediately. A result of these procedures was that personnel and other resources were established to meet all possible levels of demand. The adoption of **objective b** indicated that the admission of some patients should be delayed in order to stabilize demand so that the labor resources of the hospital could be reduced to a level consistent with the steady state need for these resources. In Baker Hospital, analysis indicated that demand was equal to or greater than the physical facilities (beds) of the hospital. Yet, the hospital was operating at approximately eighty-five percent census. There were empty beds in the hospital even though the demand was available to fill the beds. Since there was a physical constraint as well as other constraints imposed by the operating procedures of the hospital, the variations in demand were quite low. The accomplishment of the objective required improving the hospital operating procedures and then determining the size of the nursing staff and service staff so that when the beds were all full the quality constraint would not be violated. In the two facilities the objective was the same, but the technical requirements differed depending upon the relationship between demand and whether or not the demand was constrained by a physical or nonphysical constraint.

A technically optimal solution must also be a complete solution. Developing parts of an innovation is easily rationalized as "allowing full participation" but leads to wasted effort and ill will. A proposed change in radiology scheduling should not only include technically correct solutions for the radiology department, but also for the interfacing of these changes with nursing units, the outpatient department, and other hospital units which form the environment of the radiology department. We have found it quite common to dispose of such a connective as "a minor detail," only to discover upon investigation it is neither minor in the technical difficulty of solving it, nor in the consequences to the success of the innovation. It is not necessary or desirable to have the organizationally best solution, a point which will be developed in the following section. It is both possible and necessary to identify obvious connectives of a new procedure with other hospital systems, and to determine the technically correct method of information, patient, or other flows between the systems.

To summarize, if an innovation is well devised in a technical sense, it will be referenced to an explicit statement of objectives, will be the soundest technically available solution, will be complete in covering observed connections with other parts of the system, but will not contain the compromises and adjustments necessary to make it the organizationally best solution. This is the initial requirement for successful change, but only one of three requirements.

## The Attitude of Critical Actors Be Favorable

The problem of securing favorable attitudes from system members is important only for those system members with a relevant basis of power. It is nice to have favorable attitudes in everybody, but it is necessary to have them only in those whose support determines the success or failure of an innovation. Our understanding of the relevant literature suggests that many supporters of participation claim too much, seeking to prove that participants with little power have much power in determining productivity.[3] We will consider later the practical problem of defining who counts, after we have discussed the mechanism of attitude change.

Resistance to change rarely arises from mindless opposition to everything new. It is usually a reasonable response to avoiding one or more of three problems. Change may cause a member to lose status, influence, or valued relations, in short, to lose something of value.[4] The "may" (the uncertainty) is as much a part of the problem as what will be lost. Second, a specific change may simply not fit within the complex social and technical networks that bind any organization together.[5]

Finally, a change requires a person to raise "why am I here?" type questions, to rethink relations between means and ends, and therefore to consider whether some hitherto unexpressed purposes are in fact legitimate.[6] A reasonable approach to overcoming resistance to change will deal with these causes.

The most direct method is to involve the system members in the change, fully engaging them in the development of the innovation. Only by this involvement can a system member learn enough about the innovation to decide how much it will add or detract from the balance of benefits he receives under the status quo. If the member suffers a clear loss, he rationally must either oppose the change or seek modifications in it. In our experience the individual gain or loss is less often a basis for resisting change than a well based conviction that it will not work. Drucker is correct in suggesting that General Motors executives (or hospital head nurses) will find many compromises with the technically correct solution, but one must recognize that these people are true experts in defining nontechnical but very important elements of the constraint set that will fit an innovation to the existing procedures, status relations, and other attributes of that part of the organization which the innovation affects.[7] Compromise is bad only if one is inflexibly commited to the innovation, rather than the results it is intended to achieve. In problems of fitting the innovation to the system, the technically qualified experts are the novices, and cannot match the knowledge base of the system members.

When two groups with different but equally relevant expertise are interested in the implementation of an innovation, a clear basis for conflict exists. If one thinks of resolving this through "participation," an implicit assumption is that one group (with power) is allowing another group (without power) to participate. But relevant knowledge is a basis for power, and it is more reasonable to think of resolving the conflict through negotiation. A rough equality of power and interest in the outcome, and a symmetry in the relation between groups is acknowledged in calling a process a negotiation.[8] We offer below several examples of this distinction between participation and negotiation.

In the initial development of an information system for department heads, it was necessary to define units of output for each department. Department heads participated in providing information that allowed such output units to be defined. The developed information system required department heads to use forecasts of output to make staffing adjustments for a future four-week period. At this point negotiations began, for department heads criticized the requirement, pointing out they had inadequate information from payroll. This "rather minor detail" led the research team into a forest of problems which has taken nearly twenty-four months to clarify, and to develop (but not yet implement) a reliable and timely reporting system for department heads.

The operating room supervisor in one of the hospitals found it unpleasant to contemplate a shift in scheduling procedure that would reduce the ability of the operating room to control its own scheduling. Initially, the supervisor was able both to ignore the proposed scheduling revisions and involve some surgeons in the issue. Discussions with surgeons helped neutralize that potential source of resistance, and the use of the hospital administrator's authority legitimated the research team's proposal. In about three months the four-sided (admitting office, operating room, surgeons, research team) negotiation was completed, and the basically unmodified component of the scheduling system that affected the operating room was accepted and used. We should emphasize that our concept of negotiation is in no way limited to people sitting on two sides of a table arguing. The setting may be a board room or a hallway, it may start with a formal presentation or be concealed in a general discussion of problems, it may have two clear "sides" represented or may have a whole series of interests being asserted or defended, it may be restricted to verbal exchange or as in the case of the operating room supervisor, be communication through action. The example below also illustrates how effectively action, in this case by admitting physicians, can be used to communicate a negotiating position.

The final illustration comes from the implementation of the original admitting/discharge model.[9] In this hospital physicians in a medical staff meeting participated in (approved) the final design of the patient scheduling system. When implemented, however, physicians who were asked to delay admissions began admitting patients to another hospital, a bargaining tactic which so impressed the administrator that he considered eliminating the whole program. The controller, drawn into earlier negotiations because the innovation used computer facilities under his control, supported a compromise which would reduce the financial benefits of the innovation but minimize the number of admission delays experienced by physicians. The outcome of this, and a rather similar negotiation with physicians about the manner of securing discharge data estimates, was a substantially modified system which had cost savings much less than the initial design, but a level of fit for the key actors which allowed it to exist. In fact, the savings were not clearly greater than the operating cost of the system, and with less psychic investment in the innovation the research team might well have suggested its abandonment. In our experience, however, we find it nearly as difficult to abandon an innovation we have labored to produce as it is for hospital personnel to abandon work methods they have come to accept as their occupational reason for being.

We should like to emphasize that in each of the illustrations, and others that could have been given, technical experts were qualified to apply current state of the art knowledge to the achievement of specific goals, and system members were qualified to adapt these proposals to the unique sociotechnical system. The experts' problem can be stated as someone else's resistance to change, but that is misleading. The true issue is whether, and in what form, an innovation will be introduced in a hospital.

The negotiations cause pain in both parties. The pain experienced by system members is well recognized; it is also experienced by technical experts. In the case of the department head information reporting system, the original innovation was discussed, explained, illustrated, and otherwise sold to a rather passive group of department heads. Only when it was experimentally introduced did the department heads begin to point out problems. When those problems were acknowledged, roles were reversed and department heads were change agents, anxious to unfreeze the research team from allegiance to the original idea and forcing them to accept the need for adaptations. These adaptations were developed and brought back, again challenged by department heads and again renegotiated, with the Bureau team facing the unpleasant possibility that funding would end before results were in. The experts experienced the pain that comes when good ideas, carefully thought out, tested, and refined in discussion, commited to paper and asserted in talks, publicly presented as evidence of competence and accepted as such, are threatened by the very people who must make them work if the experts are to make good on their promises.

The symmetry in this relation of technical experts and system members is important to understand and often ignored. Unless those who design the change recognize that system members are also experts, properly credentialed to require change in the outsider proposals, then expert efforts will be directed toward manipulation of the system members, forcing them to accept ideas, and in other ways denying the valid basis of system members' expertise. Among academicians this is called (incorrectly and pejoratively) "overcoming resistance to change." Only when the symmetry in the relation is recognized is it possible to recognize that successful system member inputs are the assertion of additional constraints to the original set, and to evaluate that new constraint set which the innovation must now be designed to fit.

Recognizing the symmetry of the change process permits system members to adapt the innovation to fit their system; it also forces both technical experts and system members to repeatedly distinguish between the purpose of an innovation, and the mechanism (the innovation itself) designed to achieve it. The system member faces greater difficulty than the expert in giving up a focus on means and refocusing on ends, though the problem exists for both. Inevitably, genuine negotiations turn to issues of what will work, and finally to why do anything. The honest confrontation of this latter question is fortunately difficult to avoid in the negotiations, and is a central part of refocusing on goals. The negotiation/renegotiation process between technical experts and system members pictured in figure IV.1.2 encourages a constant review of purpose, and thus protects the attainment of purpose for which the innovation was designed.

Neither experts nor system members speak with one voice. The status quo in either group is in reality an often delicate balance of opposing interests that many may find unpleasant, but none finds intolerable. Internal negotiations are a continuing process in any complex organization, and have been made a central part of several theoretic models of the firm.[10] An important part of the attitude change process is to establish mechanisms for bargaining between system members which are appropriate to the social system of the organization. Open discussion is always a preferred

**FIGURE IV.1.2**
The negotiating process

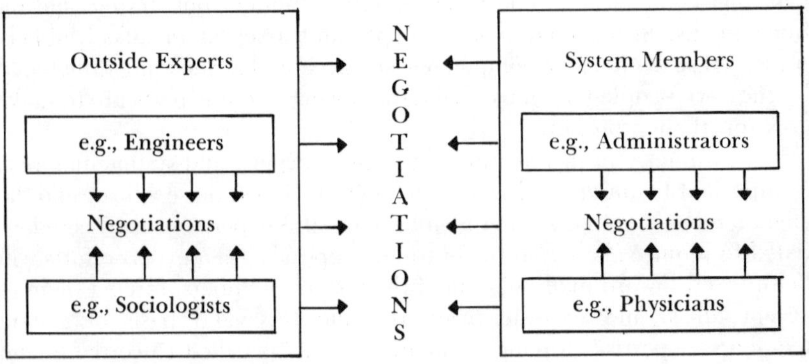

method, but both the status system of the hospital and the occasional existence of deep mistrust or hostility may make it impractical. We have found it helpful to assign individual members of our group to be contact persons with key system members, both to keep them fully informed and also to develop alternative methods of hammering out compromise between system members when open negotiations are initially not possible.

A brief summary may help reemphasize the focal role we give to the negotiation/renegotiation process. Recognition of the symmetry of the change process between change designers and system members encourages honest negotiation and renegotiation. This process, by acknowledging the expert role of the system members, permits their meaningful participation in the design process, and this allows them to:

• Clarify the consequences for them of adopting the innovation; therefore to know whether they will gain or lose something of value.

• Fit the innovation to the system by requiring the change designers to accept the additional constraints needed and modify the innovation to meet them.

• Rethink relations between means and ends, and thus become open (unfrozen) to the possibility of new means being more appropriate. The negotiation/renegotiation process, in short, deals with the causes of resistance to change that apply to both system members and technical experts.

## Learning To Perform Required Actions

Contrary to some beliefs about human nature, it is not the natural state of man to resist new ideas. It is natural to resist useless or troublesome information, and equally natural to be curious, problem solving, and anxious to experiment. The first step of learning is motivation, to be in a setting which evokes the second response set. It is sometimes (in our experiences often) necessary to provide this motivation by troubling people when they continue to use their present repertoire of skills. Providing feedback of bad current results often troubles people enough so that they wish to find new methods to achieve better results. Simply requiring a new task performance may trouble people enough to want to learn how to perform it. Fortunately, most persons have aspirations which already exceed their achievements, and the problem is to show them that alternative methods will narrow that gap. For example, two key physicians in one of the hospitals were already troubled by excessive lengths of stay: it was only necessary to show them that a proposed change in the admitting process could reduce length of stay for some patients by as much as one day, and their interest was assured. It was less easy to show admitting office personnel that maintaining several new records was important; their aspirations did not place high value on improved holiday scheduling or reduced cancellations, which in the past had been no part of their concerns. Thus it is often necessary to establish a setting in which new behaviors are required before there is sufficient motivation to learn them. The system actors may deal with a proposed change by ignoring or otherwise delaying it unless it is actually introduced. To provide teaching and to assume learning is to ignore the need for motivation. When motivation exists, learning is possible and teaching becomes relevant. The simple need to train in specific behaviors is the most important aspect of this step. Unthinking adherence to a practice is not good but is bliss compared to the chaos of an "it will become clearer as you go along" approach to training. Refreezing is a central requirement of successful change, and few things hinder it more than significantly increased error rates, angered employees, irate doctors, and similar results which a badly operated new system produces.

In the introduction of a department head information system directed toward staffing control, the three training requirements appeared to be:

• What department heads should expect to receive (forecasts, cost reports, etc.).

• What they should do (compare with prior period report and with budget, determine current and expected staffing, adjust forecast to expected local and specific causes of variation in future volume).

• What search process and decision rules they should use (with lower expected volume: review scheduled overtime, check with nursing administration to see if an employee can be loaned, etc; select an alternative that balances hours with expected requirements).

These requirements are applied in different ways to department heads and higher levels of administration, and to those in the hospital who would be generating the information and interfacing with the computer. The tendency to "train by results," telling system members to achieve a result rather than training them to perform a task is perhaps natural (it substantially reduces what the trainer must understand) but leads inevitably to problems. System members, when asked to perform in ways that are new to them, become heavily dependent upon the outside experts to provide them with precise information on what to do next in order to perform the new functions. Since many of these requests for what to do may be considered unimportant details by the expert, he may not readily have the answers. Operating people then become less secure, and may also wish to return to previous procedures. The outside expert must have thought about as many of the questions regarding the required actions by the operating people as possible to be able to answer promptly and with authority questions regarding the actions necessary to implement the system. We are currently experimenting with simulation of the admitting process to see whether it is possible to offer direct experience with the search and decision component of training. This method may avoid the stress which accompanies experimenting in the live situation, arising from the anticipation of the real consequences of poor decisions.

Whether by classroom instruction, on-the-job training, simulation, or other methods, the key to the skill acquisition step in learning is the concentration on specifics. This is both because tasks cannot be completed with generalities but only with specific behaviors, and because confidence grows fastest as specifics are mastered and how-to knowledge becomes recognizably complete.

There is a fine but significant distinction between knowing how to do something and actually being able to do it. It is the distinction between swimming with and without a supporting hand, the distinction between knowing and using a skill. Often it is not certain whether a skill has been acquired until live application begins. A complicating factor in this step when implementing new control systems or similar organizational changes is that only rarely are the recently acquired new skills both appropriate and complete. As we have earlier indicated, negotiations continue during the initial introduction. Therefore, modifications continue to be made in the innovation, and necessarily in the required behaviors.

The first trial of the new behaviors is not only a key step in the learning process, it is also a key one in determining how well the initial requirement of a technically complete solution is met. An example is in an early implementation of the admission scheduling system. In this case, the admissions officer was given a computer output and instructed that when the physician called he was to admit patients subject to the constraints of admission given to him through the computer output. The problems arose when the physicians' offices called to have patients admitted and were also asked by the admissions personnel to give an estimate of the length of the stay of the patient. This was the first time that this type of information was ever requested. The reactions of the physicians varied: some physicians were willing to give estimates; others asked what the estimates really meant; and others flatly refused to give an estimate. In addition, the technical experts did not anticipate that in many cases the physicians' secretaries did the calling. During the introduction of this system, there were repeated questions by the admissions personnel as to how to handle these situations. The implementation of the system was hurt because the research team had not anticipated many of the questions and did not have answers readily available. In later implementation more thought has been given to this stage, and to the need for gradual transition from constantly present to readily available support, and from there to eventual disengagement of the technical experts from the ongoing process.

Meeting this third requirement of having system actors to perform the required actions is closely akin to the Lewinian change model. In Table IV.1.1 below we summarize this relation.

**TABLE IV.1.1**
Stages of the change and learning process

| | | |
|---|---|---|
| Frozen | – Precondition | – Stability |
| Unfreeze | – Motivation to learn | – Rethinking goals, considering alternatives |
| Move | – Skill Acquisition | – Learning new methods, feelings of insecurity |
| Refreeze | – Skill application | – "I like it! It really works!" |
| Frozen | – Postcondition | – Stability |

## Handling Negotiations

What we have called the negotiation/renegotiation process is important in meeting all three criteria for successful implementation. Its formal purpose is to make the required refinement in the substantive content of the innovation to turn the technically optimal into the organizationally feasible solution. The sequence of repeated negotiations gives time and opportunity for attitudes to change, and the nature of negotiation makes learning the new skills natural and necessary. We conclude this chapter with some issues we have identified in making negotiation work.

### The Need for Internal Committees

An innovation which affects many sets of actors requires either many sets of negotiations, or more complex negotiations between technical experts and system members with potentially conflicting modifications to propose. It is in such cases that internal committees have their greatest value. System members' ability to influence the change designers is maximized by giving organizational recognition to such a group. Most important, an explicit arena is identified for the internal negotiations that are required to allow each system member to unfreeze and gradually move toward acceptance of the new consensus required by the (modified) innovation. We have said earlier that the technical experts must sometimes assist system members in making these internal negotiations genuine. The nursing department in one hospital had difficulty developing such a group, though the need was clear. Our practice is gradually turning to the initial identification of key members, and attempting to treat them as an entity. Where mistrust is high this is not feasible at the start, for people who mistrust each other will not communicate honestly. Dealing with groups also means delay in scheduling discussions, but on balance it is better to build groups and accept delays than to fail in developing a group of the key members which permits honest negotiation.

## The Need to Negotiate with the Right Group

The centrality of an innovation to a member and his ability to determine its success will determine the importance of involving him in the negotiation/renegotiation process. An innovation which touches everyone in the organization could have negotiation costs which far outweigh its estimated benefits. Given perfect knowledge about the centrality and power of each member, negotiations would be limited to that group of members which would result in the highest net advantage of the innovation. Perfect knowledge does not exist, and decisions must be made which make assumptions about the centrality and power of each member; negotiations would be limited to that group of members which would result in the highest net advantage of the innovation. In introducing the admitting system, for example, no effort was made to involve each admitting physician directly, and in one of the study hospitals only two representative physicians were involved in initial meetings. They were present in the discussion with the executive committee of the medical staff, and at the medical staff meeting in which approval was requested from all admitting physicians. By contrast, in the staffing control innovation, all cost center heads were directly involved. In practice, we discover additional system members as they become powerful at different stages of the innovation. (This element of a successful implementation program came to our attention in the evaluation of service unit management programs.)[11]

## The Need for Open Communication

We have alluded to the internal negotiation which takes place in the hospital as a feasible solution is being generated. Internal negotiation also occurs among the technical experts. Sociologists and engineers, for reasons mentioned at the beginning of this chapter, do find issues on which communication is difficult. Yet curiously this is not the most important problem. If the sociologist is the one who has developed an innovation and is carrying it to the hospital setting, it may be the engineer who helps him recognize that system members have the right, and the power, to force changes upon him if the changes make the innovation fit the system better. Much internal negotiation has taken place in the quite supportive environment of our Bureau research group.

## The Need for Protecting System Members

The fact that in our own group changes were negotiated in a basically friendly environment has helped us recognize that negotiations need not be antagonistic, and that once system member involvement is secured, the negotiation process in the hospital can provide a nonthreatening environment in which real issues can be faced, including uncertainty about ability to perform, and questions about goals. ("Does cost really make that much difference? After all, most patients are covered by insurance.") One of the desirable methods of securing the joint products of the negotiation/renegotiation process is to implement early on a pilot basis, and then to proceed with modifications and training. The explicitly tentative, experimental setting is itself a protection from organizational criticism, and from a sense of failure when things go badly. Our experience is that additional protection sometimes is required when the results of an innovation are strongly desired by a powerful system member (the hospital administrator). In such cases the experts have either joined with system members to resist excessive pressure, or developed in advance with the administrator the necessary protection from an early demand for results.

## The Common Need to Change the System

A fortunate, though problem causing, byproduct of negotiation is the uncovering of clearly bad practices. Three examples will suffice. A part of the evidence adduced by a system member to prove that a department's output could not be forecast by conventional techniques was the (accurate) assertion that some physicians who rotated through the department would significantly increase the number of tests requested when they personally were receiving the fees. Another department challenged the possibility of developing an output measure by the (again accurate) assertion that many of the supplies issued were not recorded in departmental records. Finally, much trouble in resolving inconsistencies between different sources for manhour reports was eventually tracked down to a reporting practice that showed for example, 100 overtime hours as 150 hours worked. The reporting of on-call hours and pay was equally confused. The elimination of such practices is of course desirable as an end in itself, but their identification through the negotiation/renegotiation process gives further evidence that system members are indeed experts at identifying what has to be changed in the hospital environment, as well as in the innovation, before the latter can be fit into the system and frozen into place.

## The Need to Recognize that People Need Time To Change

One great advantage in acknowledging the negotiation/renegotiation process is that we have become more sensitive to time as a variable. We recognize that for others, like us, time needs to pass for ideas to become acceptable. An order can be followed in seconds; an idea cannot be accepted so quickly. In one hospital the controller was not enthusiastic about the admitting system for two months. Yet when the first challenge came from the physicians, he was among its strongest supporters. By treating negotiation as a part of the implementation process we have recognized that time is needed for attitudes to change, as clearly as it is needed to design the technically correct method.

## The Need for Managerial Resources

We occasionally find administrators who cannot accept an obvious corollary of our experience, that if the three requirements (excellence of the innovation, supportive key participants, and their ability to act) are really requirements, then we have specified a demand on managerial resources that cannot be avoided. In the study hospitals the Bureau research staff made up some of that required resource, but outsiders have limitations as well as advantages, and the absence of internal hospital resources to support the change process has caused significant delays in several of the innovations. We now believe that a hospital with a thinly staffed management structure may find it nearly impossible to introduce significant structural changes without major damage to the morale and effectiveness of the institution.

The resources requirements are varied. Technical assistance in data processing, sophistication in adapting forecasting models, assisting in budget preparations, advice on dealing with recalcitrant or insecure subordinates, technical training, facilitating open communication during internal negotiations—these are some of the skill requirements which can be supplemented by outsiders. But the competence and depth of a strong department head group cannot be replaced by consultants, for the possibility of using task forces or ad hoc committees to be the internal change group cannot come from outside the organization. It rests on having management personnel with the competence to perform in such a group, and with backup that allows them the time to do it. Our interest is in the implementation of control systems, not the introduction of new management structures, yet we must say that a hospital which wishes to improve its control or any other system should first invest in its human organization.

## Summary

Our experience in implementing change in the study hospitals has taught us that three requirements are sufficiently important and identifiable to warrant their use as a focus of review and evaluation by those concerned with the implementation process. The first requirement is the excellence of the innovation itself. Our present feeling is that excellence is best reached by starting with a complete and technically optimal method for reaching a given purpose, and modifying it to meet local conditions only after that optimal definition is made. The second requirement is a favorable attitude on the part of key participants. This has required us to think carefully of which participants are key, and what demands they will make on the innovations. Third is the ability of the participants to take the required actions; and there we have learned to accept training, whether achieved through programmed instruction, simulation models, formal lectures, the provision of incentives, hands-on guidance, group discussion, feedback of results, or any other training method, as a key obligation of the change designers.

### Process

It has become clear to us that it is dangerously easy to slip over into a manipulative mode in our relations with system members, and that an explicit acceptance of a negotiation/renegotiation model helps avoid that danger. It becomes the key process by which the technically optimal solution is transformed into an organizationally feasible solution, and also becomes the key process in identifying and dealing with the (usually sound) reasons of system members for opposing the innovation. The learning which takes place in a negotiating as opposed to a manipulating or persuading context has proven to be more lasting and effective, though it by no means replaces the need for explicit training programs when the major modifications in the innovation have been hammered out in the negotiating process. We have also come to recognize and deal more explicitly with the need for internal negotiations, both within our own research group, and among the key participants within the hospitals.

### Time Dimension

The negotiations have produced innumerable illustrations of the Lewinian proposition that organizational change is a process made up of attitudinal changes in individuals and groups. These changes take time, and a later step in the process (refreezing) cannot take place until the prior step (moving) has been passed. Therefore it is a gross error to ignore the probable time requirements for such attitude change. It is erroneous to assume that if resources are allocated, the intended change will take place. An intensive training session is a resource allocation, not the achievement of a step in the attitude change process. Needless to say, without the skilled human resources which can train, facilitate communication, find compromises, provide technical and social support, and perform the other tasks necessary to meet the three requirements, the prospects for successful change are very poor.

In the following chapter we report research carried out by a member of the research team which focuses on the probable long-term stability of efforts to change the information feedback to department heads in order to increase their effectiveness in controlling costs. Some of the difficulties identified in this chapter are reinforced, and some long-term requirements for avoiding system deterioration are specified.

## NOTES

[1]Adapted from Fred C. Munson and Walton M. Hancock, "Problems of Implementing Change in Two Hospital Settings." *AIIE Transactions*, December 1972, pp. 258-266.

[2]K. Lewin, "Group Decision and Social Change," in G. E. Swanson, T. M. Newcomb, and E. L. Hartley (eds.), *Readings in Social Psychology, Second Edition*. New York: Henry Holt, 1952, pp. 459-473.

[3]L. Coch and J. R. P. French, "Overcoming Resistance to Change." *Human Relations*, I, 1948, pp. 512-533.

J. R. P. French, Jr., J. Israel, and D. As, "An Experiment on Participation in a Norwegian Factory." *Human Relations*, XIII, 1961, pp. 3-19.

Rensis Likert, *New Patterns of Management*. New York: McGraw-Hill Book Co., 1961, chapters 4 and 8.

George Strauss, "Some Notes on Power-Equalization," in Harold J. Leavitt (ed.), *The Social Science of Organizations*. Englewood Cliffs, NJ: Prentice-Hall, 1963, pp. 40-84.

Dorwin Cartwright, "Power: A Neglected Variable in Social Psychology," in Warren G. Bennis, Kenneth D. Benne and Robert Chin (eds.), *The Planning of Change*. New York: Holt, Rinehart and Winston, 1962.

James Q. Wilson, "Innovation in Organization: Notes Toward a Theory," in James D. Thompson (ed.), *Approaches to Organizational Design*. Pittsburgh: University of Pittsburgh, 1966, pp. 193-218.

Rensis Likert, *The Human Organization: Its Management and Value*. New York: McGraw-Hill Book Co., 1967, chapters 3 and 4.

[4]Chester Barnard, *The Functions of the Executive*. Cambridge, MA: Harvard University Press, 1962, chapter 11.

Wilson, "Innovation in Organization."

[5]E. L. Trist and K. W. Bamforth, "Social and Psychological Consequences of the Longwall Method of Goal-Getting." *Human Relations*, IV, 1951, pp. 3-38.

Joan Woodward, *Industrial Organization: Theory and Practice*. London: Oxford University Press, 1965.

Likert, *The Human Organization*.

[6]Robert K. Merton, "Bureaucratic Structure and Personality," in Robert K. Merton (ed.), *Social Theory and Social Structure, revised edition*. New York: The Free Press of Glencoe, 1957, chapter 6.

Herbert A. Simon, "On the Concept of Organizational Goal." *Administrative Science Quarterly*, IX, 1964, pp. 1-22.

Richard M. Cyert and James G. March, *A Behavioral Theory of the Firm*. Englewood Cliffs, NJ: Prentice-Hall, 1963.

[7]Peter F. Drucker, "The Effective Decision." *Harvard Business Review*, January-February 1967, pp. 92-98.

[8]Dorwin Cartwright, "Influences, Leadership, Control," in James G. March (ed.), *Handbook of Organizations*. Chicago: Rand McNally, 1965, pp. 1-47.

[9]Galen P. Briggs, Jr., "Inpatient Admissions Scheduling: Application on a Nursing Service." Doctoral dissertation, The University of Michigan, 1972.

[10]Cyert and March, *Behavioral Theory*.

James D. Thompson, *Organizations in Action*. New York: McGraw-Hill Book Co., 1967, chapters 9 and 10.

[11]Richard C. Jelinek, Fred C. Munson, and Robert L. Smith, "SUM (Service Unit Management): An Organizational Approach to Improved Patient Care." A study report for the W. K. Kellogg Foundation, 1971.

# IV.2

# Long-Term Responses to Control Systems

*by M. David Ermann*

## Introduction

While the various control systems were being installed in Baker Hospital, the author was working independently of the Bureau team to evaluate department head response to external information demands of all kinds.[1] In this chapter he uses data gathered by himself and others to analyze the stability of changes in department head reporting procedures. These changes had several noteworthy characteristics:

- They were intended to produce a higher level of performance in the department generally and the department head specifically.
- They relied on data generated by the department to monitor its own achievement.
- At least in the study hospital, they were not reinforced with specific external requirements or sanctions. (These might be created in the future by competitive pressures, prospective reimbursement, tangible rewards for good departmental performance, and other devices.)
- They were devised and installed principally by the Bureau team, who are referred to as "technical experts" below, and who clearly had no permanent position in the organization.

The combination of these conditions makes it relatively easy for a department head to avoid coming permanently and realistically to grips with the changes. Further evidence that this is so can be adduced from the case studies of specific projects presented in the three chapters which follow. While the conclusions here may appear bleak, they serve to emphasize the difficulty of introducing innovations which must rely primarily on attitude changes, and the importance of making other changes in the organization which will support these attitudes. The author outlines the steps necessary to make progress permanent.

## Requirements for a Control System

The preceding chapter (IV.1) outlined requirements for technical experts to introduce a control system successfully. This chapter will outline the requirements for such a system to accomplish its goal after it has been introduced and technical experts have departed: to influence hospital behaviors in desirable ways over the long run.

Two major prerequisites for accomplishing this long-term goal will be explained here. The first is that attitudes of key actors must be altered in the process of introducing a new system. Lacking these attitudinal changes, there is reason to believe that key actors will seek, and find, ways to defeat the system. They usually will have little difficulty defeating the system when they are no longer constrained by a need to negotiate with outside technical experts.

The second prerequisite for long-term behavioral influence is that the system be capable of constraining the key actors when their attitudes have not been changed (or when their vested interests have overcome their new attitudes). As with weak attitude changes, we will argue that weak system constraints will permit system degeneration after negotiations with technical experts have ceased.

Two traits of the type of control system described in this study enhance its potential for long-run degeneration. First, many of its components rely on information supplied by the very people who are to be controlled. This creates the opportunity for the nonsupply of information after the technical experts have departed. More importantly, it creates the motive and opportunity for reporting departments to distort in their favor the information they do supply. Technical experts will not long be available to assess the quality of information departments provide.

Second, this type of system relies on hospital personnel to use it to control themselves and other hospital personnel. A project such as ours is concerned, not to use the system for its own purposes, but to insure that the hospital itself uses it. The project thus will have neither long-run sanctions nor long-run legitimacy to influence department head attitudes and behaviors. This creates the opportunity for long-run indifference to the controls, and the possibility that key actors will change the system to defeat its purposes.

The reader should not infer from these prefatory statements that we feel that key actors are recalcitrants who will invariably respond to innovations by trying to defeat them. Rather, he should recognize that the absence of attitudinal changes and system constraints will make innovations that appear frozen into behavior patterns when technical experts are present, begin to thaw after they have left. Often there is no thaw; too often there is.[2] Control systems introduced by technical experts (especially systems based on in-house data collection and in-house control) are notorious for their tendency to degenerate over time, particularly when the experts devote all their energy to introducing the system, and none to building the internal technical competence to support it. Therefore, long-term desirable responses to control systems can be secured only if the attitudes of key actors and the traits of the system preclude long-term undesirable responses.

The balance of this chapter will use our experience as a basis for discussing the role of attitude change and system design in preventing long-term degeneration of control systems.

## Attitude Changes and Long-Term Responses

There are many good reasons to have expected our newly instituted system to change the attitudes of those using it, even without manipulations by technical experts. Our system gives key personnel information quicker than they previously got it, and gives them much that they never received before. They therefore can be expected to ask questions that the system now has prepared them to answer.

Looking at budgets, Cyert and March come to essentially this conclusion, proposing broad changes that budgetary systems can cause. A budget, they say,

> tends to define—in advance—a set of fixed expectations. Although budgets can be flexible, they cannot help but result in the specification of a framework within which the firm will operate, evaluate its success, and alter its program.[3]

A similar case can be made for periodic reporting in general, whether we view hospitals as hierarchies or coalitions. We can view hopsitals as coalitions of semi-independent departments with only minimal communication between them. In this case we see that periodic reports initiated by technical experts will require communication between departments which previously were insulated from one another. Such information is potentially threatening, and can disrupt many established relationships.

On the other hand, we can view hospitals as hierarchies, where those on the top want information to use to control their subordinates. Here we see that periodic reports will permit superiors to establish objectives whose attainment they previously could not measure. The conventional wisdom supports this view, suggesting that preparing periodic reports serves to remind each subordinate that he must meet certain standards of performance. It postulates that personnel want to look good to their superiors and that they therefore will emphasize whatever is evaluated. Hence, it is argued, merely having poor performance in any area opened to exposure is often sufficient to make subordinates want to improve on that performance.

However, our project's experience indicates that, even with apparently successful introductions of information systems, the relevant attitudinal changes in the area we studied were minimal. We studied most rigorously attitude changes related to budgets. Here we will discuss two studies, done two years apart, beginning in the project's second year.[4] These studies evaluated the extent to which the new control system in fact changed the attitudes of department heads.

Department heads, the key actors in Bureau attempts to use budgets to change attitudes and behaviors, understandably were not cost conscious before the onset of the project. Until around the time the project began, they were not receiving information on their departments' costs and budget performances, and had been uninvolved in budget construction. However, the project expected, based on the literature, that they would become cost conscious (and therefore cost controllers) after they were given the needed cost-related information.

Somewhat to our surprise, our first study found that our new budget system had produced no attitudinal changes. No department head interviewed indicated, either directly or indirectly, that his goals for his department included the problems of cost control. In fact, a few explicitly denied these goals without even being asked. One said that his goal was to improve quality regardless of cost. Nevertheless, we continued to feel that these attitudes would change as department heads became more familiar with the new budgetary control system and the new responsibilities it implied.

Our second study, two years later, appeared at first to indicate that the budget system had been accepted and that it had resulted in changed attitudes. Department heads were quite conscious of the budgeting system. And they said, when discussing budgets, that, yes, cost control was indeed part of their responsibility. With some minor reservations with regard to specifics, they were unanimous in the opinion that the budgetary system was proving beneficial.

Unfortunately, this did not show that department heads' attitudes related to their whole jobs had changed. Before we asked them questions about their use of and attitudes toward budgets, we had asked them their general goals and objectives for their departments. And, after three years of effort by us and the hospital's administrator, only two of them included cost control (they used the word "efficiency") among their departmental goals, while one volunteered that cost control was irrelevant because of Blue Cross cost-based reimbursement. The budget system had not moved overall goals far from their earlier emphasis on quality at almost any cost.

We conclude from these divergent responses to questions about goals versus questions about budgets that attitudes on cost control became compartmentalized. Cost control was accepted when specifically talking of budgets, which is the context in which it was introduced. But it was not accepted when overall departmental goals were discussed. That is, acceptance of the budgetary system as a means of controlling costs was internalized—but the need for cost control was not.

Our implicit belief that what key actors accepted in the context of budgets they would also accept in other contexts has been called into question. Attitudinal changes have not spilled over from their narrow confines in the budget.

Therefore, we must question the long-run efficacy of installing a budget system to increase cost consciousness, where other attitudes and pressures do not support cost control. The budgetary system can simply become compartmentalized when it is not supported by other attitudes and by rewards. Given cost-based reimbursement, there are still too few incentives for genuine cost consciousness to replace the compartmentalized and somewhat ritualized concerns now displayed when talking about budgets. Compartmentalization is a rational response for department heads who lack deep commitment to cost control, but are proselytized for, and made to work with, a budgetary control system.

We read these findings to suggest that budgetary and perhaps other control systems are no more than tools, influencing attitudes and behaviors only when those in positions to use them desire to use them. Hospital department heads, in our experience, will not become cost controllers simply because they have cost information. They must have reasons to use the information. Otherwise they can, and probably will, compartmentalize control systems from their other activities. Encouraging cost consciousness in lower level personnel cannot be done by mechanical systems, budgetary or otherwise. These are the tools, but top management (and Blue Cross) must provide the reason or motive to use them. Attitude change is easier to advocate and predict than to implement.

## Control System Traits and Long-Term Responses

Even if attitudinal obstacles can be overcome, these attitudinal changes nonetheless would have an uncertain future as influences on behavior. Personnel change, situations change, vested interests change. As a result, attitudes change. Effective control systems must insure that these attitudinal changes will not negate the effects of the controls. That is, control systems themselves must be designed so that they can be used for control after technical experts have left and attitudes have changed.

Put more succinctly, desirable systems must maximize the probability that department head responses over the long run will be consistent with the goals for which the systems were established. They must continue to provide top management and department heads with the types of information that make it most probable that desired behaviors will continue. To do this, they must avoid four ways in which systems can deteriorate.

Information systems deteriorate when, rather than responding with desired behaviors in the long run, personnel: cease to collect the information called for; collect it but ignore its implications for change; collect it and recognize its change implications, but distort information that would make the control system change their behaviors; or collect it without distortion, but alter their own behaviors in ways that defeat the system's goals. Examples from our work can illustrate each of these undesirable response options.

The first of these responses—ceasing to collect information—occurred in the admission scheduling proposals for Able Hospital. There, the system proposed by the Bureau, though technically feasible, was ultimately dropped because many physicians refused to supply the information they were asked for. In fact, there were pressures in Able to stop participation in the project entirely.

To prevent this type of deterioration, to insure continued information collection, a control system must be backed by sanctions or legitimacy, or both. A significant proportion of innovations disappear once technical experts have left, or even before they leave, because their innovations lack needed sanctions and legitimacy.

These sanctions may be positive or negative: rewards for continued participation, or penalties for nonparticipation. In the case of the Able Hospital physicians' nonparticipation in the admitting system, the hospital could not apply penalties against those who took their patients elsewhere. Nor could it offer tangible rewards to those who participated in the system. In the case of Baker Hospital, in contrast, the hospital had a waiting list, so the Bureau could offer to reduce the list, and reduce cancellations for all physicians if they cooperated.

With sanctions absent, a control system can nevertheless continue to collect information if it has legitimacy; that is, if those responsible for using the system, though they do not benefit from it and would not be adversely affected were it dropped, continue to believe that it is right and proper to collect this information. The budget system described earlier, which was accepted without being consistent with departmental goals, is such a case. It was accepted partly because those who advocated it enjoyed some legitimacy, and partly because the budget notion itself has legitimacy.

Even lacking sanctions and legitimacy, however, a control system can continue to collect information if the collection is done by specialized departments (particularly medical records and the business office) whose reason for being is to collect information. Specialized departments have vested interests in collecting information, they insulate department heads from the sources of control systems, and they add their own sanctions and legitimacy to the systems. This partially is why information collection for control systems often is entrusted to specialized departments.

**In sum, to ensure that information continues to be collected, control systems must have sanctions or legitimacy, or they must rest on specialized information collection departments.**

The second undesirable response—collecting information while ignoring its implications—occurred when the Bureau instituted a system to encourage department heads to vary their manhours used based on forecasts of departmental activity levels. The manhour information also was intended for use in preparing budgets and evaluating performance. The key actors acquiesced in collecting the manhour information for this system, but they ignored its implications. Despite concerted efforts by our staff, one-third or more of the department heads did not understand the program, its procedures, or its stated goals, nor did they value the negotiation process involved in reaching decisions relating to it. None understood the problem we, the technical experts, had set out to solve, and none felt pressure to use our solution. As a result, no one was using it. Thus, this particular effort, though it produced information and had some surface appearances of a functioning system, made only a small dent in the behavior patterns of key actors.

In this example, the control system lacked constraints against ignoring system information. It was not sufficient that information be collected for an internally operated control system; a control system must be able to judge behaviors and must be supported by rewards for success and penalties for failure. It must have standards that are known to department heads, measurable by the control system, tight enough so that failure is possible, and related to activities controllable by those held accountable.

**To ensure that the behavior changes implied by control systems are not ignored, the systems must have sanctions and measurable standards that are valid indices of controllable activities.**

The third undesirable response—distorting the information supplied—occurs differentially by type of information. For instance, it occurs differentially for financial versus nonfinancial information. Information was distorted in the admitting procedures when some physicians at Baker Hospital, not impressed by a system which delayed elective admissions, declared all their cases to be emergencies. Such distortion of qualitative nonfinancial information can be detected only when it is possible to independently verify the information supplied, as for example by having the executive committee of the medical staff review emergency admissions.

By contrast, distortion is less likely with financial data because these data are easier to verify. Financial data are quantitative, and therefore usually can be crosschecked. Accounting developments over hundreds of years have provided methods of crosschecking and multiple recording, as well as rules of reporting and norms against outright falsifications, that make intentional distortions within a given reporting system relatively difficult. For these reasons, financial information appears to be more verifiable and less vulnerable to intentional distortion than nonfinancial information.

**To ensure that information supplied to control systems by those controlled is not distorted, data must be verifiable by those running the system.**

The fourth and final undesirable response—changing behaviors in undesired ways to evade the control system—can be illustrated with a problem commonly encountered in using full time equivalent position control.

Given a large department such as nursing, with full and part-time personnel in several classes and shifts, the usual absenteeism, and authorization to use overtime and replacement personnel, it is always possible to meet an FTE budget, while exceeding the equivalent dollar expense which would occur if all FTEs actually worked the stated hours. The "explanations" for the average, once detected, are usually complicated and varied enough to confound the controller for several periods, or perhaps indefinitely. It was this problem, encountered at Baker, which led to the reporting of actual manhours worked, rather than FTEs employed.

Another example of changed behavior involves an attempt to increase productivity of a hospital's physicians, with productivity measured by the reported number of patients seen per day. Doctors could not respond by ceasing to collect the information, because those asking for it had strong bureaucratic sanctions. They could not ignore its implications because unchanged patient loads were likely to be considered unfavorably, and there was a likelihood of sanctions for reported poor behaviors. They could not distort the information because it was simple to understand (and possibly asked for on a standard form) and easy to verify.

However, doctors were able to change their own behaviors (in undesired ways), at little cost to themselves, by reporting on behaviors which they had altered to make their productivity appear favorable. Instead of seeing patients for the lowest number of visits clinically appropriate, they made patients return when they otherwise would not have. This increased the ratio of patient visits per day without increasing their productivity. It was particularly undesirable because many of the patients were poor people who were away from home and lacked adequate overnight shelter. What the doctors in this case lacked was a set of vested interests, attitudes, and training that directed them—when confronted with pressure for behavioral change—to change in desired ways.

**To ensure that behavior changes that do occur are desirable, the attitudes, backgrounds, and interests of those being controlled must be consistent with the desired change, or the control system must preclude evasive changes.**

Thankfully, not all control systems are failures. The desirable response—changing behaviors to those which the system was intended to produce—occurred in the admitting procedures of Baker Hospital, where a modified system was successful in transferring admission decisions from nursing to the admitting department, and in increasing the occupancy rate from eighty-seven to ninety-five percent. The nursing department, which opposed the change, was not powerful enough to refuse to supply needed information. It could not ignore the implications of the new system; control of the system had been given to admitting. It could not distort admitting or discharge information, which by its nature was readily verifiable. And it did not have the power to alter patient lengths of stay.

Thus, though nurses had operated an admission system in their own interests, a new system was able to change this organizational behavior without first changing nurses' attitudes. The control system provided effective control.

## Summary

This chapter has suggested that to assure long-run influence on behaviors, control systems using internally generated data for control of hospital activity by hospital personnel would be helped by, but cannot rely on, long-run desirable attitudes of key actors. In addition to trying to change attitudes and organizational environments that influence attitudes, they must have built-in safeguards against four types of deterioration that can happen after technical experts leave. By recognizing the specific causes of deterioration, it is often possible to design such safeguards. Where such safeguards are clearly not possible, it may well be appropriate to reconsider the design of the system.

## NOTES

[1]M. David Ermann, "Asking Organizations About Themselves: A Case Study of the External Information Demands on One Hospital." Doctoral dissertation, The University of Michigan, Ann Arbor, 1973.

[2]Often, also, this thaw is justifiable. As indicated earlier in the previous chapter, the vested interests of key actors and technical experts may conflict. The technical expert with a demonstration project succeeds when the quantity and quality of his successful innovations are high, with few penalties for innovations that fail. The department head has different responsibilities. He succeeds partly by keeping the quantity and importance of failures and false starts low. He cannot accept the failure rate that would be acceptable to a technical expert, nor can he afford to stick with a questionable project as long as an expert would prefer him to. For these reasons, he may want to unfreeze an innovation long before the experts would want him to.

[3]Richard M. Cyert and James G. March, *A Behavioral Theory of the Firm.* Englewood Cliffs, NJ: Prentice-Hall, 1963, p. 111.

[4]Ermann, "Asking Organizations," chapter 7.

William L. Jackson and Nancy Teague, "Evaluation of a Budget Process." Unpublished paper, Program in Hospital Administration, The University of Michigan, 1973.

Gary R. DeLisle and William E. Welton, "The Process of Change: An Evaluation of the Social Consequences of a Technological Innovation." Unpublished paper, Program in Hospital Administration, The University of Michigan, 1972.

# IV.3

# The Failure of Admission Scheduling at Able Hospital[1]

*by Kurt R. Student*

## The Setting

Able Memorial Hospital is a 287 bed, voluntary hospital, one of three in a city of 70,000. Its medical staff is composed entirely of allopathic physicians, most of whom also maintain active privileges at the 201 bed Martin Hospital. The community is also served by a forty-four bed osteopathic hospital, but there is little interchange between the allopathic and osteopathic physicians.

The community rate of utilization is 957 per thousand population which is below the average for the state of 1,223 per thousand; this was not due to a shortage of beds. In 1969, the average census in Able was eighty-three percent; in Martin the average census was seventy-one percent. A study in late 1969 estimated that thirty adult medical-surgical beds were in excess of current requirements of the community. There were possibilities for reducing the bed needs in obstetrics. At the same time, there were shortages of psychiatric beds and shortages of long-term care beds at the basic nursing care level.

In a series of six meetings between October 1969 and March 1970, project personnel from The University of Michigan Bureau of Hospital Administration and the Able administrator confirmed the willingness of the administrator to have his hospital participate in the demonstration, and identified the scheduling of patient admissions as the first major project.

These initial discussions supported a prior conviction of the University team that a service area planning study should be undertaken. During this initial period a presentation to all hospital department heads and supervisors was made by the administrator and the Bureau team. Funding, which also was approved during this period, was followed by a publicity release in the community paper. Based primarily on the opinion of the administrator, no formal discussion was deemed necessary with either the board of trustees or the medical staff. Some previous research by others from the University had involved collecting data from Able's medical staff. In the opinion of the medical staff, these data were not properly fed back and, as a result, the staff was somewhat reluctant to participate in another research program.

## The Admission Scheduling Model

The original suggestion to work on admission scheduling came from the Bureau team. It was chosen on the basis of evidence of wide variation in daily census at the hospital. The initial thrust of the project was to control census by forecasting emergency admissions and discharges and controlling the scheduling of elective and urgent admissions. The initial quantifiable savings were expected to come from reduction in nursing staff. Intangible benefits were seen by the University as reducing the probability of serious overload upon nursing personnel and in providing firm future dates for elective admission to both the physicians and patients. It was envisioned that a second round of savings might come from the further refinement of nurse staffing needs once census had been stabilized and from the use of admission and discharge forecasts in work scheduling, and planning manpower needs in social service, dietary, housekeeping, and pharmacy. The project was begun in January 1970.

A doctoral candidate in industrial engineering was assigned the task of review of the existing literature, and the construction of a practical scheduling system. With guidance from two senior members of the Bureau team, he worked for the next two months to devise a theoretical model, analyze the historical variation in census, and establish the goals of a new scheduling system.

The initial work by the Bureau team established a number of postulates which appeared desirable in an admission scheduling model. The admissions office performs three principal functions, the *scheduling* of patients for admission, their *assignment* to specific beds or units, and the completion of certain legal, financial, and clerical tasks associated with the patient's physical *admission* into the hospital. While many admitting offices have a variety of other tasks, these three are central. An ideal admission system would develop appropriate measures of performance of each of these three tasks and also give the admitting officer mechanical aides to complete the necessary work and make the necessary decisions. It was clear that the most cost-effective area for study was in the scheduling portion of the activities. The average occupancy on the four medical-surgical floors during 1965 was 82.6 percent, and average weekly occupancy ranged from 52.4 percent to 95.3 percent. Except for obvious seasonal fluctuations, the variation did not appear to be predictable.[2]

It was clear to the Bureau team that the goal of the admitting office should be to handle the scheduling decisions in a manner which optimally used the resources of the hospital without interfering with the medical needs of the patient. This desired goal statement was different from the actual goal of the Able admitting office, "to keep the hospital full." The actual goal meant that any patient would be scheduled immediately as long as a bed was available and not reserved for possible future emergency. The desired goal under the proposed system was optimal use of beds and other resources. Patients could be deferred for three reasons: the lack of a bed; the lack of nursing staff; and the lack of necessary ancillary services (principally on weekends).

Implementing this scheme would require an assessment of overall demand, forecasts of likely admissions and discharges, and an analysis which changed these data to a daily guideline for the number of elective patients to be admitted. Guidelines for several days into the future would be given the admitting officer each day. Whenever the guideline was reached for a given day, elective patients would be deferred to a later day. Thus, the proposed guide would inevitably introduce short delays for some patients, but would, at the same time, eliminate the "feast or famine" characteristic of occupancy and of nursing workload.

It soon appeared that the critical technical problem was the forecast of occupancy, and the critical policy question was the trade-off between dampening occupancy swings and delaying elective patients. If the forecast of discharges could be made accurately, not only in terms of the number of patients to be discharged but also the identification of patients to be discharged, then the next process of the admitting office, assigning patients, could be facilitiated by such information. This led the study group to conclude that estimates provided by physicians with revisions as the individual patient's stay progressed would be most likely to yield the necessary accuracy.

## Presenting the Model to Able Staff

This formulation of the admitting office problem (in expanded detail) was reviewed in April 1970 with a key group consisting of the hospital's administrator, director of nursing, controller (and supervisor of the admitting office), and the chief admitting officer. On their acceptance, more intensive work was begun with them in weekly meetings aimed at establishing the specific procedures to be used, developing the necessary information to measure potential achievement, and establishing the desired occupancy levels. From April first through June of 1970, meetings were held weekly with most of the members of this group. The administrator attended occasionally; the controller and the admitting officer were the most frequent participants.

These meetings were generally well received. The controller and the admitting officer were clearly interested in the project from the outset. They and the Bureau team contributed substantial amounts of work on their own between the meetings. The director of nursing was cooperative, as were members of her department, although their role was not large at this point in the project. A number of important findings and outcomes came from the discussion at these meetings and the analysis of relevant data. These were: 1) *There was at the time essentially no constraint on the admitting decision by the admitting office.* Except in periods of extreme crowding called "emergency conditions" which occurred about ten days a year, any patient was accepted and usually admitted the same day as the request. 2) *There was substantial variation in daily census and in nursing hours per patient day.* Variation was caused by both day-of-the-week and seasonal cycles in demand and also by random factors. 3) *The opportunities to improve control of the occupancy level differed in the various parts of the hospital.* Obstetrics, pediatrics, intensive and coronary care were felt to have almost entirely emergency admissions; orthopedics and psychiatry were specialized floors with different occupancy patterns. Eliminating these six units left four nursing units of varying size serving essentially the adult medical-surgical population. 4) *Data were developed which showed high variation in census and in nursing hours per patient day in these four floors.* These data, a portion of which are shown in the attached figure, were used to explain the goals of the project to both other members of the hospital staff and the medical staff. The justification was explained in terms of the opportunity to eliminate peak periods of census by deferring some elective admissions to the future. As a result, other periods when the census was low and nursing capabilities were underutilized would be reduced as well. 5) *Studies of the demand for beds in the hospital's service area confirmed that there were more adult medical-surgical beds available in the area than were necessary to meet present or near future forecasts of demand.* This finding verified the impression that the administrator and others in the community had had for some time. 6) *There was considerable uncertainty about the exact bed count on the four floors of interest.* The admitting officer treated the private rooms as available for two-person occupancy whenever necessary to follow her prac-

**FIGURE IV.3.1**
Comparison of actual nursing hours and hours needed for uniform hours per patient day, fifty weeks Able Hospital

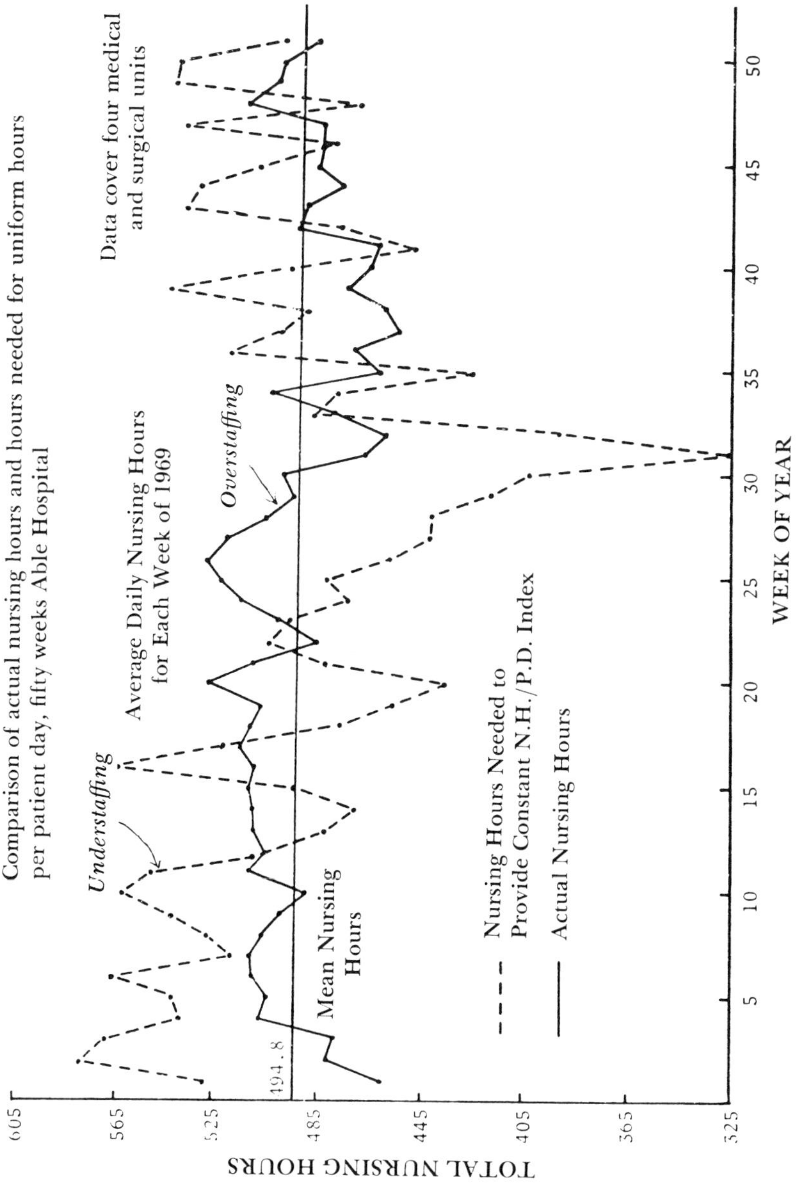

tice of accepting any patient for whom a request was made. The "ideal" capacity of these floors was 133. This could be increased when necessary to 144. The result of this policy, of course, was to heighten the possibility for variation in census and for overtaxing the available nursing supply. The guideline for establishing an emergency condition was not precise but was approximately a census of 140. The remaining capacity was felt necessary to handle true emergencies which might occur. 7) *Although the hospital had clear policies for defining emergency, urgent, and elective patients, the fact that this classification was only applied in peak occupancy periods resulted in a lack of accurate data on distribution of emergencies.* A special data collection effort was necessary by the admitting office to gain this distribution which was critical in the design of the scheduling model. 8) *Elective surgical patients were accepted by the operating room, not by the admitting office.* The admitting office was notified of these bookings with varying lead times before the patient's arrival and processed them in the usual manner. The operating room functioned well below its physical capacity but was also staffed below maximum levels. When the "emergency" condition existed, it was necessary to cancel prior surgical commitments for some elective patients. 9) *There was no advance notification of discharge given to the admitting office.* In emergency conditions, the admitting office sought out additional information on discharges. At other times the admitting office was notified after the patient had left the building by means of a discharge slip left at the admitting office by a ward aide who escorted the patient to the door.

After considerable discussion, the appropriate manual and telephone systems for coordinating scheduled admissions between the admitting office and the operating room were arranged and it was agreed that the system of obtaining discharge estimates from physicians on the nursing floors and delivering the information to the admitting office was feasible. It was also agreed that the admitting office could obtain estimates of the approximate length of stay of patients from physicians at the time the admission request was made. It was determined that the hospital computer, an NCR Century 100, could be used to implement the model of a desired occupancy level and provide the admitting office with guidelines on the number of admissions for each of the next eight future days. The program could be fit into the accounts receivable routine of the computer and could use the in-house computerized accounts receivable file as a data base. By June 1970, the hospital management and the Bureau team were convinced of realistic opportunities for smoothing occupancy on these four units. The next steps were to gain the support of the medical staff for an experiment in scheduling elective patients and to begin development of the necessary computer programs and new procedures for implementing a scheduling model.

The key role of the physicians in the admitting scheduling system had been recognized in general, but only in April and May of 1970 did the specific changes required of them in their hospital practice begin to take shape. Specifically, physicians needed: to accept delays in their elective admissions when the desired occupancy level was reached; and to provide estimates of when their patients would be discharged. They obviously would need explanation of why they should do these things. Strategy was discussed by the Bureau team with the hospital administrator. He favored a discussion with the key leaders of the medical staff rather than a formal presentation by the Bureau team to the executive committee of the staff. He held a luncheon meeting for six doctors representing the medical and surgical services and pathology, and containing the chief of staff as well as several present or former elected officers. This group heard the presentation and were cautiously favorable. They, rather than the Bureau team, made the presentation to the staff executive committee, which agreed to support the project on a trial basis. In September (1970), the matter was presented by the chief of staff as an informational report from the executive committee to a quarterly meeting of the full staff. The project director made a presentation of the goals and methods and identified the two key elements of interest to the staff. There were questions and some misgivings about the discharge estimates: (1) the doctors did not always know, and some were reluctant to guess, when their patients could be discharged, and (2) some doctors worried that their estimates would somehow be used against them by the utilization review committee, or even by Blue Shield. They were not completely reassured by promises of confidentiality. (Blue Shield had no access to the estimates, nor any legitimate reason to request them.) The discussion was brief, however, and the chief of staff and chairman of the meeting moved on to other items without a formal vote, reemphasizing the trial nature of the proposal.

## Computer Problems

Acceptance by the medical staff left only the technical problem of producing the printout which would provide the basis for requesting physician discharge estimates, and the policy issue of determining current occupancy levels. The data processing requirements were in principle easily interrelated with an existing inpatient billing routine which was part of the software package of a recently purchased small computer, adding about ten minutes to a four-hour daily run updating patient ledgers. Unfortunately, an employee hired to install the computer packages proved to be unfamiliar with both the language and with the hospital billing systems. By October, the hospital was falling behind in inpatient billings, and some three months behind in outpatient billings. Such delays caused the controller and the administrator to feel a natural concern for the hospital's cash position, and the admission scheduling system was given little attention. In November, the Bureau team finally proposed that their personnel assist in catching up in the billing, simply to provide computer time to debug the scheduling subroutine and to provide a current data base for the scheduling system. One member of the Bureau team spent much of his Christmas vacation helping to work down the backlog, learning the computer language, and debugging the scheduling subroutine. By then, two months had passed since the nurses had been informed that they would shortly be receiving training on when to request discharge estimates from physicians, and three months since physicians had been told of the impending experiment. In December the planned training of the nursing staff was again postponed, while the Bureau team learned a great deal more than they ever had wanted to know about the internal storage, disc capacity, unidimensional arrays, and other interesting features of the hospital computer and its software. The project director pressed the administrator to seek a data processing manager skilled in the equipment. He was hired in December and spent most of January familiarizing himself with the packaged routines. In the meantime, the Bureau team completed the debugging. In February 1971, nearly six months later than the September 1970 estimate, the first pilot runs of census data were produced.

## Implementation

The continuing expectation that the computer problem would be solved "soon" had led to a decision to start securing an expected length of stay estimate at the time a patient was scheduled for admission before the system was ready to utilize the estimates in setting the number of admissions required to stabilize occupancy. This procedure had some unexpected problems because the admitting request was often made by the doctor's secretary who did not know the estimated length of stay. Also, a clear explanation of why the unused estimate was being requested proved difficult for the admitting staff. The intended use of estimates, to accurately predict bed supply so that elective admissions could be scheduled (delayed) to stablize occupancy, required considerable physician interest in stable occupancy in order to be effective. During early 1971, the admitting officer indicated she was experiencing considerable pressure. The design and preparation for introducing the system had caused tension with the nursing department, but by now the controller was anxious to see the system get started and appeared unsympathetic to reports of additional problems from nursing, the physicians, or their secretaries. All of these problems were traceable to the Bureau team, but only rarely did the admitting officer show irritation with them. Like the controller, she had become an active proponent of the system.

When all elements of the admitting scheduling system were finally started at the end of February 1971, two members of the Bureau team were on hand full time to help the hospital personnel keep things running as smoothly as possible. One team member was based in the admitting office to assist in using the scheduling allowances and other admitting oriented tasks. The second team member circulated among the four nursing units in the system, to deal with questions and problems in collecting discharge estimates from the individual patients' physicians. Much of the time on the nursing units was spent attempting to persuade nursing unit personnel both that the system would actually work and that when it did there would be significant advantages to them and the hospital. The understanding of the physicians was a key element to their accepting and participating in the system, but achieving that understanding in individual physicians was a time-consuming, difficult, and often frustrating assignment. These difficulties prompted the Bureau team to supplement individual contacts with a more formal communication effort:

> In answer to specific questions which had been raised by members of the medical staff, a four minute slide-tape presentation was assembled in the latter part of May. This presentation, in addition to addressing specific questions, again reviewed the value of accurate discharge estimates and the need for the acceptance of some non-emergent delays in admissions. A small projector and screen which could be easily operated were placed in one corner of the physician's library daily and many observed the presentation.[3]

One must remember that a key feature of the admitting scheduling system was that it explicitly connected one aspect of medical need (admission on request) with one aspect of efficiency (stable occupancy) in a trade-off relation. An increase in stability could be achieved by lowering the desired occupancy level, but only at the cost of increasing the probability that a requested admission would be deferred. The key policy decision was setting the desired occupancy level, agreed upon by the administrator in December 1970, at 135 (ninety-five percent occupancy, ten percent probability of a delayed admission).

Late April and early May was a period of unusually high admission requests, and it was apparent that the admission scheduling system was not working as well as hoped. The census of the whole hospital, including the four units controlled by the scheduling system, was lower in the last week of May than it had been for several years. Further, the total patient days of care rendered since January were down and, except for the three-week spurt, had been down consistently during the five-month period. Patient days are a critical factor in the revenue of a hospital, and the Able administrator and the controller were quite sensitive to any possible loss of inpatient revenue. At the same time, some members of the medical staff were becoming more vocal in their complaints.

## Physician Discontent with Admission Scheduling

The effort to constrain the occupancy level which occurred in the early part of May resulted in deferring the admission of about thirteen elective patients. A number of doctors involved announced that they would take those patients to Martin Hospital, and at least nine of the thirteen patients were admitted to Martin. The doctors also were annoyed at the requests for advance notification of discharge; this annoyance was experienced most directly by the head nurses, staff nurses, and ward secretaries responsible for securing estimates from the doctors. The original director of nursing had been replaced several months before for reasons highlighted perhaps by the Bureau team activities, but not directly connected with them. Rather difficult problems of communication between the former director and other members of the administrative group had been experienced before the study team arrived. The new director was more supportive of the admitting scheduling system, and with some encouragement from a team member, she began to visit the four units several times a week to talk with nurses and encourage them to continue asking for estimates. But the problem was acute for some nursing unit staff who were not comfortable requesting the doctors to provide estimates and who became very upset when doctors attacked them for doing so. A study team member also would visit the units regularly and would regularly find one or two nurses ready to abandon the requests because of treatment received from physicians when requesting discharge estimates. In spite of this, some head nurses appeared to honestly support the system, and tried to make it work.

Exaggeration and rumor generation occurred in late May. Some doctors cited instances of thirteen-day delays for elective patients, eight-day delays for urgent patients, and the routine delay of elective patients even when there were "empty beds all over the house." These statements were inaccurate in substance, but fairly represented physician annoyance with the system. Patients were actually deferred because of scheduling model constraints for less than two weeks in early May. After that time demand had slacked off and the admission scheduling limits were not reached. No emergency patient was ever deferred; no urgent patient was ever deferred longer than three days. On June 2, the administrator and project director met and agreed to review the general situation with both the hospital and Bureau groups and also to meet with the full medical staff at their quarterly meeting in the evening of June 8. There was substantial question as to whether the system could be made to work.

At the meeting of the medical staff, the administrator encouraged wide-ranging discussion which touched upon the relationship of Able and Martin Hospitals and the doctors' obligation to assist in the control of the cost of hospital and medical care. The project director reviewed the goals of the admitting project and asked for continued support of both the discharge forecasts and the short delay of elective admissions. The discussion was animated. In addition to reiteration of several of the rumor statements, it revealed several aspects of the impact of the system as seen by the physicians. One physician cited a case of a middle-aged man with alcoholism and a bleeding ulcer whom he thought might exacerbate his ulcer to the point of an acute hemorrhage by drinking if he could not be admitted to the hospital immediately. The doctor was annoyed because he had to reclassify the patient as emergency when in his mind the patient's condition at the moment was only urgent. His definition of emergency clearly was limited to those conditions which were immediately and directly life threatening although the staff's formal definition, and the one assumed by the Bureau team, was much more lenient. Another doctor remarked that if he had to wait to admit elective patients he forgot some of the details of the workup he completed in his office, and thus was forced to repeat parts of the history and physical when the patient was admitted two or three days later. This remark drew some nodding heads. Another doctor added that since physicians were in short supply the community owed it to the doctors to meet their needs. The physicians were not more enthusiastic when it was pointed out that reducing the variation in nursing census would reduce the costs of hospital care for the people of the community. The implication was quite clear that the system should optimize physician convenience and whatever extra cost was involved should be paid.

Other comments were directed to the forecasts of discharge requested at several different points during the patient's stay. The doctors felt that repeated requests three days, two days, and one day prior to expected discharge were unnecessary. Some commented that they were frequently asked for a discharge estimate before they had a chance to work the patient up and others noted that they were at one point being pressed for discharge dates on patients awaiting transfer to nursing homes when they in fact had no control over discharge dates. (This had been corrected several weeks before the meeting). Another level of concern was indicated by the remark: "Blue Shield might get hold of these estimates and not pay our fees if we do not discharge the patient on the estimated day." This appeared to be a serious concern to at least a few physicians. Several doctors indicated or implied that they were deliberately giving long forecasts because of this possible danger, a fact which was obvious by comparing their patients' estimated and actual discharge dates. The restatement that these estimates were not even given to the hospital's own utilization review committee did not noticeably reassure these doctors. The team director again asked for cooperation on an experimental basis and the meeting closed without action by the medical staff.

## Reconsideration of the System

Very shortly after this meeting the nursing department noticed a new wave of complaints, with some doctors promising to eliminate the system and routinely refusing to supply discharge estimates. These remarks and actions were sometimes made in a manner highly upsetting to the nursing staff and ward secretaries. On June 16 the operations group, consisting of the administrator, controller, associate administrator, director of nursing, admitting officer, supervisor of ward secretaries, operating room supervisor, and assistant administrator, met with three members of the Bureau team. The administrator had requested the meeting to consider whether or not the system should be continued. Both nurses reported very serious concern with the attitude of the physicians. The director also noted that the response rate to the discharge requests was falling despite constant reminders by ward secretaries and nurses. The operating room supervisor reported some additional problems with the scheduling of surgery which appeared to be independent of the admission scheduling system. The admitting officer reported little problem, either in getting the initial discharge estimates or in managing the system from her point of view. The supervisor of ward secretaries reported that his people were increasingly reluctant to ask for estimates. Discussion moved to the competitive position of Able and Martin Hospitals. There was extensive discussion of the rumor that Martin Hospital was quite full of patients and of the problem of low occupancy which had plagued Able for most of the year.

In the course of the discussion it became clear that the general census loss had been from floors not involved in the scheduling system and that there was a lack of data on exactly what the impact of the scheduling system had been. The administrator again indicated that it might be better to discontinue the system and requested members of his staff to comment. The controller and admitting officer were strongly in support of continuing the system with modification for thirty days, with further discussion at that time. The administrator agreed to this, and decided to meet with the administrator of Martin Hospital to permit verification of rumors about their census and of the transfer of patients whose admission had been delayed. It was also agreed that the nursing staff might themselves supply estimates when they were reasonably sure of the accuracy. Finally it was agreed that the administrator, director of nursing, and team director would meet with the head nurses, ward secretaries, and ward managers of the four floors involved to attempt to counter the rumors and to communicate both management's understanding of the burdens being placed on these people and the decision to continue the system for an additional thirty days.

The meeting with the Martin Hospital administrator occurred on June 22. She confirmed that the hospital had renovated and improved inpatient accommodations and added a chemotherapy service. Martin Hospital had also installed new dictating equipment in the past year. This equipment could be reached by ordinary telephone and used to update medical records. She also noted that Martin did not check specifically for history and physical within seventy-two hours of admission, but relied instead on postdischarge review by the appropriate medical committees on the quality of care as a whole. This policy, she noted, was much more popular with the doctors, and she believed that they recognized the other advantages to the use of Martin Hospital.

She agreed to release data on census and to trace the patients who allegedly changed from Able to Martin admissions and also agreed to provide data for a study of the potential cost reduction of sharing services between the two hospitals. She declined to participate in any admission coordination procedures.

The meeting with members of the Able nursing staff was held late in the same day. One of the hospital's most senior head nurses said that the doctors on her floor were now supplying discharge estimates and that she felt their attitude would improve as time went on. Another senior head nurse noted that it was difficult to supply a reasonable estimate for some kinds of patients (particularly the aged, chronically ill). A ward secretary pointed out that estimates were being requested on the day of surgery when the patient, the doctor, and the medical record were all off the nursing unit. This made compliance very difficult. Several versions of what appeared to be the same rumors as encountered among the medical staff were brought out.

It became clear that there were two concerns among the people present. One belief was that the hospital was taking a series of actions which invaded the prerogatives of the physician, such as forcing him to defer emergency admissions; the second was that the system appeared to be resulting in a reduction of work available for nurses. One nurse commented that the hospital was turning patients away, but at the same time the opportunties for part-time work for nurses had decreased. The administrator noted the potential advantages of the scheduling system, and that the nursing department would avoid being overworked as it has been during peak census periods in the past. The team director stressed the new option of the nursing department to use their judgment in requesting estimates from the physicians, and in the case of registered nurses to supply estimates on their own when appropriate.

The early summer of 1971 saw the admitting scheduling system in place and operating, but by no means stabilized as a part of Able Hospital's standard procedures. The controller was a strong supporter because the analysis preceding the innovation had clarified for him the possibility of budgeting quarterly adjustments in nurse staffing, with a potential savings estimated at $40,000 per year. The simple good sense of the system appealed to the admitting officer, and the increase in significance which it gave to her own role made it attractive to her. The pressures she experienced had come fully three months before the problems of securing estimates had hit the nursing floors, and in a sense were investments she had already made in the system. Floor personnel, notably nurses, saw few benefits, some level of irritation if it continued, and some degree of job insecurity and usurping of doctors' prerogatives if it were successful. Only a minority felt it made sense and were truly willing to support the system. The administrator had a vivid memory of the emotions generated in the medical staff during the two weeks when the system seriously constrained admissions. He also recognized that the cost savings of the system were proportional to the number of delayed admissions. Among physicians there was now a vocal minority that opposed the system in principle, a minority which would probably increase in size if admission delays were experienced again.

Analysis of Martin data by the Bureau team showed no evidence of a significant shift of patients to that hospital. Martin had had two near-capacity weeks with the adult medical-surgical service in May and June, but like Able, its occupancy was subject to wide and unpredictable swings. It was not true that it had been "crammed to the gills" after the Able scheduling system had been installed. Analysis of the revised and less demanding discharge estimate system showed that accuracy had not declined, and that the response rate was somewhat better. The data were reviewed with the administrator and his key personnel, and again there was consensus that continuance of the system required that the desired occupancy be set at a level which generated very few patient delays. In fact only three patients were delayed during the last half of 1971.

## Failure

By midsummer of 1971 it became somewhat easier for the Bureau team to assess the implications of a continuing desired occupancy level that generated very few delayed admissions. Among these implications were a rather low return on the bad will and emotional strain that the repeated requests for discharge estimates were producing. An August meeting with the medical staff's executive committee had confirmed that the executive committee did not think it appropriate for them to help make the discharge estimate system work, but that further revisions in it might reduce the irritations it caused. The executive committee determined that the medical staff should be polled on the continuation of the system at its September meeting. The result was enough continuing criticism that the initial request for a discharge estimate was dropped, and only a single estimate, to be provided voluntarily by the doctor twenty-four hours before discharge was retained. The last collection of data to estimate the accuracy of estimates had been done in July, and there seemed little reason to collect further data.

At this point the system was functioning at a level scarcely different from the original admissions procedures. A minimal control of overcrowding was in effect which would eliminate the highest five percent of daily census values. Even assuming that the nursing department could adjust staffing uniformly, this would result in insignificant savings, little different than the added cost of maintaining the system. The reason for retaining the system was because the costs of reinstalling it were great, and it was hoped that attitudes might change over time.

Instead, the opposite happened. An article appeared in *Medical World News*, January 7, 1972. This brief and rather inaccurate article confused Able Hospital with other programs in other institutions, even to the point of placing the Able administrator in the wrong hospital. At least one member of the medical staff was highly offended, apparently because the article failed to give sufficient recognition to the amount of work and support the Able doctors had given the project. He also served as a hospital trustee, and in this role he urged that the program be discontinued. The medical executive committee recommended discontinuance, and the admitting scheduling system was dropped in February 1972.

## NOTES

[1]Chapter IV.3 and the following two chapters record detailed histories of the implementation process as the Bureau team observed and experienced it. The reports were written by members of the research staff, and therefore are not impartial. The authors were consicous of this problem, and three steps were taken to overcome it. A member of the project team who had no responsibility for achieving results within the hospital guided the preparation and in two cases wrote the reports; multiple reviews of draft reports were made by members of the research team not directly responsible for the innovation; and a guideline for writing emphasized reporting sequences of events, rather than plausible explanations for them. In many cases daily notes, working memos, and similar documents by team members were the principal sources of information. The guidelines for report preparation also emphasized the protection of persons, and incidents which might have added color but would have embarrassed hospital personnel are not recorded.

[2]Galen P. Briggs, Jr., "Inpatient Admissions Scheduling: An Application to a Nursing Service." Doctoral dissertation, The University of Michigan, 1971.

[3]*Ibid.*, pp. 62-63.

# IV.4

# The Success of Admission Scheduling at Baker Hospital

*by Kurt R. Student*

## The Setting

Baker Hospital is a modern 290 bed facility which serves a number of industrial communities on the outskirts of a major urban area. Baker is one of four general community hospitals controlled by a hospital authority. Baker has neither internship nor residency programs. Some of the medical staff are active at other hospitals located in nearby communities. Some are specialists, but most are general practitioners. A small number are osteopaths. Baker has neither an associate administrator nor an assistant administrator; all department heads report directly to the administrator. (See organization chart, figure IV.4.1.) One reason for this is that some functions such as planning, public relations, purchasing, and some accounting are centralized in the office of the hospital authority to whose executive director the Baker administrator reports. Such an organizational structure requires the administrator to be involved in all major interdepartmental decisions because the organization is linked together only in the top management position.

Admission scheduling was introduced in Baker in early 1972, after several other activities initiated by the University of Michigan Bureau of Hospital Administration team were underway. There were significant differences between the admission scheduling system designed for Baker and the one implemented at Able. The Able system was designed to

**FIGURE IV.4.1**
Baker Hospital organization 1972

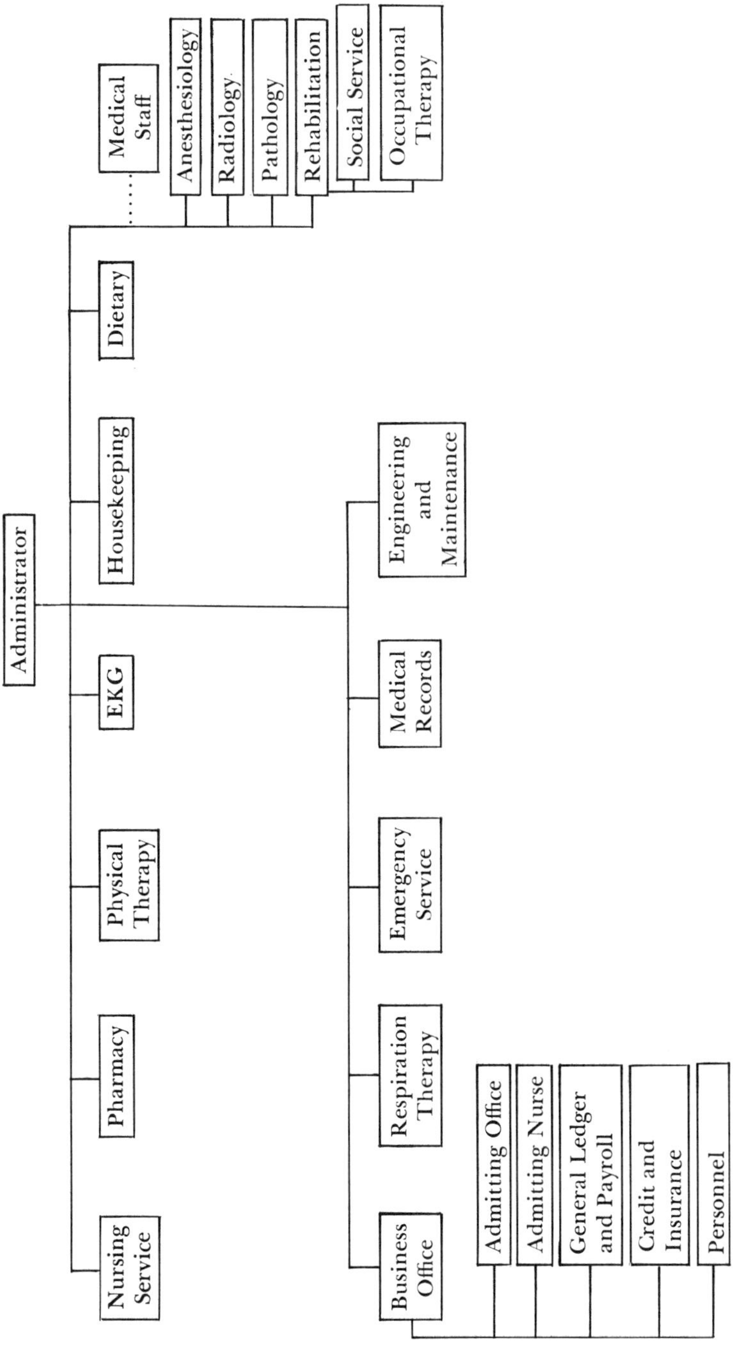

stablilize occupancy at a level below the bed capacity of the hospital. At Baker, the occupancy and the demand for beds in the three medical and surgical units covered were already stable at relatively high levels, and a Bureau planning study indicated demand would increase. The threefold objective of the Baker admission scheduling system was: (1) to reduce cancellations and transfers under the conditions of high and stable census levels; (2) to control the mix of medical and surgical patients in the hospital; and (3) to schedule a significant number of medical admissions so that preadmission testing could be performed.

Prior to the scheduling system development, physicians scheduled surgical admissions with the Baker operating room supervisor and the admitting office held beds open for these surgical patients until about 3:00 P.M. Any beds not assigned to surgical patients by that time were then filled, if possible, by medical patients. Four or five admitting office clerks telephoned patients on the medical waiting list and requested that the patients come in for immediate hospitalization. Frequently, these prospective patients could not arrange for their hospitalization on such short notice, and beds remained unfilled. For that reason the occupancy level was somewhat lower than the demand for services would indicate, and the variation and inconvenience were borne mainly by the medical service. The initial settings of the medical and surgical admission allowances for Baker were based on the hospital's historical data so that there would be no change in the balance between medical and surgical admissions.

In 1970, the Bureau team conducted a long-range planning study which indicated that the demand for inpatient beds at Baker was high and that this demand would increase. By July 1970, community demand required that Baker operate at an approximate occupancy level of ninety percent, while the planning study determined that the expected twenty percent increase in Baker's service area population over ten years would decrease Baker's share of admissions from its service area unless inpatient beds were added or the occupancy level was increased. Since there were no immediate plans to increase the number of Baker's inpatient beds, there was pressure to increase the hospital's occupancy level to offset as much as possible Baker's decreased potential to serve its growing service population. This desire to maintain high occupancy without increases in admission cancellations and organizational stress was a primary factor in the decision by the Baker administration and the Bureau to design and implement an admission scheduling system for the hospital.

## The Admitting Nurse Role

In February 1971, the Baker administrator had established the position of admitting nurse within the admitting office. His motivation for doing so was primarily the success he had experienced with such a position in his former hospital. Initially, her purpose was to expedite the admissions process for scheduled surgical patients, so that they could receive the necessary tests and exams on the day of admission (in anticipation of surgery the following day). Although there were certain routine presurgical tests, the admitting nurse normally contacted the admitting physician to obtain specific orders for each patient. Since surgery was performed essentially on a Monday through Friday schedule, the admitting nurse position was staffed five days a week. Because of the strong nursing orientation of the admitting nurse function, the position was initially established so that she was administratively responsible to the director of nursing. However, she performed her job geographically and functionally within the admitting office (which is a component of the hospital's business office). A number of conflicts arose. The situation was resolved within a few months by making the admitting nurse directly responsible to the business office manager, while retaining professional liaison with the director of nursing.

Preparatory activities for the implementation of the admission scheduling system began in November 1971. The Bureau staff analyzed PAS data on patient discharges in order to establish a basis for the historical discharge estimating system used to establish "flag dates." The analysis indicated that patients' age and service categories were the best explainers of length of stay; the attending physician was the third best explainer.

## The Early Testing Trial

One of the early efforts was to determine the feasibility of sending medical patients to the laboratory and to radiology for diagnostic testing early in the morning of their day of admission prior to going to the nursing floor. The test results could be made available to the attending physician on his visit the day after admission instead of two days after admission, thereby possibly reducing the length of stay of adult medical patients. The experimental results indicated that patients had to be at the hospital by 9:00 A.M., that fifteen minutes of laboratory time was needed for the usual blood sampling, and that seventy-five percent of the adult medical patients required radiological tests, usually chest x-rays or flat plates. Two conclusions were reached as a result of this trial: (1) early testing was feasible and should be presented to the hospital for consideration, and (2) successful implementation of early testing, as well as of the admission scheduling system, would require much greater coordination between the admitting nurse, the admitting office, the laboratory, radiology, housekeeping, and the nursing unit personnel.

## Improving Coordination

In late January 1972, the Bureau team discussed the lack of coordination evidenced in the early testing trial and the coordination which would be required for implementing an innovation as encompassing as the admission scheduling system. The Bureau favored an internal steering committee to plan a series of meetings which would establish the required interdepartmental coordination at Baker. On February 2 a conference was held with the administrator. The Bureau staff explained that during the early testing experiment, patients had appeared on the nursing floors without any knowledge by nursing personnel as to what was occurring. The nursing department had been notified, but communication to head nurses and staff nurses was failing. The need and value of several coordinating meetings was clear, and the first meeting was scheduled for February 17.

The chief of the internal medicine department, a prominent surgeon representing the surgical department, the chiefs of radiology and pathology, the administrator, the business office manager, the director of nursing, and four members of the Bureau team attended the first meeting.The Bureau team reviewed the admission scheduling proposal and stressed the meeting's importance for its success. The early testing trial was reviewed to illustrate the need for coordinated cooperation. A particular effort was made to seek comments and support from members of the medical staff.

The internist was particularly enthusiastic about implementing early testing. He stated he had long favored better screening of medical admissions, and he realized that scheduling diagnostic tests in a medically preferred sequence would have great potential for reducing patient length of stay. The surgeon was also enthusiastic about the proposal. The radiologist and the pathologist made no comment about the admission scheduling system and were concerned only in their departments' involvement in early testing activities. The acceptance of the Bureau's proposal by the internist and the surgeon made quite clear to the others attending that they believed the medical staff would want to implement the innovations quickly. When the Bureau's staff explained that the requests for discharge estimates were based on analyses of Baker's PAS patient discharge data, both the internist and the surgeon indicated they wanted to use these analyses for medical staff utilization review purposes. However, the Bureau cautioned that releasing the data for this purpose might be viewed as threatening by some of the medical staff and might result in their reluctance to provide estimates and to cooperate in implementing the system. It was agreed, with some reluctance by the surgeon, that the discharge estimates would be used solely for admission scheduling purposes. The meeting ended with agreement that the admitting nurse would meet with the chief of medicine and doctors from pathology and radiology to establish the preferred diagnostic test sequences. The Bureau agreed to assist her in compiling these lists and arranging their distribution. It was also agreed that the admitting nurse should attend the next task force meeting.

The second meeting held on March 9 included those attending the first meeting, the admitting nurse, and the housekeeping department manager. Prior to the meeting, agreement had been reached on the role of the admitting nurse for administering the early testing sequences, and at this meeting it was decided to implement early testing concurrently. Agreement was also reached to start up the admission scheduling system on April 10. The director of nursing voiced some reservation about getting the physicians to cooperate with nursing personnel in securing the discharge estimates; she stated that some members of the medical staff were well-known for their lack of cooperation with nursing. The chief of medicine replied that he would personally "straighten out the troublemakers;" the surgeon also agreed to help secure medical staff cooperation. This outspoken support by two influential members of Baker's medical staff set the stage for initiating the implementation activities. Although the director of nursing voiced some lack of conviction and lingering reservations about the nursing department's role in securing discharge estimates, there was a strong desire from the doctors to begin implementation as soon as possible. The medical staff executive committee met on April 6 and approved the beginning of the admitting scheduling system.

## Admitting Office Reorganization

In January, Baker's admitting office was found to require extensive reorganization in order to raise its effectiveness to the level required by the admission scheduling system. The Baker office received intensive attention from the Bureau staff during February, March, and April. It should be remembered that the office had been given expanded responsibilities only a year and a half earlier. Well developed traditions and even written protocols were missing. Communications within and from the office were incomplete. Both the employees and first line supervision seemed unclear as to their full responsibilities.

The general admitting procedures and the specific admitting clerk tasks were studied in detail for all three shifts. As a result, the procedures were categorized into three activities: direct patient admission activities; patient transfer activities; and census activities. A detailed work flow was made for each of these activities, and three major problem areas were identified: there was a lack of job definition on the afternoon and midnight shifts; there was too great an overlap in responsibility between shifts for the performance of many of the activities; and there was need for greater communication from the admitting clerks to the admitting office supervisor and the business office manager. On March 1, the Bureau recommended strengthening supervision of the second shift as well as a number of changes in office procedures and work flow. The admitting office's second shift was deemed particularly crucial to the admission scheduling system because second shift personnel were to input Baker's data. Because the second shift admitting clerks were less experienced than the first shift clerks, the admitting office's second shift received particular attention from the Bureau's implementation team. An experienced second shift supervisor was hired, and several clerks were trained to operate the terminal. The adoption of these changes proceeded slowly and required the extensive involvement of Bureau personnel.

Start-up occurred April 10, 1972. Four broad and interrelated problem areas developed almost immediately and consumed major efforts of the Bureau team for the next two months. These problem areas were the discharge estimating system; the communications between nursing, admissions, lab, and x-ray; surgeons' dissatisfaction with allowances; and resistance from the operating room supervisor. These problems were simultaneous and interconnected but are described separately below for clarity.

## The Discharge Estimating System

The Bureau team was familiar with the resistance which physicians had to making discharge estimates for their patients, and considerably modified the system which had been used in Able. A study of historical data indicated that patient age, diagnosis and admitting physician were the best predictors of length of stay; they were used to determine a probable discharge date for each admitted patient. Three or two days before this date each patient's record would be flagged, and the physician would be asked to estimate a discharge date for the patient on this "flag day." Such a system relies on a computer for three functions: to identify the flag day for each patient (for about twenty percent of the patients each day); to provide printout for discharge estimate requests and to process the estimates obtained from the physicians; and to provide the scheduling guidelines for the admitting supervisor's use. A computer terminal was installed to support the dynamic system, and the data collection and the processing system were begun in April.

Initially, the computer output was not used for scheduling decisions. It was understood that discharge estimates would be difficult to obtain, and the initial results would not be sufficiently accurate to provide a stable system. Beds available through discharge were calculated manually, based on the average number of expected discharges for each day of the week. The intention was to change over to the dynamic system once it proved stable.

The provision of patient discharge estimates soon proved troublesome. On April 21 a meeting was held with the head nurses and ward clerks to review the discharge estimate situation. Two of the clerks attending were quite negative; one stated that she believed the system would not work and that she would not participate in securing estimates. The percentages of requested estimates actually supplied were forty-seven, forty-nine, and sixty-one percent, respectively, for the medical, medical-surgical, and surgical units. The head nurse on the surgical unit was more receptive when the physicians visited the unit. She was more interested in making an effort to ask each physician personally for the required discharge estimates, and she also felt that estimates were easier to obtain on her unit.

During the middle of May, the overall discharge estimate response rate on the three nursing units declined, and varied from ten percent to forty percent, indicating an apparent lack of interest on the part of both nursing personnel and physicians. During a period in July, the overall physician response rate was twenty-two percent with an accuracy rate of thirty-four percent.[2] Since previous research indicates that if physicians are asked to provide an estimate of discharge one day prior to a predicted discharge based on historical data for the patient's service classification, the accuracy rate can be from eighty-five to ninety-five percent correct,[3] an accuracy rate of thirty-four percent suggested an apparent unwillingness on the part of Baker's medical staff to cooperate with implementing this aspect of the admission scheduling system.

The Bureau was dealing with two problems simultaneously, the problem of improving the physician response and accuracy rate, and the problem of making the manually based scheduling system work. There was a shortage of resources to handle both problems thoroughly and an inevitable tendency to concentrate on the scheduling system, which was producing real decisions, and therefore had to work if the hospital was going to admit patients. It was argued that heavy emphasis on getting the physicians to do better on estimating would cause further antagonism. Moreover, there was no readily available mechanism to reach individual physicians in order to get them to do better. The manual system of estimating available bids was adequate, and after several months of indecision, the effort to secure physicians' estimates was terminated.

## Coordination and Communication

Shortly after the start-up of the admission scheduling system, it became clear to the implementation team that greater coordination was needed both within the nursing department and between nursing and the other departments involved in the system. Unwittingly, problems were being created simply because one department lacked knowledge of the impact of its actions on the other departments. One example of such problems involved the assignment of a specific bed to a specific patient prior to or at the time of admission. Traditionally, it had been the responsibility of nursing unit personnel to assign surgical patients to beds based on the list of patients scheduled for surgery the following day. With the need for bed control in the admitting office in order to make the scheduling system work well, the Bureau team tried to have the bed assignment function switched to admitting office personnel. However, because of the feeling among nursing personnel that the admitting clerks would not be able to make "good" assignments based on both the personal and medical considerations of the patient, they resisted giving up their control.

The computer-printed nurses' reports used to collect discharge estimates for individual patients from their physicians created other problems. The reports were produced on the computer terminal in the admitting office, and were distributed to the nursing units early each morning. Nursing unit personnel attempted to obtain the discharge estimates from the physicians, and filled in certain information on the reports. Since this information was to be input data for the next day's reports, both the format and content were crucial. In fairness, it should be noted that the entire situation was aggravated by a number of technical problems in producing accurate and timely reports. Corrections were not always completed and computed in the system.

Such problems appeared to be attributable to a lack of organizational coordination, and Bureau proposed that a communication meeting be held with nursing supervisors and head nurses, the admitting officer, and the admitting nurse. After continued urging by the Bureau an initial "gripe session" was held on May 16. This meeting had an immediate cathartic effect.

As these meetings continued to be held, they became an increasingly important part of Baker's operating structure. When the meetings began to deal with more important interdepartmental matters, decisions had to be delayed because, in the absence of an associate or assistant administrator, only the administrator, himself, could deal with these new issues coming before the communication meetings. In January 1973 the meetings were rescheduled so that the administrator could attend all the meetings personally.

## Changing the Surgical Admission Allowances

The Bureau's system of medical and surgical admission allowances helped to increase the number of medical admissions in May 1972, and there was also a small increase in the number of surgical admissions. However, during the period 1969-1971, forty additional physicians had been granted hospital privileges at Baker, and a considerable number of these physicians were given surgical privileges. Consequently, the number of procedures per physician had been decreasing for reasons independent of the Bureau's activities. For whatever reason, implementation of admission allowances became the immediate focus. This brought the Bureau into direct conflict with a powerful group within the hospital—the surgical department of the medical staff.

On May 22 a surgeon known for his volatile temper became angered because he observed a number of empty beds in the surgical nursing unit. This occurred because the operating room supervisor, who scheduled surgical admissions, had not implemented the Bureau's surgical admission allowances. The surgeon demanded that one of the nurses present write a note verifying that there were ten empty beds, and then met with two of his colleagues, one of whom was a former chief of the medical staff. These three then went to the administrator and voiced a vigorous complaint. At the next regular surgical department meeting, a surgeons' ad hoc committee was formed to review the surgical admission allowances. This committee was appointed on the spot by the chief of surgery, and consisted of the three surgeons who were most vocal in their complaints, plus the administrator at his request. Shortly thereafter, the administrator told the Bureau's project principal that he was under pressure. Some of the surgeons were apparently talking to board members and the the executive director of the hospital authority. The project principal, the administrator, and the executive director met promptly. After a thorough discussion, the executive director authorized further work with the system. He noted that the overall impact was helpful to the patients and to the doctors and that the slight slack in the summer months would give time to settle disputes and smooth the system's operations.

On June 7 two of the Bureau's investigators met with the surgeon's committee in order to resolve the conflict. The surgeons objected to the Bureau's basing the allowances for medical and surgical admissions upon historical data which did not reflect Baker's increased occupancy level, and they claimed the allowances favored the medical department of the medical staff. The allowances actually gave the surgeons a slightly higher fraction of total hospital admissions than they had held historically. However, the surgeons requested a redefinition of equity between medical and surgical admissions. According to the surgeons on the ad hoc committee, equity was equal waiting times for medical and surgical patients. Because the surgical length of stay is about thirty-six percent shorter than the medical, 7.2 days compared to 11.2 days, this would allow the surgeons to admit proportionally more patients.

At the surgeons' request, the Bureau readjusted the allowances by basing them on an arranged balance in the length of the waiting times for medical and surgical admissions. At the same time, the administrator was able to transfer six pediatric beds to the adult medical-surgical unit. (This decision had resulted from other studies.) As a result of these negotiations, the surgical admission allowance was increased by eight per week; the medical admissions allowance was decreased by two per week. The Bureau anticipated pediatric scheduling problems due to the bed reduction, and preliminary pediatric admission allowances were determined. However, the pediatric system was not implemented because both the Baker administrator and the Bureau wanted to concentrate on the adult medical and surgical units. In addition to changing the allowances, it was agreed that the business office manager would periodically review the length of the waiting lines and make admission allowance adjustments in order to maintain equity in the length of the admission waiting times. Shortly thereafter, on June 21, the new allowances were implemented. The surgical department was satisfied; the revised allowances were accepted without further resistance. Curiously, the change did not arouse resistance from the internal medicine department.

## The OR Supervisor and the Surgical Allowances

Prior to the Bureau's intervention, the Baker operating room supervisor had the responsibility of controlling surgical admissions by virtue of her surgery scheduling function. When most admission control was transferred to the admissions office, she kept this power. Moreover, the hospital had an admissions process in which surgical patients received preference. Surgical patients were scheduled first; medical patients were then called to fill whatever open beds remained. As a result of her crucial role, the operating room supervisor established close relationships with the surgeons. She viewed the Bureau's activities as a reduction in her role and in her power vis-a-vis the surgeons. She alone kept records of surgical admissions and surgery schedules. When the Bureau's representatives asked to see these data to establish the admission allowances, she claimed the data were not available. Her lack of cooperation continued; as already noted, she did not implement the initial allowances correctly. On some days she would exceed the allowances, on other days she would schedule fewer surgeries than the allowances. This practice continued after the revised allowances were agreed to on June 21. However by this time, the Bureau had arranged for the admitting office to keep records of surgical admissions. These deviations from the revised allowances were brought to the administrator's attention, and he wrote a sharply worded memo to the operating room supervisor, ordering her to implement the surgical allowances. A copy of the memo was sent to the chief of the surgical department; another copy was posted in the physicians' staff room. The memo had its intended effect and the surgical allowances were implemented properly. Shortly thereafter, the operating room supervisor became a regular participant in the communication meetings. She became an important and cooperative member of this group; on several occasions she praised the Bureau's system and stated that the Bureau had improved the operation of the hospital.

With the change of heart of the OR supervisor, the initial installation problems subsided. Three of the four—communication, the supervisor, and the allowances—were solved by specific adjustments. The fourth, discharge estimating, had been deferred.

## Termination of the Discharge Estimating System

The discharge estimate response rates and the accuracy of estimates remained at unsatisfactory levels through early September. On September 7, the executive committee of the medical staff formed an ad hoc committee of doctors who were interested in meeting with the administrator and representatives from the Bureau to discuss the discharge estimate situation. Significantly, only three doctors attended the meeting on September 20. At a subsequent surgical department meeting, the chief of the surgical department also discussed this matter with his colleagues. These two meetings produced no change; the surgeons ignored any suggestion for altering or improving the system to facilitate getting better estimates. As a result, it was decided to discontinue the discharge estimating system; this was done on October 26. Shortly thereafter, the computer terminal was removed from the admitting office. The "dynamic" system had never reached operational level, because of the estimating performance.

The success of the allowance-based system indicated that precise discharge estimates were not necessary to maintain high occupancy and low cancellations. The occupancy level of the three units involved was maintained at an average occupancy level of ninety-six percent during April to September 1972. A simple system, not requiring daily computation was found to be feasible, and with this system no computer terminal was required.

## Maintaining the Admission Scheduling System

During an eight-week period beginning in December the Bureau team left the administration of the admission system completely in the hands of Baker's personnel. This was done to determine whether they had developed the internal capabilities to administer the system without outside intervention. Prior to December the Bureau had developed a system for holiday scheduling which would minimize the expected drop in admissions during the coming holiday season. However, the Bureau learned that the holiday scheduling system had not been well implemented, and by the beginning of 1973 Baker reported increasingly serious problems administering the system. A marked increase in the number of cancellations of surgery drew ire from the physicians while nursing complained of extra workloads as a result of an increase in the number of transfers.

By mid-January the Bureau team decided to begin a series of analyses to identify problems which had arisen during the period when the hospital was solely responsible for maintaining the system. Before withdrawing from active involvement with the system, the Bureau and the hospital had agreed upon the data base required to administer the system. It was arranged for the admitting office to keep weekly graphs which plotted the following data: the predicted census and the actual census for the three units in the system; the number of emergency admissions before 1:00 P.M., the number after 1:00 P.M., and the total number of emergency admissions to the units; the total weekly cancellations; the total weekly transfers; weekly totals of the actual and allotted number of surgical patients; weekly totals of the actual and allotted number of medical patients; weekly totals of the actual and allotted numbers of both surgical and medical patients; the number of days in the future medical and surgical patients were being scheduled, and the delay (in days) for both medical and surgical admissions. Periodic adjustments to the system, as well as its daily administration, were to be based on these records. When the Bureau team asked to see these data in order to begin their analysis, they learned that the data had been collected but not regularly summarized. Without the summarized data, the system could not be administered properly. Basing the system on the above sixteen data points added administrative as well as data collection problems and was in fact a somewhat cumbersome system. Yet the data requirements were clear, and it had appeared that these requirements were well understood by hospital personnel when the Bureau stopped direct assistance in December.

At near full occupancy, the system is highly sensitive to small changes in the number of additional admissions. Usually, the hospital overreacted to immediate conditions. When occupancy was lower than expected, too many patients were called in, and several days later cancellations had to be made. The Bureau underrated the time required and overrated the organizational resources available at Baker to administer the system. It was also learned that a system so sensitive requires considerable administrative experience.

Further study identified several other factors which contributed to the problems. The most important of these was a large and unexpected increase in the number of emergency admissions. The emergency admission allowance in the initial admission scheduling system was based on historical data which indicated am average of six emergency admissions per day, about three of which occurred after 1:00 P.M. However by the spring of 1973, the emergency admission rate had risen to an average of eleven per day. This near doubling of the number of emergencies was responsible for much of the increase in cancellations and transfers.

A health records analyst was hired in November 1972 and was asked to study the increase in emergency admissions. He learned that three physicians accounted for approximately half of the hospital's emergency admissions. The admissions of the three doctors were studied and given to the executive committee of the medical staff for review and possible action. The three physicians were brought before the executive committee in order to defend their practices. Two of the three did not receive specific sanctions. The third was suspended for the month of April and placed on probation for the remainder of 1973.

The January analysis also identified two secondary factors which suggested that refinements in the system would bring the admissions process under greater control. The initial allowances for the three nursing units did not include a provision for transfers from the hospital's intensive care units (ICU/CCU) to units in the system. This factor would not be important with lower occupancy levels, but when occupancy approaches 100 percent, transfers into and out of the units in the system became critical. At near capacity, the system would not have been able to absorb what equaled two admissions per day without very serious problems had it not been for an offsetting factor which had also not been included in the initial allowances. It was learned that some patients coming within the surgical allowances who were admitted for clean gynecological surgeries, were placed instead on the obstetrical unit. These admissions did not completely offset additions due to transfers from the intensive care unit, but they did help to reduce the number of potential cancellations.

The various implementation problems were not minor, and it was by no means possible to say as of May 1973 that the system was stable and permanently a part of the admission process at Baker. It was reasonable to assess the introduction as successful, both in economic and organizational terms. The role of the admitting nurse had been expanded, and this increased the effectiveness of the admitting process. The admitting office was reorganized, strengthened, and made more efficient. The communication group created an important new organizational mechanism for improved problem solving and decision making as well as for better interdepartmental communication. The admission allowances enabled the hospital to provide firm future admission dates, an important benefit to both patients and physicians. The Bureau's activities resulted in strengthening the hospital's supervisory staff, not only by employing a more experienced second shift admitting office supervisor and a health records analyst, but by increasing the skill and competence of those who came in contact with the system. Finally, the overall system allowed the hospital to operate at near full occupancy without the organizational stress that existed prior to the introduction of the system. By May 1973 the situation was viewed as favorable for future work. Among the encouraging signs were the decisions to look at emergency admissions and approach physicians who were responsible for excessive emergency admissions, and to look at the admitting office's practice to determine if they were following the revised procedures. An alternative to either would have been to blame the system. The shared willingness to look for other explanations of difficulty suggested that key actors in the system had begun to acknowledge an investment in the innovation, and that it was on the road to acceptance, if not there yet.

## NOTES

[1]Connected to the University of Michigan computer. Had the hospital been using conventional accounts receivable programs, the computer requirements could have been modified to fit these routines.

[2]Response Rate = Number of responses ÷ Number of times asked

Accuracy Rate = Number of patients accurately estimate ÷ Number of patients with estimates provided.

[3]G. H. Robinson, L. E. Davis, and G. C. Johnson. "The Physician as an Estimator of Hospital Stay." *Human Factors*, 8, 1966, pp. 201-208.

# IV.5

# Baker Hospital Nursing Department Accommodates to Change

*by Edwin H. Tuller*

The two preceding chapters described the multiple effects of introducing a single change, the admitting scheduling system. This chapter reports how multiple changes affected a single department, the nursing department at Baker. The focus on a single department's response to a variety of changes makes a clear chronology important to understanding the events and reactions to them, and the material is presented in eight-month segments, time periods which seem to fit the continuing flow of events during 1970-73.

## January-August 1970

The total staffing of the Baker nursing department in early 1970 was slightly over 300. The registered nurse employment was approximately 100, licensed practical nurse employment seventy, and aides and orderlies 145. The staff was distributed by shifts as follows:

| | | |
|---|---|---|
| Day | 125 | ( 7:00 A.M.— 3:00 P.M.) |
| Evening | 100 | ( 3:00 A.M.—11:00 P.M.) |
| Night | 90 | (11:00 A.M.— 7:00 P.M.) |

The department was organized by shifts, with the nursing supervisors responsible only for the operation of their units on the day shift. This organization structure was questioned very early, as a result of initial work on the development of responsibility centers for the budgeting process.

Twelve separate nursing responsibility centers were proposed to provide for the accumulation of financial, activity, and other data useful in future budgeting and managerial control. One responsibility center for the department of nursing was simply too big for purposes of control.

The research staff recommended establishing responsibility centers across shifts, on a nursing unit basis. This recommendation was consistent with the goal of continuity in patient care and required a major increase in responsibility for nursing supervisors, and some decrease in responsibility for the house (shift) directors. The director of nursing did not feel so major a structural change was appropriate. Because she did not delegate financial matters to her assistant, the director now handled the increased paperwork for dealing with twelve cost centers instead of one.

On May 1 the new administrator began his work at the hospital. One of his first actions was to order an increase in the occupancy level, from seventy-five to approximately eighty-five percent. A higher occupancy level would increase the overall operating efficiency of the hospital if the budget, specifically the manpower complement, did not increase accordingly. The result of the new administrator's policy was indeed an increase in occupancy, which during mid-1971 averaged just under eighty percent.

## September 1970-April 1971

An August attitude survey to secure base line data for the project was viewed with some irritation by the nursing department, as it required releasing each employee for forty-five minutes at a specified time to complete the questionnaire. Moreover a number of nursing and other personnel worried about how the results might be used against them by the new administrator. A brief summary of results was prepared and made available to the nursing director and others, but neither the Bureau team nor any member of hospital administration urged that feedback be arranged for all personnel.

The policy of increasing occupancy was in full force, and the census moved from about eighty to ninety percent, exceeding that figure in two of the fall months. This increase in occupancy meant a substantial increase in workload for floor nursing personnel. If one assumes seventy-five percent to have been the norm, then ninety percent occupancy represents a twenty percent increase in workload in a period of less than six months. Moreover, high occupancy meant a disproportionate increase in transfers to accommodate the extra patients, which further added to nursing workloads. Occupancy declined in December, but only to about eighty percent.

During this period, the research staff began to study employee turnover. Although this project was based in the personnel-payroll office, there were several questions about record keeping in nursing. In this "backdoor" fashion, the director learned of the turnover project. Her reaction was one of cautious cooperation; as with the attitude survey, she was uncertain how her department would compare to other units and how the turnover information would be used. In any event, she was more interested in solving the problem of absenteeism within her department. She asked the research staff to assist her with this problem, especially in suggesting methods to reduce absenteeism. At this time, the study of absenteeism was not on the agenda for the research staff, and her suggestion was not taken up.

In early 1971 the pace of activity in the nursing department picked up considerably. Not only did the research staff want to implement some of their ideas, especially in the area of budgeting, but the new administrator also wanted to make some changes in nursing. Complicating the picture somewhat was the fact that during this period the director of nursing was out of the hospital on an extended sick leave.

Preparation of the next year's budget began in January. Department heads had not participated in the budgeting process before, nor did they have a well developed sense of their managerial responsibilities and areas of managerial concern.

A member of the research staff was assigned to work in the hospital on a full time basis as a budget officer. His first activity was the collection of historical data about each of the departments and nursing units: the number of units of output per month; and the number of manhours worked per month. These data were necessary to assist in the forecast of departmental activity for the fiscal year, and to determine the appropriate number of manhours per unit of output.

In the department of nursing, the unit of output was "patient days" although it was recognized that nursing had output other than patient days, and that all patient days were not equivalent because some patients required more care than others. The statistical forecasts of patient days were increased by the administrator to represent his target occupancy rate for each nursing unit.

The director of nursing was formally introduced to the budgeting activity at a department head meeting called by the administrator. As she was on sick leave, the director came to the hospital only for the meeting, at which the purpose of budgeting, the budget procedure, and the timetable were explained. She left the meeting with a department head package containing forecasts of work volume, manpower use data, written instructions, and forms to be filled out.

In part because the assistant director of nursing was already carrying a heavy load, the director chose not to burden her further with a budgeting assignment. Furthermore, the director realized that this budget would be the one she would be responsible for meeting through June 30, 1972. The budgeting process seemed quite complicated to the director of nursing, as well as to the other department heads. She was unsure, for example, of the implications of the "volume forecasts" on the number and classification of personnel which would be approved for each nursing unit.

The budget officer worked closely with the director of nursing throughout this period, and they developed a healthy rapport. When they worked on the budget, the director came to the hospital solely for that purpose. Occasionally, they worked on Saturdays. While the budget was in the process of preparation, it became clear that the limited time available would not permit the use of the more sophisticated techniques which had been planned and presented to the department heads. The administrator agreed to carry forward the existing personnel complement with only a few exceptions. This decision sharply diminished the importance of the budget negotiation sessions which each department head had with the administrator; there was little left to negotiate.

In February a second attitude survey was administered. This time only a sample of employees was taken, and it was somewhat easier for nursing to comply with the administration schedule. Because nothing dramatic resulted from the previous survey, department heads and employees alike were less apprehensive. The feedback of results and a comparison with the previous survey occurred several months later. The comparisons indicated that satisfaction in the nursing department had declined significantly in the interim. The clearest single explanation appeared to be the increased occupancy; both oral and written comments from nurses emphasized the problems associated with more patients and more moving of patients. To some degree, the problems were attributed directly to the new administrator. Curiously, the workload comments came only from registered nurses, although licensed practical nurses' satisfaction had also decreased.

In February and March two changes in the nursing organization were made: the position of admitting nurse was created in the nursing department, and two additional nursing supervisor positions were authorized on the day shift. In addition, the assistant director of nursing resigned; the vacancy was filled by a transfer from within the department. The admitting nurse, a position suggested by the administrator, was responsible for expediting the admission process for scheduled surgical patients. The nursing supervisors were responsible for the quality of care in their areas, but this did not mean a responsibility for staffing, or other activities on the second and third shifts. The supervisors were to have more responsibility than in the past, yet the division of responsibility between supervisors and second and third shift house directors had not been changed. In any event, the issue of defining formal accountability on a shift rather than area basis was being overshadowed by other major problems. For the director the problem of dealing with absenteeism with a continuing high census remained acute.

## May-December 1971

Mid-1971 was a period of considerable pressure for the director. The pressure of higher occupancy was felt throughout nursing, and though the pressure experienced may have peaked earlier in the year, it was still pronounced. Occupancy was holding close to ninety percent, down slightly from early 1971 but fully ten precent above the comparable period in 1970. The close working relationship which the director had experienced with the former administrator had not been reestablished with the new administrator, and the director indicated some difficulty in adjusting to the new situation.

During this period two major activities of the research staff involved the nursing department: the development of the manpower input decision (MID) planning report; and development of a patient classification instrument for the nursing staff allocation project.

In May the concept of the manpower input decision or MID was formally presented to the department heads. The MID was in fact an alternative to a time study based work standard. The research team saw little value in (and even less possibility of) developing engineering standards which would replace department head judgments. Bureau interest was in formalizing this judgment as an explicit part of the cost control process. The process began with the follow-up and expansion of data collection begun during the budgeting work, and the compilation of a thirty-three month listing of units of production and manhours worked. The Bureau staff worked directly with the department heads involved, analyzing the data collected and asking them to judge the appropriate manpower input per unit of output. The same data were presented to the administrator for review and analysis. The department of nursing and the laboratory were selected as prototype departments. Thus the director of nursing along with the chief laboratory technician met with the budget officer prior to the introduction of the MID to the other department heads. Even in this small session, the MID concept was difficult to communicate. It was explained that an MID would be selected by the department head for each responsibility center, based on the past thirty-three months of data. This MID would be presented to the administrator in a negotiation session at which an MID would be agreed to, for use in short-term manpower planning. Specifically, a forecast would be made of responsibility center activity over a two-month horizon; based on this forecast and the MID the department head would know how much manpower to schedule.

The questions were many. Was the patient day the best and most complete measure of departmental activity? How did the MID relate to the recently negotiated budget? How accurate were the forecasts? Was the director of nursing responsible for the accuracy of the forecast, since in the end her performance would be judged on the actual ratio of manhours to patient days? How could the MID be used in the emergency room or obstetrics where some of the output is "standby capacity?" How did the MID affect the mix of nursing personnel (RNs, LPNs, and aides)? How did the MID help in day-to-day assignment of personnel? Did the MID recognize that employees come in eight-hour increments, and in a certain job classification, on a certain nursing unit, on a certain shift? A number of these questions raised issues the Bureau team had not considered, and no further effort was made to implement the manpower adjustment part of the project until more progress could be made in resolving some of the problems raised.

In June another member of the research staff began meeting with the director for the purpose of developing a patient classification instrument which would be used in a nursing staff allocation project he was heading. The director assigned one of her supervisors to this project. Over a period of six weeks, the supervisor checked off daily forty-six items for approximately fourteen patients a day. She also indicated for each patient her professional opinion regarding his nursing care requirements; was the patient a "high," "medium," or "low" care patient? As with the other projects, the explanations provided seemed to leave the director unclear of the implications of this activity on her department.

In November when the results of the patient classification activity were reported to the director, several discussions took place which again suggested that problems were being framed differently by the research staff and the director, resulting in continued misunderstandings. In brief, the original problem was a simple one, how to have the number of nurses on a shift match the need level of patients. The research staff approached the problem by defining need as the number of patients, modified by an index of care requirements, and then proceeded to gather the data required. The director in effect replied, "Very interesting, but we know how sick patients are; our problem is getting the nurses where they are needed." The research staff then developed a scheduling model using the patient classification system which could schedule registered and practical nurses and aides. Again, the director replied, "Very interesting, but we know who we need where. Our problem is getting them to show up—our problem is absenteeism." The research staff felt they had acknowledged the presence of the absenteeism problem by developing a scheduling model which optimized whatever staff was available. The director did not wish to schedule around absenteeism, she wanted to solve it. The director viewed absenteeism by nurses as irresponsible behavior, which made discussion of alternative solutions difficult. Nevertheless, it remained true that none of the research staff wished to apply their analytic tools to the problem of reducing absenteeism, although occasional efforts were made to analyze data that might cast light on its causes.

The MID activity attracted several members of the research staff to the director. Two men were examining the reception of the MID by the department heads and attempting to explain this reception in terms of change theory. Another man was trying to develop an MID in central supply where output data were not readily available. Other members of the research staff were continuing cost containment work in the laboratory and elsewhere in the hospital. Also during this period, the admitting office began preparation for implementing the admitting scheduling system. This project, too, involved occasional meetings with the director. This was the fourth major project underway at the hospital at this time. The research staff had not fully appreciated the time demands being placed on the director until she said in exasperation one day, "I can't meet with you on that day; I have three other meetings scheduled with you people. When can I get my own work done?" From this point on, the research staff tried to keep a log of meetings with the director of nursing and other key department heads.

In November the business manager resigned, and his replacement was the business manager from the administrator's former hospital. This switch had a considerable impact on the director of nursing. Under the previous administrator she held the position of unofficial second in command. Although relations with the new administrator had not been easy, there had been no clear indication that this unoffical status was changed. Now came a young, aggressive, cost-conscious man who obviously was held in high respect by the administrator. Within a month, the admitting nurse was transferred out of the nursing department to the admitting office, which was to maintain a "professional liasion" with the director of nursing. To the director, this liasion meant little more than having to provide a replacement for the admitting nurse when she went on vacation, which the director was required to do over the Christmas and New Years holiday.

## January-August 1972

During the first eight months of 1972 the tempo of activities placed severe strains on Baker's nursing department. Three major and several minor projects required significant time from nursing personnel, and some of them caused direct conflict between nursing and other departments. The director's preferred style of leadership required her to stay fully abreast of and involved in all the projects, which both focused the burden on her and limited the ability of her staff to share confidently in the process of modifying and implementing the changes.

Budgeting for the next fiscal year was required, and though the use of the manpower input decision for short-term staffing adjustment decisions had been delayed, the administrator and Bureau team planned to use it for budgeting. The intention as before was to make department heads responsible for a sound budget proposal, which would then be argued out with the administrator, the outcome being a final budget subject only to board approval. Substantial work, primarily by the director, went into a manpower budget which increased considerably the manpower authorized for nursing. The assistant director and two house directors were involved more actively than during the prior year, and were also present during the final decision meeting with the administrator. The administrator was open in his praise for the work they had done, his concern for quality patient care, and his approval of their recommendations. He noted that cuts might have to be made if the board finance committee would not approve the required money. Though the steps were different, the final result was the same; the board-approved budget which came back several months later reflected last year's budget far more closely than it did the one proposed by nursing.

One purpose of the budgeting project had been to involve department heads more fully in budget preparation; another purpose was to secure closer adherence to the approved budget. Early problems with the MID had shown the need for, in the research team's parlance, "closing the feedback loop," that is, letting department heads know how well they were doing. A manpower control program was being devised to provide information to responsibility center heads regarding hours worked per twenty-eight day reporting period; this could be compared to the forecast man-hours requirement for the same period. In addition, the manpower control report would contain information regarding overtime, sick leave, and vacation time. Unfortunately, the business manager was implementing at the same time a position control program administered by the payroll/personnel office.

The first direct conflict involving these two programs involved the department of nursing. The director had requested the posting of a new position, which, in her understanding, was within her budget authorization. She was told by a personnel clerk that the responsibility center was presently in excess of its authorized FTEs for that job category and that the position could not be posted. The director was incensed; she felt this refusal by a clerk was demeaning, and she also felt that the research staff, business manager, and administrator, though perhaps not in collusion, had set up conflicting standards to be selectively used against her. There was considerable difficulty and delay in sorting out the confusion, and clarifying with the personnel clerk, business manager, and administrator the inconsistency of the position control program as developed by the business manager, and the manpower control program that had already received approval.

The feelings of pressure were not reduced by a thorough review, required by the manpower control program, of nursing practices in assigning nursing costs to responsibility centers, and a special study initiated later when a new "Analysis of Operations" report showed major discrepancies with the conventional monthly expense statement. The discrepancies were identified as weaknesses in accounting method rather than management practice, and both the director and her staff become more convinced that many complexities of budgeting and manpower control were poorly understood within administration and in the business office.

This period was also a time of major activity for the admission scheduling project. One distinct failure of communication occurred in January with a small trial of the early diagnostic testing of medical admissions. Although the laboratory and radiology were well informed of the date of implementation of this trial, the nursing floors were not. Imagine the surprise and consternation of the head nurse when the first early tested patient arrived on the unit unannounced at 10:00 A.M. and said, "Here I am, which way to room 527?" Not only was the bed not yet ready for this patient, but the present occupant was still in the bed, awaiting transportation home at approximately 11:00 A.M.

The task force formed to oversee the admission scheduling project gave the director a chance to express her reservations about the early diagnostic testing experiment and the location of the admitting nurse (and therefore the patient assignment decision) within the admitting office. She also predicted considerable difficulty with securing discharge estimates from physicians, and registered her distaste for having the nursing department made responsible for collecting them. The difficulties did in fact arise and affected everyone in nursing. Securing discharge estimates added paperwork for the nurses, was irritating to physicians, and caused unpleasantness for those in nursing responsible for collecting them. Although many of the problems were on the day shift, the afternoon and night shifts were also affected.

After about a week, the research staff held a meeting with head nurses and ward clerks regarding the discharge estimating activity. Complaints appeared to arise from two factors: the increase in paperwork the discharge estimating activity required, and the manner in which some members of the medical staff reacted to requests for estimates. Both securing the discharge estimate and the arrival of early diagnostic tested patients on the units occurred during the busy morning hours. This is also the period when doctors make their daily rounds and patients are being discharged. Clearly, the admitting scheduling system was adding stress to the relations between nursing and the medical staff, between nursing and admitting, and inevitably between nursing and administration.

In January and February the nursing department was also engaged in a study of the times of physician rounds at the hospital. The goal of this project was "to minimize the length of time between the writing of an order and the receipt of results by the physician." Ward clerks and head nurses cooperated with these studies, although they took offense at inadvertent implications by the research staff that there were long delays in the process. To the nursing personnel, they were being harrassed once again about the administrative trivia attached to their job.

Occupancy remained at a high level during early 1972; the highest sustained occupancy during the whole study in fact occurred during February-June 1972. Thus although the scheduling system was designed to minimize the ill effects of high occupancy, its start-up problems were experienced while the nursing department was under a severe strain.

In an attempt to resolve these problems, the research staff proposed a communication meeting be held with nursing supervisors, head nurses, the admitting officer supervisor, and the admitting nurse. The director of nursing was not enthusiastic about such a meeting. Would it really be worthwhile? Her initial reaction was to postpone the meeting because of the heavy overload on supervisors and head nurses.

Continuing problems with handling early diagnostic testing patients and securing discharge estimates, disagreements between admitting and the operating room supervisor, and a proposed shift in beds from pediatrics to the surgical unit made the need for better communication critical. It was finally agreed to set up weekly meetings between nursing supervisors and the admitting nurse and her supervisor. These meetings facilitated direct and open discussion between members of the research team and what at times had appeared to be hostile factions within the hospital. The shift in beds from pediatrics, for example, had at one point become an argument about where beds (the actual hardware) were, should be, or should have been. In late May, partly because of the success of the communication meetings, the research team again raised with the director of nursing the possibility of redefining the nursing structure to allow some of her responsibilities to be delegated to her supervisors. She asked that nothing be done which would raise the issue. She felt that she was preparing her staff carefully and discretely for such a move, but that open discussion at that point would be harmful.

The latter part of May and early June was a period of unusually high tension in the hospital and in the nursing department. The surgeon discontent with the scheduling model was unresolved, and the director was faced with considerable staff dissatisfaction because of the heavy patient load and the number of transfers. The shift of beds from pediatrics, the loss of authority over the admitting nurse, the closer required liaison with ancillary departments which was in part being handled through unconventional channels (the communication meeting)—all of these were new, direct, and essentially uncontrollable pressures on the director. In early June she spent a week at a nursing conference and returned with fresh perspectives, one of which may illustrate the change. In a conversation in mid-June, she indicated that a number of the patient transfers were more for nurse or physician convenience than for patient welfare. Discussion with her supervisors, she was confident, would help reduce this component considerably. Both the acknowledgment of the fact, and the willingness to discuss it openly with the research team and her supervisors, suggested a renewed confidence that she could cope with the problems which earlier had appeared to engulf her. The resolution of the surgical allowance problem, in the week following her return from the conference, and the subsequent decision of the operating room supervisor to cooperate fully in the admitting scheduling program contributed to a marked dissipation of tension, no doubt aided by a drop in occupancy which continued in July and August.

Meetings continued on a weekly basis, coming to be generally known as communication meetings rather than gripe sessions. They began to serve a useful organizational purpose beyond that of coordinating admission scheduling activities. They were particularly effective in connecting the nursing supervisors and some head nurses with other departments, and thus reducing the misunderstandings which had become a major problem during previous months. Membership was expanded to include the business manager and the assistant director of nursing. The department heads of radiology and the laboratory attended on an ad hoc basis as the particular agenda dictated. Occasionally, the physician members of the task force would attend, and the operating room supervisor became an important and cooperative member of the group.

In late June, a series of meetings were held regarding the nurse staff allocation project. The research team had completed phase one, the patient classification instrument, and now wanted to proceed with phase two. This would involve extensive data collection. During these meetings with the director and the nursing supervisors, the research staff received several helpful suggestions. Some required more work on the part of the nursing staff, others less. The director and supervisors wanted to make sure that the data collected would be a fair representation of the work done on the nursing unit, and there was discussion of providing a refined unit of output for use in the MID, in place of the simple count of patient days. The Head Nurse Form provided for a day-to-day and shift-to-shift check on the adequacy of nursing hours per patient. Until this time discussions of the "daily MID" had been in quite general terms. The research staff stressed the importance of the professional opinion of nurses to this work; this was quite a different thrust from the typical time study approach which might have been used in this study. On the whole, the director and the supervisors were supportive of this work, despite the large amount of data collection involved and the fact that there was already much activity on the nursing units where the data would be collected.

Throughout data collection, the research staff visited the LPNs and head nurses on all shifts of each unit providing data for this study. These visits served two main purposes: to keep the nurses accurate and timely in the completion of the required forms; and to maintain cordial relations despite the added workload. Many questions on procedures were asked and answered, and it was emphasized that the project would terminate in seven weeks.

The patient classification activity required a computer-generated form which included the most recent census. The research staff incorporated into this form a daily message from "the computer." Those communications occasionally related to the project itself, but more often they were banter and jokes, the butt of which were the computer and the research staff. By the end of the seven weeks, the LPNs who worked with these forms, as well as the others on the unit who did not, looked forward to these messages. Frequently, the LPNs wrote responses and general comments on the forms. They nonetheless continued to point out to the research staff how time-consuming and onerous was the task of classification.

During midsummer there was again a clear increase in tension in nursing. The director and the nursing supervisors felt that the discharge estimating activity was destroying the physician-nursing relationship. They felt that too many administrative duties were being placed on the nursing units. Finally, they felt that there were too many meetings involving supervisory nursing personnel—so many meetings that they found it increasingly difficult to get "their own" work done.

In late August, the nursing supervisors demanded a meeting with the administrator; they asked that the director and the assistant director be invited. During this meeting, the supervisors vented their frustrations. They emphasized that their feelings were not directed against the research staff or the director, but that whatever the underlying cause, something had to be done. The supervisors were not fully satisfied with the responses of the administrator, and later submitted to him written minutes of the meeting signed by each of the supervisors; they even waited a week before submitting the minutes so that it could be signed by one supervisor who had taken a brief vacation. Overall, the supervisors felt that the administrator was unconcerned or unsympathetic with significant problems at the operating level of the hospital.

## September 1972-May 1973

The primary activity of the budgeting project during this period was the preparation of the fiscal year 1974 budget which was done during December; this was at least one month earlier than in previous years. The budget procedure had been revised (for the third consecutive year) and was based on desired staffing patterns for a given level of occupancy. Once these patterns had been approved by the administrator, the budget would be calculated by a specially designed computer program. As in the past, the research staff worked with the director in preparing for these negotiations. In the negotiations, the administrator approved only a few of the director's proposals. However, there was considerable and vigorous discussion regarding staffing levels and job assignments in the various responsibility centers. This session contrasted sharply in spirit and approach with the MID negotiations during the previous January. When the session concluded, both administrator and director remarked, "We'll have to see what the monster [the computer] makes of this!"

In October the discharge estimating activity was ended; no member of nursing lamented its passing. The prescheduling of medical patients continued, although at a rate of less than twenty per week; with a functioning discharge estimating activity that number might have been doubled.

Nursing participation in the communication meetings terminated abruptly in late November. In a memorandum to the chairman (the business manager), the director stated:

> Several incidents directly relating to the quality of nursing care have recently been brought to my attention. On closer investigation by myself, it is apparent that nursing unit management requires new impetus. It is therefore logical at this time that nursing supervisors concentrate their efforts in the area of immediate responsibility. Their physical presence on the nursing unit is imperative. As a consequence, I am requesting that these supervisors be excused from the Communications group meetings unless the subject is directly related to the nursing care of the patient.

Clearly these incidents provided a timely vehicle for ending nursing participation in these meetings which seemed less oriented to the needs of the nursing department than to business-related matters on the day shift. The chairman suspended meetings for a few weeks, after which they resumed with full nursing participation.

In November the research staff reported briefly to the director and nursing supervisors regarding the August data collection for the nursing allocation project. This report to nursing provided information on the number of high, medium, and low care patients; the number of transfers, admissions, and discharges; and the number of forty-eight hour postoperative patients. During the meeting, there was considerable discussion about the data presented, where in the study it had come from, what it meant, and what comparisons could be made. This report seemed to "validate" the work of the research staff in supervisors' minds; that is, the findings seemed to confirm their own impressions of activity on the nursing unit. No further use was made of this information as other issues had higher priority. The nursing staff, however, expressed appreciation for the report.

At an early January communication meeting, the nursing supervisors reported serious deterioration in the medical staff-nursing relationship. At their suggestion and with the concurrence of the administrator, the professional services committee of the medical staff began to hold bimonthly meetings with them regarding this problem. These meetings, begun while the director of nursing was on vacation, succeeded in providing a basis for improved relationships.

In February the research staff received permission for a one-month trial of the nursing staff allocation system. This authorization was given by the administrator in the absence of the director of nursing. For the four-week period of the study, the research staff worked closely with the assistant director and director, incorporating several of their suggestions into the system. It was continually emphasized that the system was based completely on the professional opinion and judgment of nurses—most particularly LPNs, head nurses, and the assistant director. The study terminated according to schedule at the end of March.

Problems continued with interpreting the new budget and its still confusing method of translating manpower requirements to full time equivalents to dollars and back again to authorized staffing. At one point the administrator pointed out that vacation relief could not be added to the budget, and one of the house directors responded by cancelling all vacations on her shift! At another point the director, strongly supported by the assistant director, pointed to a new requirement of securing documentation from physicians for patients with inadequate admitting diagnosis. Nurses were required to do it, but staffing was based on patient days, not on the paperwork required by administration. Nevertheless, these were minor irritants, and the high tension that characterized late spring and late summer was not present.

The problems of adaptation to change in the nursing department were by no means solved. Although some of the research staff felt the director was still overly concerned with controlling all communications which took place with personnel in her department, they acknowledged she was held responsible for results and had a legitimate interest in protecting her staff from potentially conflicting demands. Poor relations with the medical staff remained a problem, apparently not improved by the discontinuation of requests for discharge estimates. A third and final attitude survey made in May 1973 confirmed the problem of tension with the medical staff, though it was not limited to nursing alone. In other respects, however, the survey results suggested that the problems of nursing dissatisfaction were less pronounced than they had appeared to be early in the project (February 1971), or during early 1972. An experimental introduction of team nursing, not part of the demonstration project, indicated that the nursing department was no longer simply reacting to or defending against externally imposed changes.

As of May 1973 the nursing department at Baker seemed to have weathered the experience of working with the research team successfully. Some of the problems which had made the three and one-half years difficult were due to ill-conceived research team projects; much wasted energy had been expended by nursing in a still incomplete revision of the budgeting system. Nor could the director be held responsible for the change in administrators, which brought a period of truly difficult interpersonal adjustments for her, complicated by her extended periods of illness. Perhaps the most fundamental source of difficulty would in other circumstances have been an asset, the nearly universal feeling within the nursing department that any activities not a part of caring for patients were extraneous, and any addition of such activities was unreasonable. The director sought to protect and nurture this attitude, but in so doing protected the incapacity of the department to understand and deal effectively with business office, ancillary department, administration, or research team perspectives, and also limited the contribution of her immediate subordinates to social support for her in the various conflicts, rather than sharing in the search for feasible solutions. Some of the high cost of this strategy appeared in the inability of the nursing department to secure support from other influential figures in the hospital when problems arose or were anticipated. Surprisingly, this rather narrow focus on patient care activities did not generate significant support from physicians, and the poor relations which the nursing department had with the medical staff toward the end of the period suggested that important problems still remained.

The most important contribution which the research team may have made to Baker's nursing department was to create such a requirement for improved interdepartmental understanding that the communication group was formed to meet it. The director was never enthusiastic about it and the supervisors often complained about the time the meetings consumed, yet it became the effective forum for problem framing and conflict resolution during the most difficult period of the project. It is a partial, but important truth, to say that Baker nursing found a structural solution to the technical and human problems they faced.

# IV.6

# Understanding Change in the Hospital[1]

*by Kurt R. Student*

The Bureau of Hospital Administration's four-year activity would be incomplete without some attempt to understand the implementation process itself. We do not seek to add one more model to the growing literature of organizational change, but have the more modest goal of developing a paradigm which helps the reader of the case studies in this section to understand some of the underlying factors in the implementation process as described in our cases. In attempting to understand our own work, we have identified five factors which appear to have been most important in our work at Able and Baker, and they are explained and illustrated in the material below.

## The Setting for Innovation

There is some evidence in the cases that the best environment for innovating is different from the setting for maintaining high morale, high quality, or high efficiency. The goal of innovation requires a shaking up, the goals of morale, quality, or efficiency a settling down. This observation is not original; Morison noted it in his study of the American Navy, and himself quoted Admiral Mahan's earlier observation that no military organization can change itself; it must have assistance from the outside.[2] More recent work by Greiner, Haire, Kaufman, and Thompson supports this basic view of a favorable setting for innovation: there must be dissatisfaction, and the only reliable source for such dissatisfaction is the external environment.[3] In Able, two critical aspects of the external environment were a force for stability rather than change. Able physicians lost the benefit of admission at will in the new admitting scheduling system, and Martin Hospital was available to permit them to punish Able for making the change. Second, Able's trustees were significantly less interested in cost savings (only a small part of which would have benefited the Able service area) than they were in good relations with the medical staff. The potential for support within the organization was present, but such support was not sufficient to overcome the problem of an environment that was pleased with things as they were.

Baker presented a very different setting. Here a new administrator had been brought in with a clear purpose of raising occupancy, and the medical staff was faced with admission delays because of a bed shortage. Dissatisfaction was present and Baker did not need to change by itself; others were quite willing to help it.

## The Pace of Introduction

There was an inevitable tendency for the Bureau to set timetables for the various activities which accompanied the presentation and introduction of their proposals. So long as a step was mechancial and required no acceptance by hospital personnel this was no problem. When acceptance by hospital personnel was required it gradually became clear that a process was at work which could not be scheduled by the calendar. Recent research by Robert Zajonc bears directly on this point.

Contrary to the popular maxim that familiarity breeds contempt, Zajonc and his colleagues hold that familiarity breeds comfort. The research deals with the effects of repeated exposure to a stimulus.[4] This work has produced interesting and unexpected results which are directly applicable to an understanding of the dynamics of the implementation process at the study hospitals. Although the nature of the experiments has varied widely, the results have been the same; the more often a person comes in contact with something or someone, the more favorable he tends to feel toward them. Zajonc observes that the exposure effect works best in connection with someone or something one has never seen before, toward which one's feelings are neutral. He notes that if one has had a childhood aversion to turnip greens or green snakes, new exposures are not likely to change it.

In our work at Baker, we experienced several examples of Zajonc's exposure effect in our implementation activities. An example was the experience of introducing early admission testing (EAT) for adult medical patients. When the innovation was first introduced there were mixed attitudes among the medical staff. One internist embraced the idea enthusiastically, but the initial response of most of the general practitioners and internists who admit medical patients was either neutral or somewhat negative. The admitting nurse reported that very few physicians furnished EAT orders willingly. Almost always, she had to call the physician's office, often again and again, before she was able to arrange for a patient's tests. The physicians resented these calls, claimed they were a nuisance and an interference with their practice. They did not want to be asked by telephone for a patient's tests while they were busy in their office seeing other patients. Initially few physicians cooperated with EAT. It is noteworthy that surgeons at Baker (and internists at other hospitals) routinely furnish the admitting nurse preoperative tests for their patients at the time admission is arranged. Initially only a few physicians dedicated to the concept of EAT arranged for their patients to receive these tests. Laboratory and radiology, in cooperation with the Bureau, developed the methodology to handle these special patients and word about EAT began to spread slowly throughout the hospital. A few more physicians agreed to try the innovation, and the admitting nurse began to report more cooperation and less difficulty in getting EAT orders from physicians. After some time, the remaining physicians decided, apparently, that the concept of EAT would not "go away" regardless of their attitudes. Nothing that we can detect changed in the system except the familiarity of it. Six months after the first EAT patient, the admitting nurse reported that EAT had become "routine" for almost all of the physicians who admit medical patients. With very few exceptions, EAT orders are routinely furnished and the physicians now consider EAT as a part of their standard hospital-based practice. Quite clearly, a professionally sound innovation had met initial negative response but had been successfully implemented in part as a result of the exposure effect dynamics.

The character of the innovation has an important bearing on whether exposure can be expected to play a role in the implementation process. This is illustrated in the differences between the EAT system and the physician-supplied discharge estimating system. Both innovations required physician cooperation; the former could use the exposure effect, but the latter could not. The feasibility and benefit of EAT were established by a small group of initial participants; over time, other physicians were exposed to the system, became familiar with it, and also became participants. The discharge estimating system, on the other hand, required initial participation by a large percentage of the total medical staff. As with EAT, a few physicians did supply estimates conscientiously after the system's start-up. However, too few estimates were received to base admission decisions on this system, and the manual system continued. Those few physicians who cooperated initially became discouraged; others who were more skeptical never were exposed to a successful system, and the Bureau was unable to overcome their skepticism and elicit their cooperation. Exposure was able to contribute to the success of the EAT system, but it was of no consequence in the physician discharge estimating system due to the different character of the latter innovation.

The pace of introducing an innovation is related to the technical as well as the human readiness of the hospital to accept the next step of an innovation. A six-month delay in getting daily census reports from the Able computer arose from an inadequate assessment of the difficulties of computer program adaptation, the resolution of a prior billing problem, and the securing of an adequate number of hours from trained personnel. Early identification of these problems would have required questioning the judgments of competent and senior personnel, and such questioning carries some risk of antagonizing people whose support is needed. The risk would have been taken had the technical preconditions for implementation been fully recognized. Such recognition is easy in retrospect, but to recognize it when it is needed, a remarkably detailed knowledge is required of the technical requirements of the innovation and the existing systems and data sources it will utilize. When introducing the admitting scheduling system at Baker several early warnings that the admitting office did not have the trained resources to manage or implement the system were heeded, and the prior (and somewhat frustrating) investments were made in improving that resource before firm dates were set for start-up.

## Influence

Participants accept change more readily if they shape both the change itself and the process of implementing it. Externally imposed change can be expected to meet resistance unless those who must accept the change and make it work have had their "say" or exerted their influence.

All of the Bureau's innovations, the admissions allowances, the EAT system, the budgeting system, and the nurse scheduling system, have been influenced by the hospitals' participants. In the opening chapter of this section we termed the expression of such influence the "negotiation/renegotiation" process. Illustrations of this process appear throughout the cases, one of the clearest examples being the implementation of the surgical admission allowances. The initial allowance was based on historical data and attempted to keep the balance between surgical admissions and medical admissions the same as it was prior to the Bureau's intervention. This way of setting the allowances neglected to take account of the increase in occupancy which resulted from the system. The surgeons viewed this as unfair and unacceptable. The surgical department formed an ad hoc committee to advise the administration. The administration agreed that the surgeons should share in the greater number of admissions, and the allowances were revised to reflect changes in the length of the waiting times. The changes were relatively modest, amounting to a scarcely noticeable change for each surgeon. Nonetheless, the surgeons had exerted influence and power which resulted in change; thereafter the revised allowances were accepted. Fortunately, they were accepted by the medical department as well as by the surgeons. Had the allowances not been changed, it is unlikely that the admission scheduling system could have been implemented.

A common explanation for the effectiveness of participation is that it reduces external control and allows the satisfactions available from the exercise of self-control to be secured directly. It allows participants to "prove" through high performance that the participative solution was a sound one. The reasoning is persuasive and has empirical support.[5] It is worth noting, however, that successful examples of participation such as the Scanlon Plan experiences do not eliminate control, but rather provide a setting in which expertness replaces authority, irrespective of who has it.[6] Authority is the typical source of influence in a static organization; the cases suggest that expertness is bound in the same close relation to successful innovation. The cases make clear the Bureau held no monopoly on expertness, particularly in devising the modifications necessary to make the budgeting, nurse scheduling, payroll-based reporting system, or other innovations viable. Participation in the discussions which modified the different innovations allowed persons who could identify problems in detail to bring this knowledge to bear on an innovation and on the strategy for its implementation. Admittedly, the power to direct (authority) was also important, as was the unquestioned power of the physicians to use or ignore the early admission testing program.

The number of influential participants in a hospital makes the mechanisms through which influence is applied of particular interest. The physician role in supporting or resisting change is often salient, but it is apparent for others as well that the mechanisms which allow participants to use their power base to stop an innovation also allow them to be coopted. Whether because of the exposure effect, rational assessment, or the alchemy of participation, detractors may become supporters of innovation. The same widespread sources of influence which make the hospital a difficult setting in which to introduce innovations provide, paradoxically, fertile opportunties to generate support for them. The power of the idea, its inherent soundness, becomes a significant factor, and those who have shaped it use their influence to help bring it to fruition.

The conclusion from the cases is not that expertness is the only relevant source of influence. The significant point is that successful implementation was most often achieved when expertness was acknowledged to be the most relevant source of influence in framing and modifying the innovation, and participants with other sources of influence then used it to support the implementation.

## Soundness of the Innovation

All of the innovations proposed in the study hospitals were worthwhile ideas; not all of them were brought to an acceptable state of technical and organizational soundness. The manpower input decision (MID) lacked technical soundness. It was not thoroughly developed, and inadequate resources were devoted to shortening the turnaround time from receiving raw data to presentation to department heads, and in developing the decision criteria and methods of applying them that would cause the MID to have an impact. The discharge estimating system both at Able and Baker was technically sound, but never achieved the modifications necessary to stabilize it within either organization. Nursing personnel were key actors in ensuring the success of the estimating system because of their role in securing estimates from the physicians. Yet the amount of criticism and conflict they experienced was directly proportionate to the energy they exerted in securing the estimates, and this organizational anomaly was never resolved.

The cases show rather clearly that key participants do test the soundness of an innovation, and also the degree of support it will receive from other key participants in the system. Outside groups such as the Bureau staff can expect some skepticism regarding proposals for change and some informal testing to see whether the proposal is a soundly conceived and seriously supported one. Change agents are often viewed as being unable to understand the "real world." When proposed changes have already been successful elsewhere, a common reaction nonetheless is: "We're different—it won't work here." Consequently, the external change agent, as well as his proposed changes, can expect to be tested. He must win the respect and approval for his proposals with each client system, each department head, each participant, anew.

The Bureau experienced such a testing by the Baker personnel. Almost all of the personnel tested the Bureau's representatives for their specific knowledge about Baker, its organization, its history, its way of doing things. Underlying all of our initial contacts was the unasked question: "Do these guys know what they're talking about?" The testing was not always so innocuous, however. Several physicians tested the reliability of the admission scheduling system by bypassing it and bringing their patients in as emergency admission. Three physicians were brought before the executive committee of the medical staff; one was suspended for a month as well as being placed on probation for a year.

The operating room supervisor tested the admission scheduling system for weeks before beginning to cooperate fully. When surgical admissions were to be based on fixed day-of-the-week allowances rather than her judgments, she lost some of her power vis-a-vis the surgeons, and she did not implement the allowances correctly when she first received them. As the Bureau implemented a more complete data collection system, it became obvious that surgical admissions were not being based on allowances. When confronted with these data, the operating supervisor claimed there was a misunderstanding about when to implement the allowances. She then agreed to begin using the allowances; again she did not do so. Clearly, she was testing the system, as well as the power she had over her activities. After some time, the administrator sent a clearly worded memo to her with copies to the chief of the surgical department and to the admitting office ordering her to implement the allowances immediately. Shortly thereafter, the number of daily surgical admissions matched the allowances, and there were no subsequent problems with the operating room supervisor's administration of the surgical allowances.

From the point of view of the participants, testing is a common sense way of confirming whether the request for change is serious or not, and whether the organization has the required resources available to implement the proposed change. Typically, such testing is the way in which participants with relatively little power (or with little power they wish to use) can determine whether they can sabotage the change simply by ignoring it. The manner in which the Baker department managers thwarted the implementation of the manpower input decision (MID) illustrates this strategy. The department managers did not resist the introduction of the MID concept, and they cooperated with the Bureau in setting the initial MID levels. However, they ignored the planning reports based on the MID, they did not alter their usual staffing methods, nor did they make an effort to help the Bureau improve the reports. The hospital administration and the Bureau were unable to commit the resources necessary to make the MID concept effective, and eventually it was abandoned.

In a sense, testing is possible because the newness of a method permits variation from it that will be troublesome to those close to the innovation, but not to others in the organization. This can be viewed as permitting a silent but effective communication between two actors, the one by his actions asking "Do you really mean it?" and the other by his reactions answering "No, not really," or "Yes, I do." It is probable that many such communications were being watched with interest by other participants in the study hospitals, and that how they responded to the innovation was affected by the outcome of the test.

## Stress

The stress factor includes both individual stress and organizational tension. The two are similar in character, but we use organizational tension to refer to "climate," the generalized stress experienced by many or all of the members of a unit or department, while stress refers to the feelings of a single individual.[7] We have described exposure, the exercise of influence, and the opportunity for testing as three processes which can help participants accept new ideas. Paradoxically, the experience of stress can also have favorable consequences for change although stress, by definition, is a painful experience. Individual stress occurs when an individual's adaptive resources or capacities fail to make a functional response to a situation. Whether a situation produces stress or a neutral emotional state depends on what the situation means to the individual; what is stressful for one person will not inevitably be stressful for another.

Closely akin to individual stress is an organization climate of apprehension and insecurity that is generally shared by participants when situations arise for which no adequate coping mechanisms exist. This can occur when the work process of a unit is changed to demand greater technical efficiency. Increased efficiency will usually require greater interdepartmental interaction and more effective coordination. Interdepartmental problems surface faster and require faster solution. As work processes become more demanding, greater management controls are implemented. These new controls tend to uncover inefficiencies which previously went undetected, and thus organizational units come under greater administrative scrutiny. In short, organizational tension occurs when slack is reduced and when the members of a department or unit are asked to work differently and more efficiently.

The probability that interventions like the Bureau's will cause stress is directly related to the amount and degree of behavioral change required for the adoption of the innovations. The relationship between stress potential, behavior change, and change method is presented in figure IV.6.1. As figure IV.6.1 suggests, the potential for stress increases as one moves from a desire to alter customary organizational interaction patterns to shifting role behaviors, to changing values and orientations, to the most stubborn variable: changing basic motives.

While stress was an expected consequence of the Bureau's intervention at Baker, the localization of stress in the role of single participants was unexpected. Stress was experienced very clearly by the director of nursing at Baker, by the admitting officer at Able, and by others as well. Individual stress is in many cases dysfunctional, but it does cause those who experience it to look for ways of escaping the stressful situation. Experimenting with new behavior is one possible escape, and it is in this sense that stress can facilitate change. As we pointed out in the opening chapter of this section, stress is often experienced when persons experiment with new behaviors; in that setting stress increases the tendency to revert to old methods.

**FIGURE IV.6.1**
Relationship between stress potential, change targets, and change method

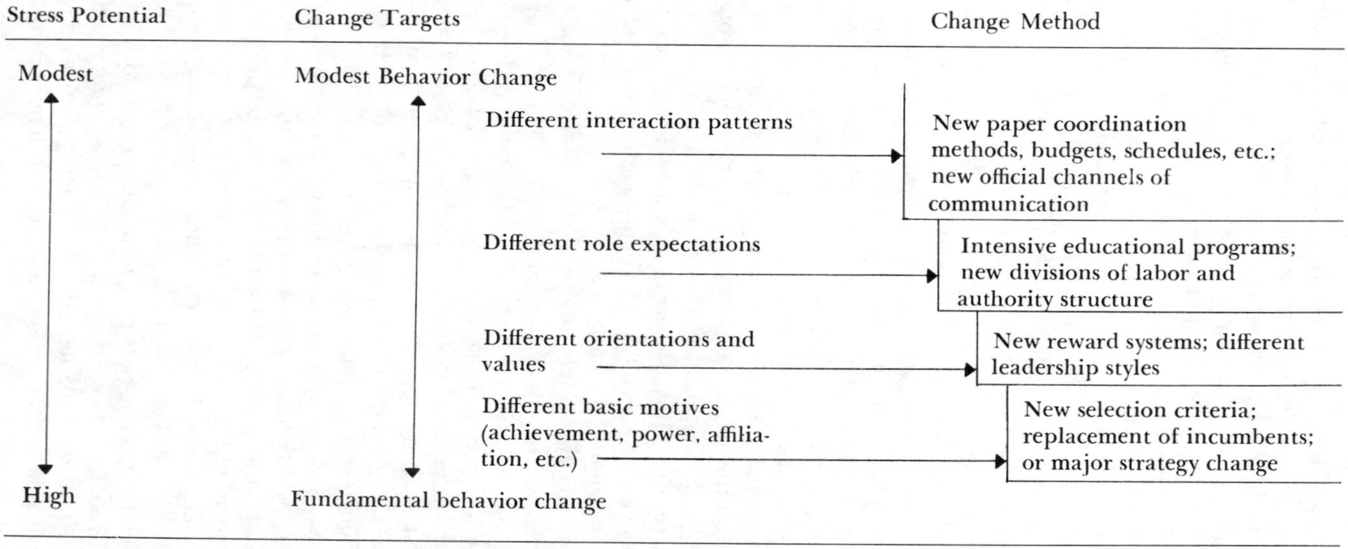


Adapted with modification from P. R. Lawrence and J. W. Lorsch, *Developing Organizations: Diagnosis and Action*. Reading, Mass.: Addison-Wesley, 1969, p. 87.

It is worth noting that Bureau personnel also experienced stress, and responded in predictable ways. When their committment to the success of the innovation was high, it encouraged them to experiment with modifications that promised to improve the chance of implementing the change. This was not always the case, and the occasional hostility and antagonism directed at Bureau personnel sometimes caused the research staff to reduce contact with the hospital and thus avoid the unpleasant situations created. Such behavior rarely facilitated the progress of the innovation, for it avoided dealing with the problems which were creating the antagonism. The close, though sometimes tension-filled relations that were maintained in the testing of the patient classification system, and the early preparation of the admitting office for the admitting scheduling system required heavy investments of time and energy but resulted in closer and more open relations in the long term. They also resulted in successful innovations.

The report on the Baker nursing department makes clear that the Bureau's work had direct impact on the nursing department and its director. As a result of the administrator's intervention, the nursing units no longer controlled their own workload by making admissions decisions; these decisions were shifted to the admitting office. The discharge estimating system also increased the department's work, and brought nursing personnel into increasingly acrimonious interactions with the medical staff. A new organizational structure, the communication group, required the participation and cooperation of the nursing supervisors. This group gave the participating nursing supervisors new responsibilities and reduced the organizational importance of the director. Some problem solving and decision making which she had previously handled alone was now being made on an interdepartmental basis. This new group also resulted in exposing some of nursing's intradepartmental problems which might otherwise have gone undetected. The EAT system created a new class of patients requiring better coordination between nursing and housekeeping so that beds would be ready for EAT patients. Finally, the admitting nurse was shifted to the admitting office where she was no longer responsible to the director of nursing, but to the business office manager. When as a result of the Bureau's activity the admitting nurse's role was expanded, the director of nursing and the admitting nurse both began to report increasingly stressful interactions.

The administrator also reported experiencing stress as a result of the dramatic way in which the surgeon's dissatisfaction with the initial surgical allowances developed. The administrator quickly consulted the chief of the surgical department and the surgeons' ad hoc committee was formed to study the situation and to "help the Bureau raise the allowances." This committee effectively neutralized the immediate situation and provided a mechanism for handling the grievance. The administrator later reported his major concern was that the surgeons would go outside the formal organization and bring the matter to the executive director or members of the board. A man as experienced as Baker's administrator would be quite used to conflict, yet the possibility of effective bypassing by the surgeons concerned him deeply, for he feared the consequences of a breakdown of the formal mechanisms for handling grievances.

Organizational tension, like stress, can act indirectly as an attention focusing mechanism. The experience of the Baker nursing department suggests that as the department searched for ways to cope with tension being caused by the several changes, they developed communicating channels (such as the communication group) and clarity about existing problems (such as the criteria for patient transfer) which provided fresh perspectives on the innovation.

Our experience in the study hospitals suggests that individual stress and organizational tension inevitably develop in a change process and that this stress has both functional and dysfunctional consequences. The presence of stress prior to change may signal the need for change. In this case, stress is functional and will elicit initial cooperation if the proposed change is perceived as a means of reducing the stress. During the change process, some stress is also functional because it will speed the acceptance of change. Individuals experiencing moderate stress will adapt to the required change, thereby relieving their stress. However, excessive stress is dysfunctional and disabling. If stress goes too high, withdrawal behavior and/or aggressive behavior results, and organizational performance suffers. We conclude this discussion of the cases with an example which draws from three of them and shows rather clearly how stress can operate both for and against change.

In early 1972 change programs in Baker hospital were moving ahead on several fronts. The early budgeting procedures were being replaced by more extensive department head involvement, an early admission testing (EAT) experiment had begun, the formal admission scheduling system had just been installed and surgical allowances were being negotiated, the program of securing discharge estimates was being pushed, work on nurse scheduling was picking up, a project identifying delays between request and receipt of radiological exam results was just concluding, discussions with nursing administration concerning a reorganization that would create greater accountability at lower levels of the department were going on, and data on absenteeism and payroll accounting procedures were being collected in two separate and somewhat unrelated projects. In a word, things were busy at Baker. In mid-May of 1972, overt hositility toward the Bureau surfaced within nursing, x-ray, and among the surgical staff. By mid-June all cause for concern seemed past, and the Bureau experienced an era of good feeling that was as unexpected as the earlier hostility. In retrospect, the reason for hostility is obvious; many of the individual activities in nursing, radiology, the admitting office, and the business office were not "in" these locations exclusively, but were in other parts of the hospital as well. No single project was enough to cause the eruption, but the interaction of several was, and the resulting tension and stress found a focus in the Bureau and its activities. One of the surgeons suggested the climate nicely when he told a nurse not to worry about discharge estimates, the Bureau staff would be out of Baker soon.

The reasons for the rapid resolution of stress are less obvious. A significant one is a somewhat exogenous event. The Bureau's nursing research program was making preparations for its hospital management summer course scheduled for June 5-9. The course was to focus on five years of research and evaluation of service unit management (SUM) and nursing organization. The Baker director had asked to attend some weeks before. The administrator's willingness to sponsor her at this particular time reassured the director about the importance of her role at Baker.

Her week in Ann Arbor brought her in contact with other directors and associate directors, hospital administrators, unit managers, and others who had had extensive experience in implementing change in nursing departments. These contacts were a stimulating experience for Baker's director. For the first time in some years, she had the opportunity to come into direct contact with some of the changes taking place in nursing; the course seemed to give her a new perspective on the problems she had been experiencing at Baker. Specifically, it seemed to alter her attitudes toward the possibilities for change in her department. The effect appears to have been more general than specific, for example, in a new openness toward nursing reorganization issues, a greater understanding of the value of hard data in planning change, and a willingness to question some prevailing nursing department practices.

Perhaps the crucial factor in resolving the stress was an immediate move by the Bureau staff into a negotiating mode for the surgical allowances. Revisions here, combined with strong support from the administrator's own superior, had the effect of mollifying the irate surgeons and strengthening the confidence of the administrator that he could still count on front office support when it was needed.

A third factor was really a payout on some earlier negotiations which had involved a number of key participants. Various nursing supervisors and other hospital personnel who had taken part in the communication group meetings were, like the nursing director, developing new orientations toward some of the changes, and the inclusion of suggestions from them in part of the nurse scheduling study produced a favorable attitude.

The reasons for the sudden appearance of favorable attitudes included a large component of coincidence. The significant point is that the stress and tension produced a setting for the director to benefit materially from her attendance at the seminar, for the nursing supervisors to value highly their inputs to the scheduling study, for the administrator to do the same with his support from the executive director and, not the least, for the Bureau to approach the surgical allowance negotiations with a distinctly conciliatory attitude.

Our summary and discussion of the cases have not distilled any single rule, which if adhered to would invariably have brought success to the hospitals' change efforts. Perhaps this is because we failed to see the rule; perhaps it is because there are sets of conditions, but no single condition, which ensure success to a change effort. We hold to the latter view, and hope that the documentation of our work will assist others in determining the necessary and sufficient conditions which will make their own efforts successful.

## NOTES

[1]A revised version of this paper entitled "Understanding the Implementing of Change" was published in *Hospital Progress*, June 1974.

[2]Elting Morison, "A Case Study of Innovation." *Engineering and Science Monthly*, April 1950.

[3]Larry E. Greiner, "Patterns of Organization Change." *Harvard Business Review*, Vol. 45, No. 3, May-June 1967, p. 122.

Mason Haire, "Biological Models and Empirical Histories of the Growth of Organizations," in Haire (ed.), *Modern Organization Theory*. New York: John Wiley & Sons, 1959, pp. 288-290.

Herbert Kaufman, *The Limits of Organizational Change*. Birmingham, AL: University of Alabama Press, 1971, pp. 41-67.

James D. Thompson, *Organizations in Action*. New York: McGraw-Hill Book Co., 1967, pp. 66-82.

[4]Robert B. Zajonc, "Attitudinal Effects of Mere Exposure." *Journal of Personality and Social Psychology*, No. 9 (Part 2), 1968, pp. 1-27.

Robert B. Zajonc and Donald W. Rajecki, "Exposure and Effect: A Field Experiment." *Psychonomic Science*, 17, 1969, pp. 216-217.

[5]See for example the research reviewed in Rensis Likert, *The Human Organization*. New York: McGraw-Hill Book Co., 1967, pp. 13-46.

[6]Frederick G. Lesieur, *The Scanlon Plan: A Frontier in Labor-Management Cooperation*. Cambridge, MA: The Technology Press, 1958.

[7]The interested reader is referred to the following for a more complete discussion of stress: S. Levine, and N. A. Scotch (eds.), *Social Stress*. Chicago: Aldine, 1970, and R. L. Kahn, D. M. Wolfe, R. P. Quinn, J. D. Snoek, and R. A. Rosenthal, *Organizational Stress*. New York: John Wiley & Sons, 1964.

# Section V

# Analysis of Results

# V.1

# An Analysis of the Results at Baker Hospital

*by John R. Griffith*°

## Background

At the outset of the demonstration project in the fall of 1969, the project team specified an evaluation hypothesis:

> Study hospitals by 1973 will show significant improvement relative to control hospitals in the cost per unit of service without significant decline in their own level of quality or human resources.

There are a number of both technical and conceptual reasons why this hypothesis was ambitious. At the conceptual level, the principal problems are that the actual reduction of unit costs (in terms of dollars per admission, per patient day, or per capita) is a function of many factors other than the technical systems which were to be the focus of the research and secondly that the interrelation between these technical systems and either quality or the human resources of the institution are ill defined at our current state of knowledge. The technical problems center around the construction of a reliable experiment and the feasibility and cost of collecting appropriate data on three different variables for both experimental and control hospitals. As a result of this combination of difficulties, we have no formal test of this hypothesis.

°Kurt R. Student Ph.D. prepared the part of this chapter on employee satisfaction.

The most central of the difficulties in the hypothesis has to do with the motivation of the institution to reduce costs. Numerous technical studies have been done in hospitals which have identified ways in which significant savings could be accrued. Rarely, however, has anyone successfully traced these savings to changes in the relative cost position of individual hospitals.[1] Two problems appear. The first is that results of suggested managerial improvements are not implemented and the second is that the savings which are accrued are expended on other activities.[2] On the other hand, it is clear that a hospital which takes cost containment as an important goal can be successful, largely without the kinds of technical improvements and systems which are the focus of this demonstration.[3] The explanation of this conundrum appears to be simply that hospitals will not reduce or control expenditures unless this is a high priority institutional goal. In the setting of the demonstration hospitals at the start of the experiment and until mid-1972, there was little environmental pressure to raise the priority of cost control. While there was considerable public attention to the problem of costs, as there has been for many years, Michigan Blue Cross and Medicare were both reimbursing at a level of 102 percent of a defined per diem cost. Enlargement and improvement of services, prestige, and the maintenance of growing financial reserves were apparently the dominant motives of hospitals at that time. In addition, most capable administrators were recognizing the ironic probabilities that incentives for cost reduction would come in the future and the hospitals who had done the best job of cost containment before the installation of these programs would have the hardest time earning the incentives.

The project team knew that the hypothesis was ambitious bordering on the foolhardy. Still, in retrospect the selection of the hypothesis was extremely fortuitous. The reason is that it gave the project team a clear "bottom line" focus. It steered the project around the pitfall of simply calculating either real or potential departmental savings without tracing these through to the point where they can be passed back from the hospital to fiscal intermediaries, presumably for distribution to the customer and taxpayer. It was this focus that led us to uncover the hierarchical nature of the cost containment problem described in section I.2. It helped us to understand that interdepartmental systems such as admission scheduling and preadmission testing are of critical importance. Finally, it helped us to identify that cost minimization is not necessarily a primary goal of a single department, even when it is the goal of the institution as a whole. Cases in point were in laboratory and x-ray where preliminary studies indicated quite clearly that there were potential reductions in expenditures on the order of $100,000 a year each, but continued examination showed the even greater importance of assessing and improving the time necessary to turn information back to the physician (see section III.5.). While this finding may seem obvious, the literature does not show serious operations research emphasis on this objective and the statistic is not commonly known in hospital management.

## Demonstration Hospital Arrangements

In assessing the overall impact of the projects, it should be noted that the kind of control over the environment normally expected in scientific experiments was lacking in the demonstration. The demonstration hospitals are created by and responsible to their communities who delegate the authority for operations to administrators whom they select. The authority of these administrators to accept or reject not only findings of the demonstration but also the direction of efforts was explicitly recognized in the project proposal. As a result of this authority, the environmental differences between Able and Baker, and the rapidly growing knowledge of the demonstration team, the two demonstrations quickly developed divergent courses. The Able demonstration eventually went in the direction of long-range planning. The time lags of action in this area are such that at this time nothing has been implemented. Work with the hospital and in the community continues, however, and we believe the eventual outcome will be both more rapidly reached and sounder than it would have been without our assistance. No data are presented on Able because we do not believe our interventions have reached the point where we could reasonably claim they affected the cost of operations. At Baker Hospital a number of shorter range activities were undertaken with the aggressive support of the Baker Hospital administrator. Thus, it is of interest to explore the original hypothesis to the extent it is possible with particular emphasis on two questions: What has been the relative cost performance of Baker Hospital? What can be said about the interaction between the systems developed, the cost performance, and the attitude of the employees? The data for these questions come from the HAS reports, the budgets, and the routine accounting and statistical statements of Baker Hospital and from two major surveys of personnel satisfaction and a third partial survey.

## Impact on Quality

On the question of the quality of services offered by the hospital, little can be said. Baker Hospital did not become a PAS member until September 1970. The medical staff has been identifying certain quality and utilization problems since that time and in the opinion of the administrator, has improved its performance despite its rapid growth. (Approximately forty new members of the active staff were added in the 1971-

73 period.) One of the most important aspects of quality of care is the ease of access to primary medical attention. It is known that this area of Michigan has a relatively low physician population ratio. The problem was identified and quantified by the project team who reported it to hospital management. The quantification showed only 0.44 active physicians per thousand population in 1972 while U.S. and Detroit metropolitan area figures were at a level of 1.2 physicians per thousand population. Management was surprised by the numbers, but it was aware of the problem and had taken action which obviously was effective to increase the number of physicians on the Baker staff. Progress on problems such as these is slow, however.

Another aspect of quality, in addition to the technical performance measured by PAS and the problem of access to a doctor, is the availability of the hospital's health care resources and the effectiveness with which they function. Data presented below and in section IV of this report show that certain of our projects maintained a high occupancy of the hospital, assisted in the reduction of length of stay, and therefore increased the number of patients through the hospital. In addition, these systems tended to reduce transfers and cancellations of admitted patients, assist nursing personnel in providing uniformly adequate coverage, and encourage rapid return of laboratory and x-ray data to the physician. While the exact relationships of all of these factors to community health is complex and unclear, they do seem to be in a direction which is supportive of high quality. Thus, it can be argued that the direction of movement of quality indicators in all three areas—technical quality, access to primary medical care, and availability and organization of hospital resources—is upward. There is no evidence that demonstration activities either threatened quality of care at Baker Hospital or were inconsistent with a variety of simultaneous efforts aimed directly at the quality problem. In fact, we would argue that the demonstration systems provide a firmer foundation for quality improvement than exists in most hospitals at the present time.

## Summary of the Baker Projects and Their Results

Figure V.1.1 shows the major studies and changes which occurred at Baker Hospital during the period January 1970 through September 1973. A quick overview of this figure shows three general conclusions about the impact on the demonstration hospital. First, there were a great many more preliminary and investigatory studies than there were actual procedural revisions. Second, there was only one procedural revision until two years into the demonstration, and the pace intensified after January 1972. Third, changes of key personnel and procedures continued at Baker Hospital without clear and direct relation to the demonstration project, and the pace of these also accelerated after January 1972. By the conclusion of the period shown in figure V.1.1, the identifiable changes were as follows:

1. The system of preparing the annual budget had been substantially revised twice with the active participation of the Bureau team in both revisions. The second revision appeared to be satisfactory and was scheduled for use in the budget cycle of January 1974.
2. Control of the bed supply had been removed from the nursing department and firmly installed in the admitting office by the administrator and supplemented with an ongoing admission scheduling system devised and installed by the Bureau team.
3. The successful development of an admission scheduling system was supplemented by a program of early admission testing (that is, testing of elective patients on the day of admission) and this had been expanded to preadmission testing after completion of arrangements with fiscal intermediaries. Both of these activities had direct involvement of the Bureau team.
4. A program for the daily allocation of nursing personnel had been developed by the Bureau team and successfully field tested. There is a reasonable probability that this program will be installed by the hospital at a future date. The absence of an on-line computer terminal limits the use of this program.
5. Recommendations by the Bureau team for thirteen-period accounting and for the development of payroll-based cost reporting systems had been adopted by the hospital. Payroll reporting was in a manual mode as of September 1973, but fully automated reporting was expected within the fiscal year.
6. The medical staff utilization review committee was considerably strengthened by the administration and was taking deliberate action to discipline members of the staff with excessive lengths of stay or emergency admissions.
7. A team nursing system had been installed by the hospital administrator and director of nurses.
8. Not shown in figure V.1.1. but likely to gain implementation during calendar 1974 were systems for monitoring and controlling turnaround time for laboratory and x-ray data which would be monitored by the medical records analyst and the budget director. Thus, so far as can be predicted, the next year seems to hold a continued high rate of change of procedures.

There are three reasons why a number of the investigatory and preliminary studies have not led to procedural revisions. First, some of these such as the acute bed need studies and the attitude surveys were not designed to lead to procedural revisions but rather to be used as background in evaluating the demonstration and devising the correct

**FIGURE V.1.1**
Chronology of major events and field studies Baker Hospital

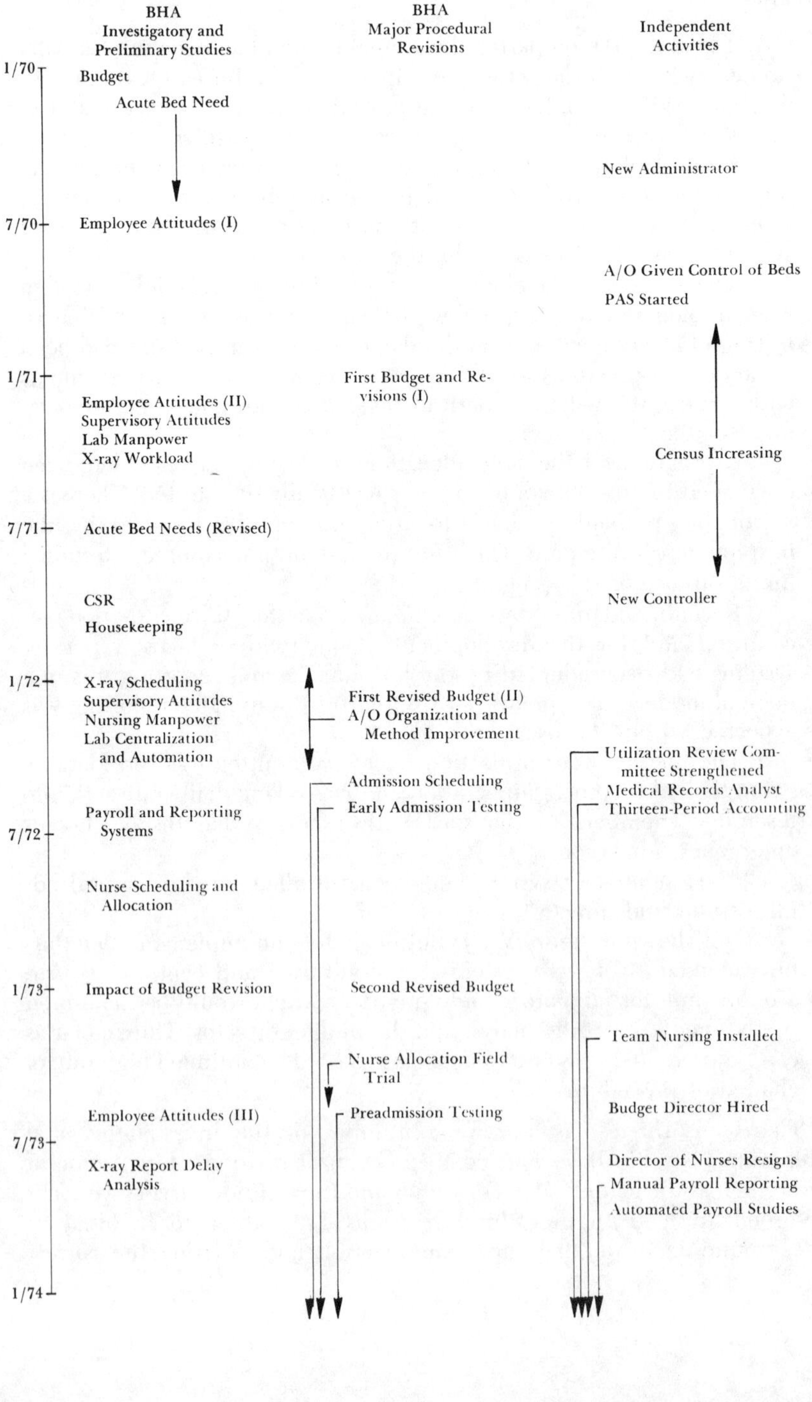

changes. Second, some of the preliminary studies, such as the laboratory manpower utilization study and the x-ray demand study led to additional studies and reframing of critical questions rather than directly to procedural revision. Third, there are distinct limits to the capability of Baker Hospital to absorb major procedural revisions. Preliminary studies of central supply services and housekeeping tended to indicate that further work in those areas was desirable but of relatively low immediate priority. Further studies in laboratory systems were sacrificed in favor of further x-ray studies because neither the demonstration team nor the hospital had resources to carry on both activities simultaneously.

Figure V.1.1. is in no sense presented as a guide or recommendation for other hospitals, but rather as a convenient way of assessing where and how the demonstration impacted on Baker Hospital activities. To summarize these, major impacts were upon admission scheduling, nursing, and financial management. Departments directly affected by the admission scheduling system, particularly x-ray and operating room, had high to moderate impact and the remainder of the departments had low impact. To specify this in terms of the initial hypothesis, one would expect: (a) an improvement in the average occupancy and a decrease in the variation in occupancy; (b) a reduction in the average length of stay; (c) an increase in the total cost and total employees, but a reduction in these measures when expressed in per diem or per discharge terms; and (d) the same finding as in (c) with regard to nursing care expenditures specifically. These will be the major variables reviewed in the following section of this chapter.

## Findings of Cost and Performance

Performance data on Baker Hospital are available from hospital internal reports, HAS[4] reports, and PAS[5] reports. Most of the analysis below is based on HAS reports because these contain current comparisons with other hospitals presented in terms of subscribing hospitals from the district in which Baker is located (without size adjustment), from 200-299 bed acute general hospitals in Michigan, and from acute 200-299 bed general hospitals in the nation. In certain of the analyses it was necessary to go to PAS data in order to get reliable statistics of the adult medical-surgical service of the hospital. Some statistics of interest were derived directly from the hospital's internal reports, and for these there is no comparison group. Finally, a few comparisons with other data were explored as a supplement to the HAS analysis.

Data were generally collected over the time period July 1970 to June 1973. HAS and PAS data were not available prior to that date. There is some evidence that the cost control posture of the hospital had already begun to change at that time (see occupancy data from section IV.2 and Michigan Blue Cross data shown in figure V.1.7) as a result of the influence of the new administrator. Thus, data from earlier time periods might have shown a larger or more significant impact. The Bureau team, however, had done only preliminary investigations prior to that time with no known impact on hospital management except that which might result from requests for information.

There are a number of problems with both Baker Hospital and comparative HAS data. Baker Hospital has an essentially manual statistical and accounting system. It is reasonable to expect at least the usual number of errors and delays inherent in handling large volumes of statistical information in a manual mode. Certain HAS reports were missing for unexplained reasons. The most likely cause of this was delay in preparing the intial submission. The comparison groups are not ideal. Most desirable would be to have a district comparison for the same size hospital, but there are insufficient subscribers in any one district to have statistically meaningful data of this kind. The district data reported by HAS, therefore, include all hospitals and the range of size and scope of services is quite large. The national data, on the other hand, include a variety of labor markets, reimbursement arrangements, and other environmental characteristics. Further, all three comparison groups suffer from some instability. Hospitals may join or leave the HAS service and in any given month some hospitals will be late in reporting and will therefore be omitted even though they are continuing subscribers.

It was felt that the Michigan size group comparison would be the most meaningful. Figures in the text generally refer to this group. Where possible all three HAS comparison groups are shown in the data tables.*

Overall, variances in the statistics presented tend to be quite large. That is, there is considerable "noise" in the data which limits the sensitivity of the analyses which can be performed and the confidence one may have in the results. Where appropriate, statistical analyses have been done to indicate levels of significance of the findings, For the most part, these are limited to investigations of the first eighteen months of the data as compared to the last eighteen months. This splits the data at January 1972, the point at which major implementation activities were noted to begin from figure V.1.1.

## Overall Cost of Operation

Figure V.1.2 shows the HAS calculation of inpatient cost per patient day (on RCCAC method)[6] for Baker Hospital and the Michigan 200 bed group. Data for this figure are shown in Table V.1.6. As would be expected, both the Baker data and the comparison data show significant increases in costs over the entire three-year period. The least squares linear regression for Baker is $y = .68\text{ (month)} + 80.36$. For the regional data, $y = .576\text{ (month)} + 84.17$. These regressions are highly significant ($p = .001$).

*Data tables V.1.6. to V.1.17 appear beginning page 423.

**FIGURE V.1.2**

Comparison of inpatient costs per patient day: Baker Hospital and Michigan 200–299 bed general hospitals July 1970–June 1974

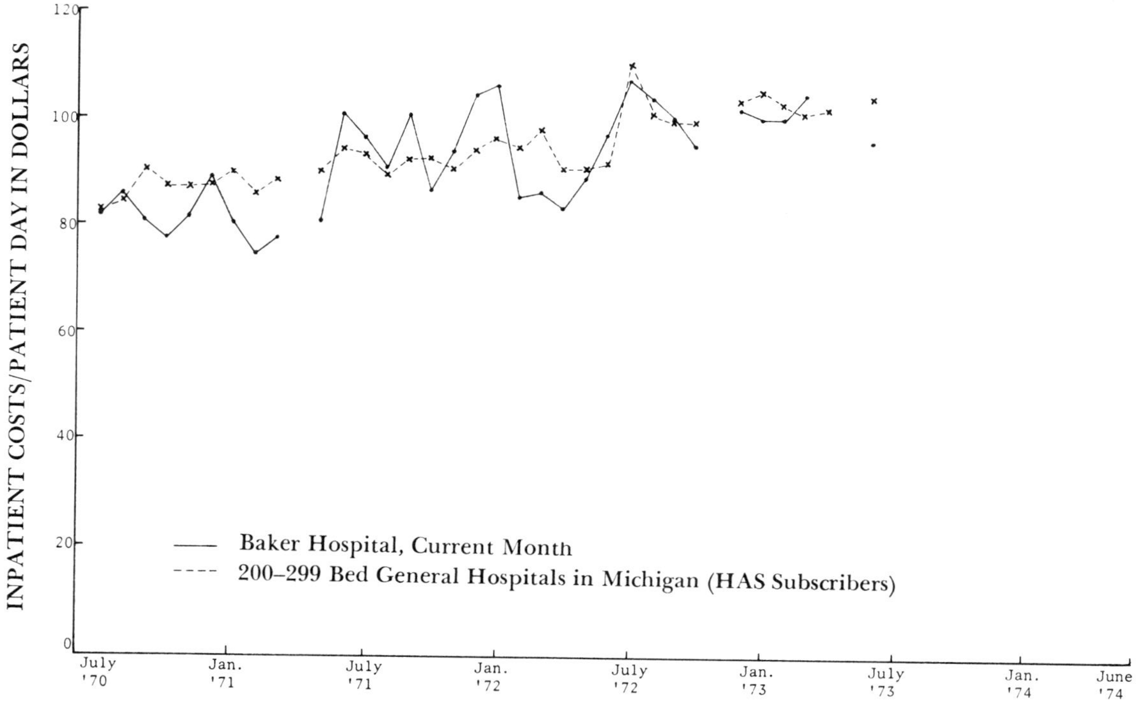


Source: HAS Monthly Reports for Baker Hospital.

(Discussions of significance of regression lines refer to tests of the hypothesis that the slope of the line is not different from zero, unless otherwise noted.) This mean cost for Baker was less than that for the comparison group—\$92.87 versus \$94.54. The rate of increase in costs (the slope) was higher for Baker than the comparison group. Differences in the means and slopes are not significant, however.

If the data are split at January 1972 and individual regression lines run for both periods, results are as follows:

| | July 1970-December 1971 | |
|---|---|---|
| Baker | $y = 1.14\ (\text{month}) + 76.72$ | $(p < .01)$ |
| | $\bar{y} = \$87.54$ | |
| Comparison | $y = .496\ (\text{month}) + 84.91$ | $(p < .001)$ |
| | $\bar{y} = \$90.67$ | |
| | January 1972-June 1973 | |
| Baker | $y = .645\ (\text{month}) + 80.51$ | $(p = .12)$ |
| | $\bar{y} = \$97.57$ | |
| Comparison | $y = .612\ (\text{month}) + 83.42$ | $(p = .10)$ |
| | $\bar{y} = \$101.23$ | |

These analyses are shown graphically in figure V.1.3. In the early time period both Baker and the comparison group had rapidly increasing costs and the linear regressions are highly significant. The Baker mean remains below the regional mean, but the difference is still insignificant. The Baker slope is more than twice as great as the regional slope and this difference is significant ($p = .06$). In the later period, the rates of increase for both Baker and the comparison group have slowed down, but much more for Baker than for the comparison. The significance of the regression lines has gone down slightly, but is still acceptable at approximately $p = .1$. The Baker mean is still lower than the comparison mean but the difference is still not significant. The Baker slope has dropped to a level approximately equal to the comparison slope (.64 versus .61, a difference which is obviously not significant). One may infer as a result that there has been a significant change between the two periods in the Baker performance versus the comparison group. From this conclusion one would further infer that the two Baker slopes should be significantly different. The later Baker slope is only half as great as the early slope. This finding can be accepted, however, only at a significance of $p = .3$. (There is only a seventy percent chance that the change is significant.)

It is possible to make a similar comparison to the cost per adjusted inpatient day reported monthly from a national panel by the American Hospital Association. Data for this statistic are also shown in table V.1.6. The three regressions of these data are as follows:

July 1970-June 1973
$y = .740\ (\text{month}) + 79.08 \qquad (p < .001)$
$\bar{y} = \$92.81$

July 1970-December 1971
$y = .844\ (\text{month}) + 78.31 \qquad (p < .001)$
$\bar{y} = \$86.33$

January 1972-June 1973
$y = .765\ (\text{month}) + 78.24 \qquad (p < .001)$
$\bar{y} = \$99.28$

This series shows the same general trends as the HAS Michigan 200-299 bed group. Means are lower, and slopes higher for the national panel, but these differences are not significant. While the significance is still questionable, it is worthy of note that the flattening which occurred in both the Michigan HAS group and Baker Hospital after January 1972 was not nearly so pronounced in the national panel. Both the Baker slope (.65 versus .77) and the Baker mean ($97.57 versus $99.28) were less than the national panel values.

Yet another standard of comparison can be found for per diem costs in the data reported by Michigan Blue Cross for participating hospitals. These data are total expenditures, adjusted for nonreimbursable elements under the retrospective cost-based contract with participating hospitals, and are reported for the southeast district of Michigan and two size groups, above and below 150 beds. Baker Hospital is compared with the larger group in figure V.1.4. Data are given in table V.1.7.

These data show a similar pattern to other per diem cost data. For the full period of available data, January 1969 through June 1973, the regressions are as follows:

Baker Hospital $y = 2.14\ (\text{quarter}) + 61.23 \qquad (p < .001)$
$\bar{y} = \$81.53$

Comparison group $y = 3.20\ (\text{quarter}) + 68.64 \qquad (p < .001)$
$\bar{y} = \$98.99$

Both the Baker mean and the Baker slope are less than the comparison group's with significance of $p < .001$. Further, with the larger time period prior to January 1972, a significant change in the Baker slope can be detected:

January 1969-December 1971
$y = 2.08\ (\text{quarter}) + 61.39 \qquad (p < .001)$
$\bar{y} = \$74.89$

January 1972-June 1973
$y = 1.25\ (\text{quarter}) + 75.47 \qquad (p = .007)$
$\bar{y} = \$94.79$

**FIGURE V.1.3**
Trends in cost per patient day Baker Hospital versus Michigan 200–299 bed general hospitals

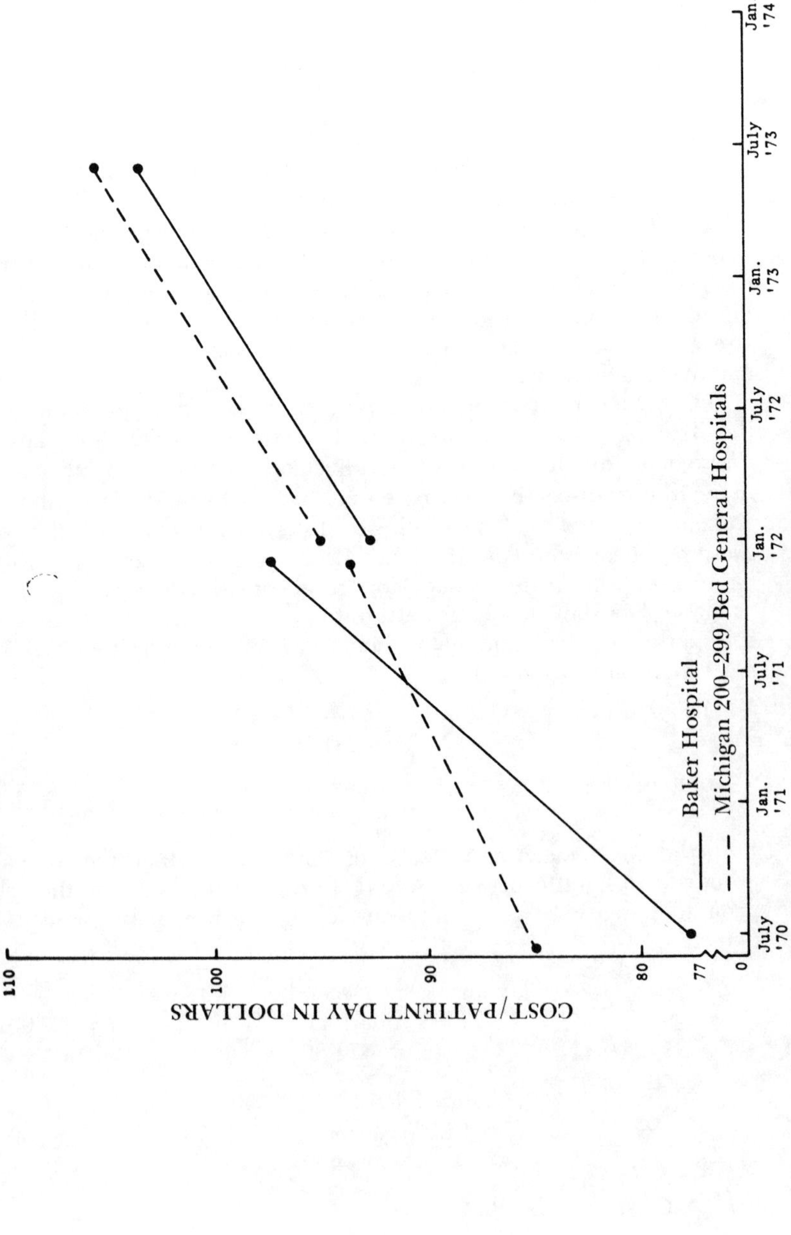


Source: Table V.1.6. Trend lines by least squares regression.

**FIGURE V.1.4**
Average per diem cost Baker Hospital and Blue Cross participating hospitals in Southeast Michigan over 149 beds

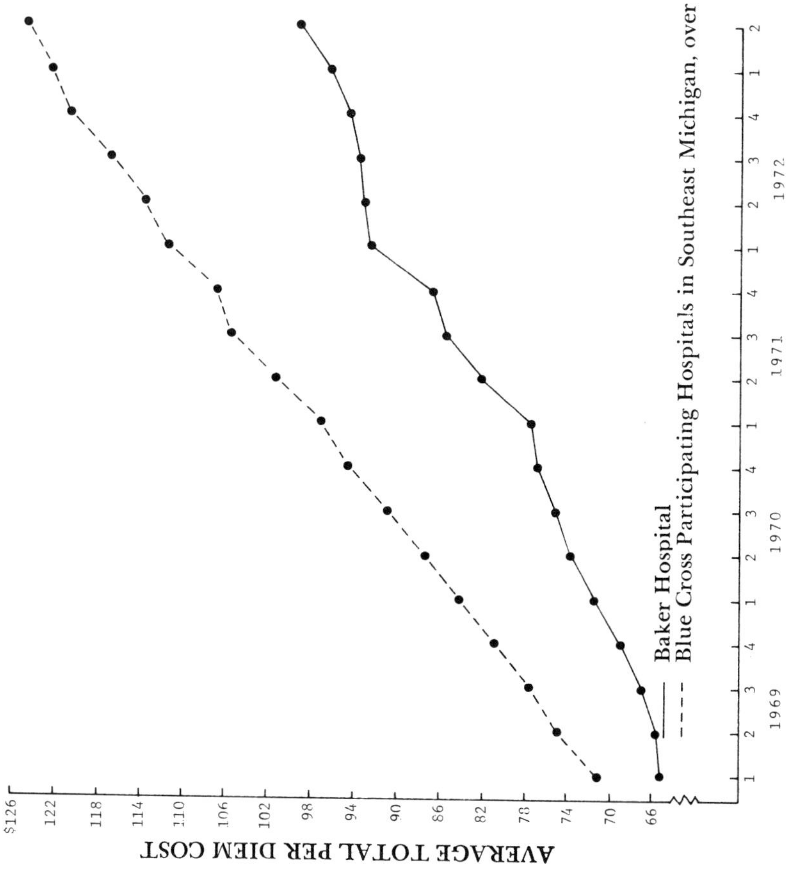


Source: Michigan Blue Cross, "Report to Participating Hospitals," issued quarterly by M.B.C., Detroit.

These changes are all in the desired direction and in addition are in comparison with a stable group of hospitals operating in a nearly identical environment to Baker. They reinforce the general conclusion that Baker Hospital performance did improve in the later months of the study, and the improvement was greater than that which might be traced to external factors operating on all hospitals.

Since nursing is one of the largest components of hospital costs and since nursing costs per patient day are at least partly a function of occupancy, one might assume that this HAS statistic would show a similar pattern to overall inpatient costs per day. The data age given in table V.1.8 and shown graphically in figure V.1.5. The results of the analysis are in many ways similar to that found with the overall inpatient cost. In this case, however, the Baker Hospital costs are consistently greater than the comparison group. Differences in the average costs at Baker Hospital and the comparison group in the early period prior to 1972 were significant ($p = .03$). In the later period, the Baker Hospital costs were still higher, but the significance had dropped to a level of eighty-five percent ($p = .15$). The slopes for Baker Hospital were also higher than the comparison slopes and the later slope was lower than that of the earlier period. However, none of these differences were significant. There was a marginal improvement in the variance of this statistic at Baker Hospital in the later period, significant only at an eighty-two percent level ($p = .18$). Of some interest is an improvement in the ratio of the Baker nursing costs per patient day to the comparison costs per patient day. In the earlier period the Baker costs averaged 107 percent of the comparison, in the later 104 percent. This difference, which is also slightly indicative of improvement, was significant at an eighty-four percent level ($p = .16$). The results of the regression analyses are shown below.

July 1970-December 1971

| | | |
|---|---|---|
| Baker | $y = .31\ (\text{month}) + 24.04$ <br> $\bar{y} = \$26.98$ | ($p = .03$) |
| Comparison | $y = .16\ (\text{month}) + 23.60$ <br> $\bar{y} = \$25.13$ | ($p < .001$) |

January 1972-July 1973

| | | |
|---|---|---|
| Baker | $y = .21\ (\text{month}) + 22.98$ <br> $\bar{y} = \$28.52$ | ($p = .11$) |
| Comparison | $y = .14\ (\text{month}) + 23.69$ <br> $\bar{y} = \$27.52$ | ($p < .001$) |

Costs per patient stay were added to HAS reports beginning in January 1972. This statistic (shown in table V.1.9) indicates that Baker costs per stay are significantly higher than those of the comparison group. This is traceable to a higher length of stay which will be discussed below. Unfortunately, neither length of stay nor cost per stay data are available for the comparison group in the early months of the experiment. Analyses of internal data on the overall length of stay for Baker do not reveal a significant trend. Thus, it can be inferred that most of the improvements which may have occurred in this dimension are traceable to improvements in the per diem cost. It seems likely that there have been slight improvements in length of stay but this problem is best approached through the case mix-adjusted statistics provided by PAS and is discussed below.

Costs per capita would be the product of the admission rate per person and the cost per admission. The admission rate for Baker Hospital has been calculated as of the 1970 census. It was below average for southeast Michigan at that time. Further calculations would have to be based upon estimated populations. It seems likely that errors in these estimates could exceed the differences in costs. Since neither cost per stay nor the admission rate could be estimated to the necessary tolerance, no calculation was made. It should be noted that if the hospital controls its inpatient costs through better management, and its admissions and length of stay through better utilization review, the impact of these three factors will be geometric. Baker Hospital is attempting to do this, but data which would indicate either success or failure are lacking.

## Occupancy and Volume of Service

Much of the thrust of the practical interventions at Baker Hospital was aimed at increasing use of facilities, both in terms of the average daily census and number of patients processed. The administrator who took over the hospital in April of 1970 had as his announced goal the increase in these activities, and the occupancy scheduling model described in section IV.2 played an important part in achieving that goal. As occupancy rose, increased attention was paid to the appropriateness of utilization and to the development of preadmission and early admission testing to shorten length of stay. In addition, as a result in part of the experimentation with admission scheduling, it was noted that the census could be increased by changing six beds from pediatric to adult use, and this occurred in June of 1972. The data and analyses below show that the average daily census for adult medical-surgical patients was increased, the variance in census was decreased, the occupancy was increased, the number of discharges was increased, and the case mix-adjusted length of stay was finally brought under control. Most of these improvements were significant at levels of ninety percent or better. It should be noted from table V.1.10 that Baker Hospital had a higher percentage of revenue from outpatient services than comparison hospitals at the start of the study and that this percentage was increasing at the end of the study. Thus, the overall utilization and volume of service generated by the hospital increased between 1970 and 1973. There were no increases in physical facilities during this period.

**FIGURE V.1.5**
Comparison of nursing direct costs per patient day Baker Hospital and Michigan 200–299 bed general hospitals July 1970–June 1974

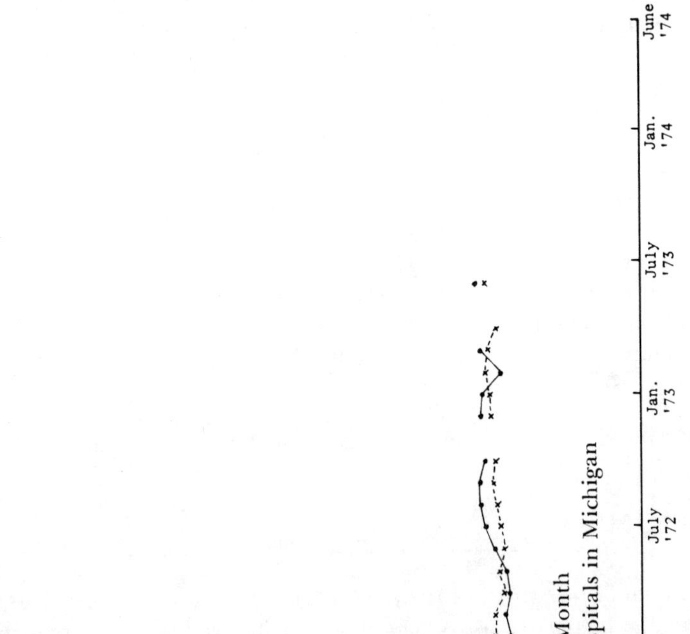


Source: HAS Monthly Reports for Baker Hospital.

**FIGURE V.1.6**
Average daily census by month adult medical–surgical service excluding ICU/CCU Baker Hospital

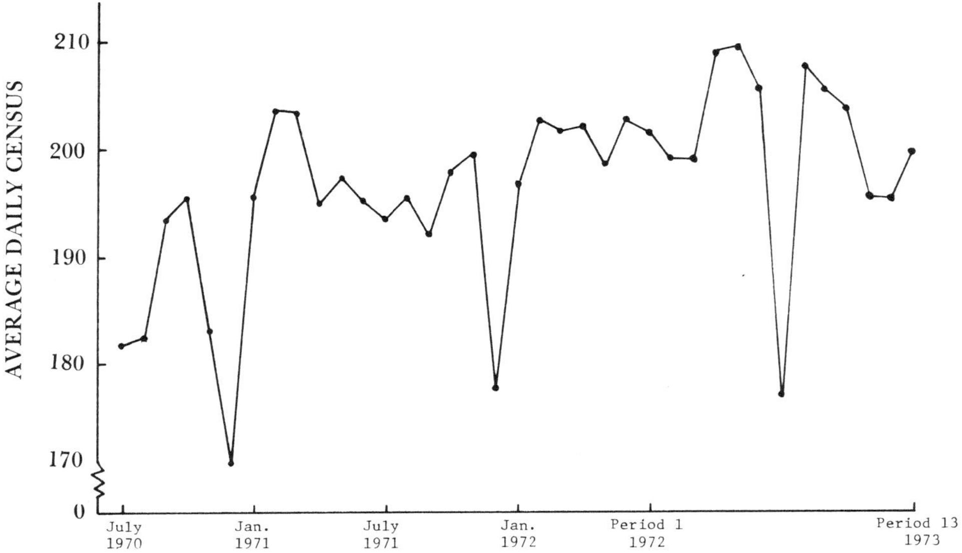


Source: Hospital Records. Occupancy based upon 208 beds May 1970–May 1972, 210 beds June 1972, 214 beds thereafter.

Figure V.1.6 shows the average daily adult medical-surgical census as derived from hospital records. Tabular data of both census and occupancy are shown in table V.1.11. The average daily census for the first eighteen months was 192 and for the second eighteen months 200, a difference significant at p = .02. In addition, the standard deviation of monthly census fell from ten patients to eight, but this difference was significant only at p = .19.

Counts were obtained on the average number of patients discharged per month from PAS Form A statistics. These are shown in figure V.1.7 with the supporting data in table V.1.12. Six-month means are indicated in figure V.1.7. These show consistent increases over the five six-month intervals with the largest increase coming in the last six months. While the interim changes are not significant, the increase from the first six-month average of 695 to the last six months of 749 is highly significant.

**FIGURE V.1.7**

Total patients discharged, adult medical-surgical

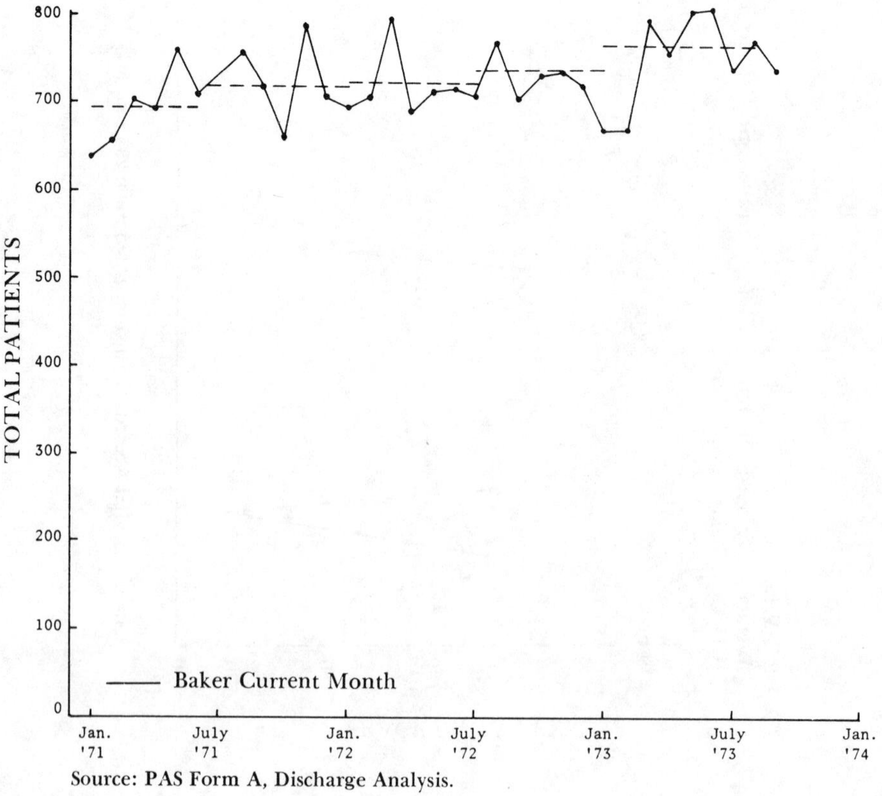


Source: PAS Form A, Discharge Analysis.

Overall length of stay calculations (not shown) show no consistent pattern. However, lengths of stay adjusted for case mix using the PAS length of stay package are shown in figure V.1.8. Because of the form of presentation by PAS, the data shown in figure V.1.8 include all services. Detail is shown in table V.1.13 for medicine, surgery, and pediatric medicine. Significance tests are provided in the length of stay package against a national matching group for the first six quarters (through December 1971) and against a regional matching group for the last six quarters. Regional stays for the Great Lakes region for these case mixes are generally higher than the U.S. stays. For the first three quarters, through April 1971, the overall length of stay was significantly higher than the U.S. average. For the last two quarters of comparison against the national data, the differences were not significant; and for four of the six quarters of comparison against regional data, the differences were not significant. It should be noted that the upward trend in the national data probably means a slight increase in the number of long stay patients being treated at Baker Hospital. Analysis of the detail between the medical and surgical service shows that the surgical service is consistently below the comparison group, although not significantly so in any specific quarter. The average stay of adult medical patients was consistently higher than either com-

**FIGURE V.1.8**
Length of stay adjusted for case mix

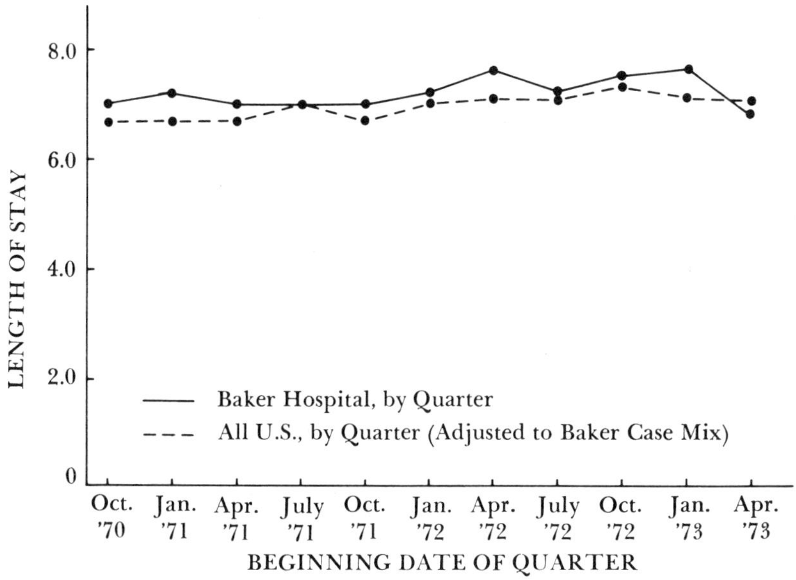


Source: PAS Form S, Summary of Services.

parison group by a significant amount until the last quarter reported, when it dropped below the regional comparison group, although still above the national comparison. The last quarter differences are not significant. Pediatric medicine showed a high variability, sometimes above and sometimes below the comparison group with significant variations in the first three quarters and three of the last eight quarters.

## Manpower Measures

The HAS service offers four measures of manpower which reflect major elements of cost in areas likely to have been affected intensively by this project. They are FTEs per bed, FTEs per occupied bed (not available prior to January 1972), nursing hours per patient day, and medical-surgical nursing hours per patient day. Given that the hospital did not change its general array of services nor expand its physical plant nor experience a large shift in case mix, one might expect that better control systems would result in a decrease in the mean and variance of these measures unless they were significantly below the comparison group at the start. As figures V.1.9 through V.1.12 show, Baker Hospital in July 1970 was at or above comparison group levels. The goals of a better management system would be reductions in the means of these statistics and also reductions in their variances. In most cases this is what occurred and the changes were significant at ninety percent levels or better.

Figure V.1.9 shows the equivalent full time employees per bed and indicates a pronounced reduction in both the mean and the variance beginning in August of 1972. This was the second period of the fiscal year. For the first eighteen months until January 1972, the mean was 2.66; for the second eighteen months, 2.60. There is a ninety percent chance that this difference is significant ($p = .10$). The early comparison mean was 2.50 and the late comparison mean was 2.40. The Baker Hospital means were thus higher than the comparison group in both cases. The probability that the difference was significant was very high ($p < .001$). The variance of the Baker Hospital performance in the first eighteen months was .0153 and in the second eighteen months .0328. This is a significant difference ($p = .07$) in the wrong direction apparently introduced by the fluctuations in the first seven months of the second interval. The variance of the last seven months is .0108. While this was less than the first eighteen months, the difference is not significant. Data are shown in table V.1.14.

Since the occupancy of hospitals varies, particularly among those in the comparison group, and since some of the improvement in employees per bed at Baker Hospital would occur automatically if the number of employees were constant and the occupancy were raised, it is of interest to look at the number of employees per occupied bed and this statistic is given in figure V.1.10 with supporting data in table V.1.15. Unfortunately,

**FIGURE V.1.9**
Comparison of equivalent full time employees per bed Baker Hospital and Michigan 200–299 bed general hospitals July 1970–June 1974

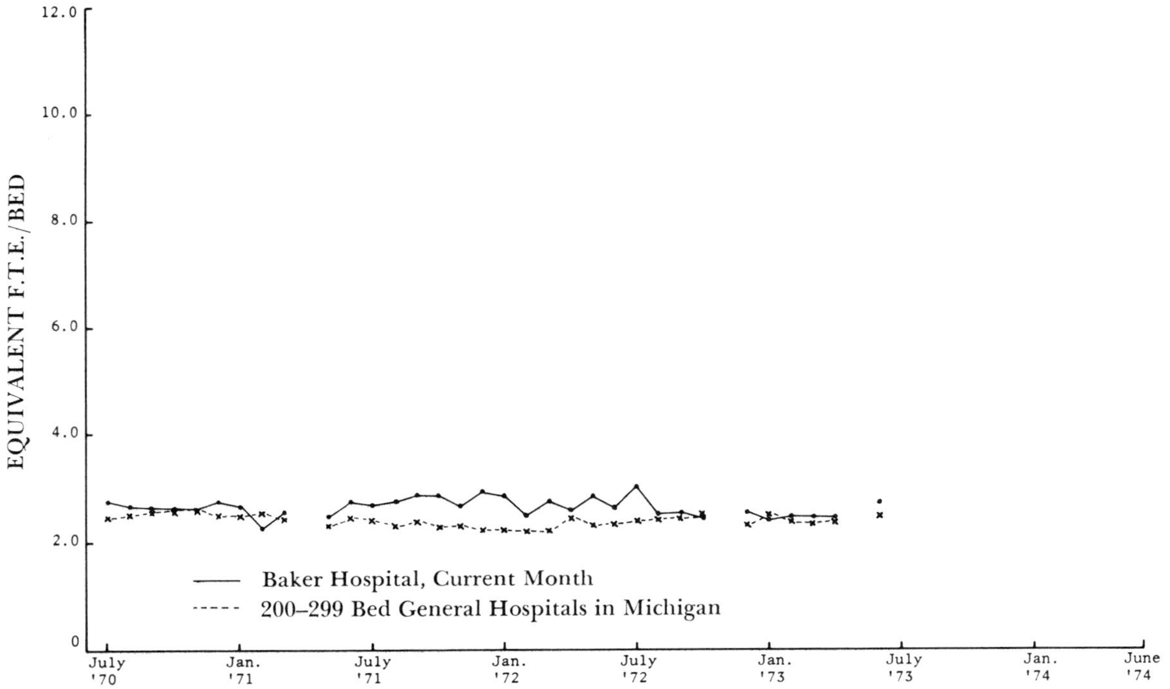


Source: HAS Monthly Reports for Baker Hospital.

**FIGURE V.1.10**

Comparison of equivalent full time employees per occupied bed Baker Hospital and Michigan 200–299 bed general hospitals July 1970–June 1974*

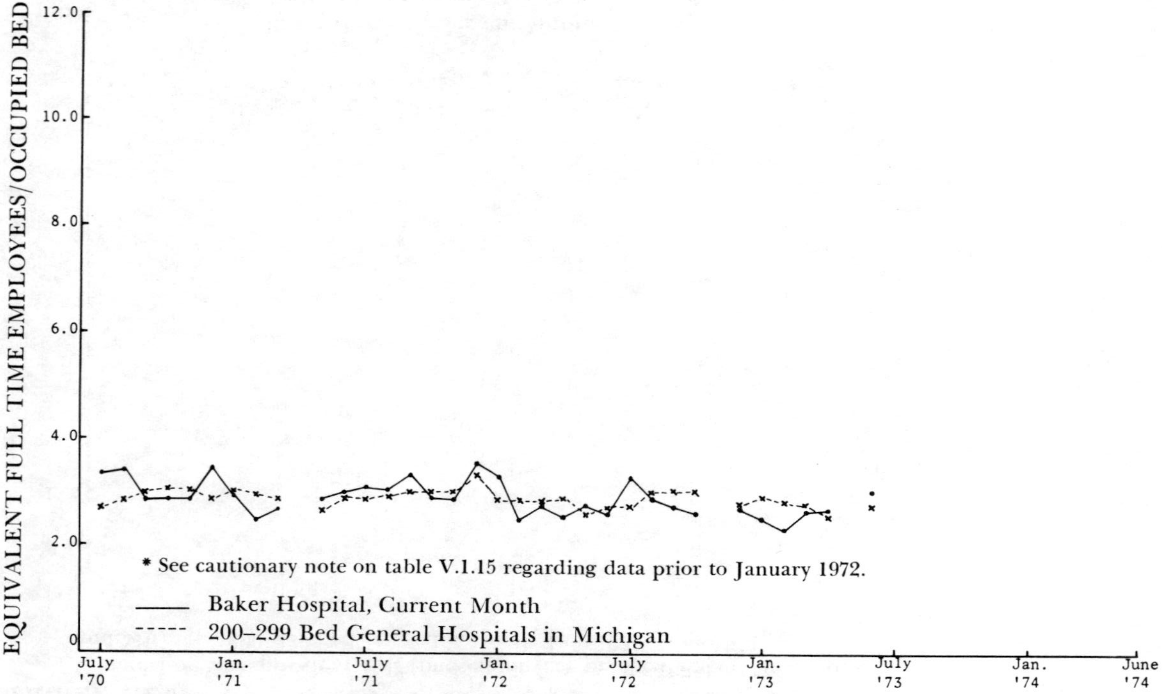


Source: HAS Monthly Reports for Baker Hospital.

HAS reports did not include either this calculation or occupancy data prior to January 1972. Baker Hospital data are calculated by dividing the data on table V.1.14 by the hospital's overall occupancy prior to that date. Comparison group data are calculated by dividing the statistic in table V.1.14 by the occupancy reported for Region 4 in the AHA National Panel data. This is admittedly very crude and it impairs the validity of the comparisons, particularly between the early Baker data and the early comparison data. However, the two Baker means, 3.04 prior to January 1972 and 2.74 thereafter, are significantly different ($p = .004$). The later variance is also lower, but the difference is not significant. There is some evidence that the early Baker mean is more than the estimated comparison mean of 2.9. Statistical tests indicate significance, but are unreliable. In the later period when the data are more uniform, the comparison mean is 2.77, trivially and not significantly higher than the Baker mean. The Baker data alone, however, show a noticeable tendency to improved control.

In the major manpower component of nursing, figure V.1.11 shows the overall nursing manhours per patient day. The supporting data are in table V.1.16. The early Baker mean was 5.90 and the late Baker mean, 5.45. The early comparison mean was 5.54 and the late comparison mean, 5.46. The late Baker mean is significantly lower than the early Baker mean ($p = .002$) and the later Baker mean is trivially and nonsignificantly different from the late comparison mean. Comparing the early and late Baker variances indicated that there was a slight but not significant increase in the variance. This statistic contains approximately half of the resources which are measured in FTE employees per occupied bed and the data were uniformly available from HAS. The evidence for improvement in the mean is quite strong.

In the adult medical-surgical area where Baker Hospital paid close attention to occupancy, there is also a relevant HAS statistic reported over the entire thirty-six months. These data, medical and surgical nursing manhours per patient day, are shown in figure V.1.12 and in detail in table V.1.17. The Baker Hospital average for the first eighteen months was 6.36 and for the last eighteen months 5.21. Comparison group averages for the first eighteen months were 6.10 and for the second eighteen months 5.66. The drop in the average for Baker was significant ($p < .001$). The early Baker average was significantly higher than the comparison group ($p = .09$) and the late Baker average was significantly lower than the comparison group ($p = .02$). The variance at Baker Hospital was reduced but not significantly. There is clear evidence of reduced cost here, although the drop in the statistic below the comparison group levels raises the question of the adequacy of quality of nursing care. Certainly any further effort to reduce nursing manhours would have to be undertaken very judiciously. However, there is little consensus on the number of adult medical-surgical nursing hours per patient day. According to data prepared earlier by HAS for the author, the distribution of medical-

**FIGURE V.1.11**
Comparison of nursing manhours per patient day all units Baker Hospital and Michigan 200–299 bed general hospitals July 1970–June 1974

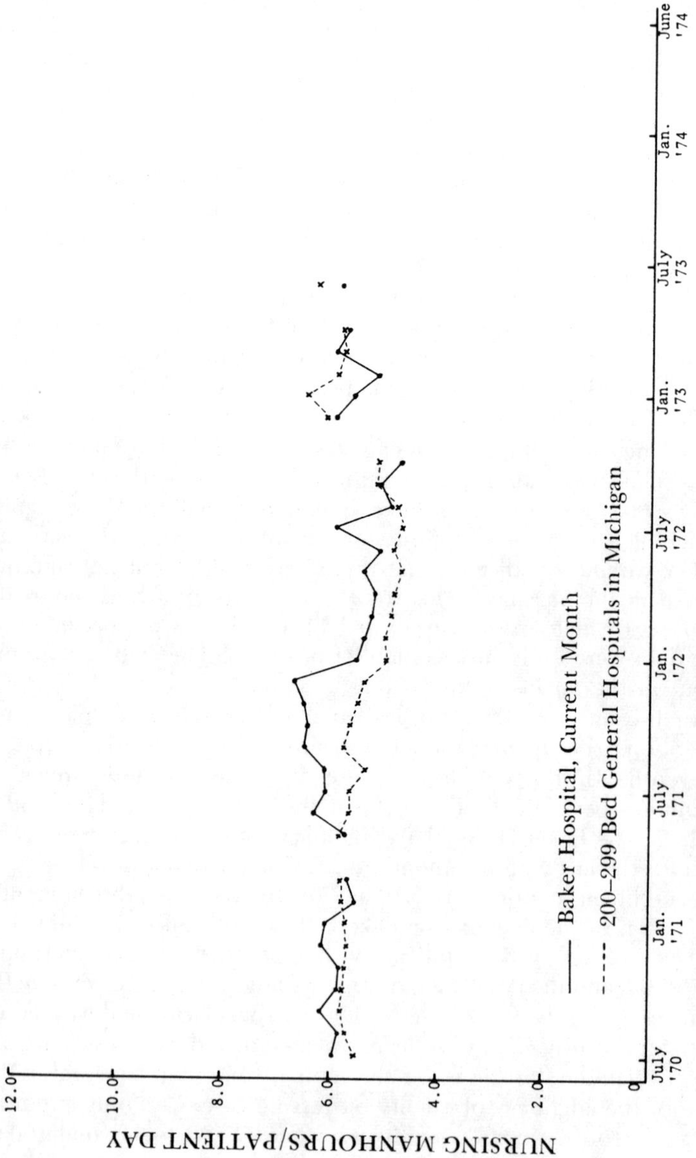


Source: HAS Monthly Reports for Baker Hospital.

**FIGURE V.1.12**
Comparison of medical and surgical nursing manhours per patient day Baker Hospital and Michigan 200–299 bed general hospitals July 1970–June 1974

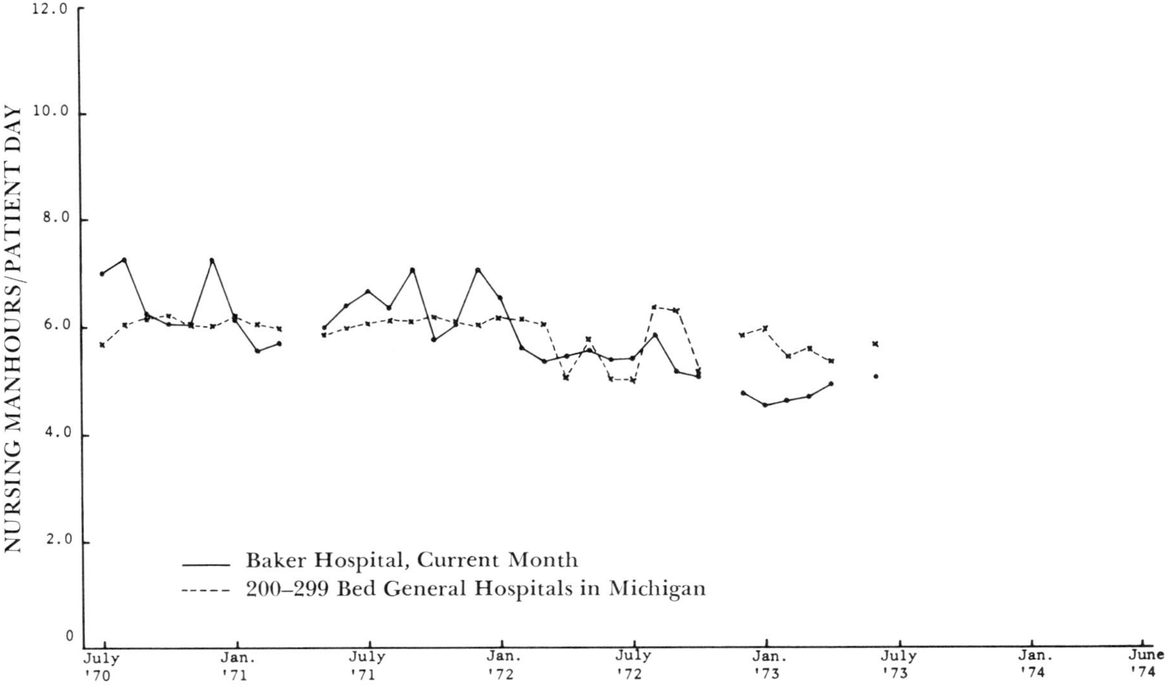


Source: HAS Monthly Reports for Baker Hospital.

surgical nursing hours per patient day for the quarter ending October 31, 1971, showed that five percent of the 200-299 bed hospitals were below 4.76 hours per patient day, twenty-five percent were below 5.51, half were below 6.04, and five percent were above 8.18. The Michigan hospitals in this size group were apparently slightly higher than the national average at that time. (See table V.1.17.) Since then, both averages have been falling. Baker Hospital, while standing low in the distribution, is not in the lowest ten percent.[7]

## Employee Satisfaction

Attitude surveys of nonsupervisory personnel were assessed by structured interviews administered to departmentally stratified samples using modified Likert-type questionnaires.[8] A seventy-eight item questionnaire was administered to Baker employees representing nineteen major departments or units in June 1970 and May 1973, and an analysis was made to determine the direction and degree of change over this three-year period. The comparison analysis focused on three major categories: satisfaction; intradepartmental activities; and interdepartmental tension (friction, strain, or conflict). Overall job satisfaction was measured by a single item question. In addition, indices were constructed to measure the level of satisfaction of five job characteristics: informational feedback; involvement in decision making; interpersonal relations; wages and working conditions; and career opportunities. Two additional indices were constructed to measure intradepartmental cooperation and intradepartmental problem solving. Interdepartmental tension was measured by asking employees in the nineteen major departments to indicate whether they had contact with any of the twenty-seven other departments at Baker or in the authority. Where contact was indicated, the level of interdepartmental tension was measured. Finally, data from an interim February 1971 questionnaire which measured only the satisfaction of registered nurses, licensed practical nurses, and nurse aides were compared to the responses from nursing personnel in 1970 and 1973.

In addition to the analysis of overall change, the Bureau studied the relationship between the selective impact of its activities and the reported changes in the nineteen departments surveyed. In some departments, the Bureau had a high impact during the three-year interval while other departments had very little or no contact with the Bureau's activities. To study this differential impact, six departments or units were classified as high Bureau impact, six departments as moderate impact, and seven as low impact. These classifications are presented in Table V.1.1.

A third analysis was conducted to study the effects of the introduction of team nursing on three of the high impact units only weeks before the 1973 survey. Team nursing was introduced on the medical unit in late March, on the surgical unit in late April, and the medical-surgical unit was receiving preparatory introduction activities at the time of the survey. To control for this confounding factor in the high Bureau impact comparisons, responses for the three nursing units were combined and analyzed separately from the remaining three high impact departments: admitting, radiology, and operating room.

The final analysis studied the pattern and the direction of change between 1970 and 1973 with data from the interim survey conducted in February 1971. The 1971 survey repeated only the satisfaction questions asked in 1970 and again in 1973, and the survey was administered only to nursing personnel. A preliminary investigation indicated that in 1971, registered nurses and practical nurses responded similarly, and differently from the nurse aides. Consequently, the former's responses were combined and analyzed for patterns of change in satisfactions from 1970, 1971, and 1973 for the combined nurse-practical nurse group, and separately for the nurse aides.

## Results: Changes in Satisfaction, 1970-1973

The results of this analysis are presented in table V.I.2 which indicates a general decline in satisfaction among the Baker Hospital employees during the 1970-1973 period. Of the six satisfaction measures, four declined significantly while the other two showed a nonsignificant declining trend. Since overall satisfaction showed only a declining trend while satisfaction with specific job characteristics declined more sharply, the data suggest

**TABLE V.1.1**
High, moderate, and low Bureau impact departments/units at Baker Hospital

| *High Bureau impact departments/units* | *Moderate Bureau impact departments/units* | *Low Bureau impact departments/units* |
|---|---|---|
| Medical-surgical | Laboratory | Obstetrics |
| Surgical | Emergency room | Nursery |
| Medical | Pediatrics | Delivery |
| Admitting | Intensive care | Collections |
| Radiology | Housekeeping | Dietary |
| Operating room | Accounting | Personnel & payroll |

**TABLE V.1.2**
Changes in satisfaction at Baker Hospital: 1970–1973

| | | | Changes in satisfaction | | | | | |
|---|---|---|---|---|---|---|---|---|
| | *1970 sample size* | *1973 sample size* | *Informational feedback* | *Involvement in decision making* | *Interpersonal relations* | *Wages and working conditions* | *Career opportunities* | *Overall* |
| Total Baker Hospital | 388 | 436 | *DOWN* | *DOWN* | *DOWN* | (–) | *DOWN* | (–) |
| High Bureau impact departments* | 150 | 163 | (–) | down | *DOWN* | 0 | *DOWN* | (–) |
| Moderate Bureau impact departments* | 121 | 122 | (–) | 0 | (–) | (–) | 0 | (–) |
| Low Bureau impact departments* | 82 | 85 | (+) | 0 | (+) | (–) | (–) | (+) |
| High Bureau impact departments–nursing | 97 | 116 | down | down | *DOWN* | 0 | down | 0 |
| High Bureau impact departments–nonnursing | 54 | 47 | 0 | 0 | (–) | 0 | down | down |

* High, moderate, and low impact departments less than total because several small departments were excluded.

*CAPS* – 95+% significance
Noncaps – 90–95% significance

(+) or (–) – direction of change, not significant
0 – no change

that the specific dissatisfactions did not generalize to a major decline in morale. The data also indicate a relationship between the Bureau's activities and the decline in satisfaction. The low impact departments showed a trend toward increased satisfaction and the moderate impact departments showed significant declines on three satisfaction measures as well as a declining trend on two of the remaining three measures. Finally, table V.1.2 indicates greater dissatisfaction among the high impact nursing personnel than among the other high impact personnel. This difference may be due to the greater effect of increased occupancy on the three nursing units. Spontaneous comments on the questionnaire by nursing personnel made reference to increased workloads as a result of higher occupancy. Also, nursing personnel, more than other Baker employees, spoke to the Bureau staff about the problems of high occupancy during implementation activities. Although this explanation cannot be proven, it is consistent with our data and is supported by our own subjective assessments as well as by comments on the questionnaire.

## Changes in Intradepartmental Activities: 1970–73

The results of this analysis are presented in table V.1.3 which indicates a divergent trend in intradepartmental activities: cooperation did not change while problem solving declined significantly. It should be noted that problem solving measured the emphasis of a team goal as well as a willingness to listen to problems and to solve problems, and it is also noteworthy that this significant decline in problem solving occurred in both types of high Bureau impact departments, nursing and nonnursing. The divergence between intradepartmental cooperation and intradepartmental problem solving appears, also, to result from increases in occupancy. With greater workloads and greater job demands, employees will have less time and be less willing to help others solve problems. However, employees may continue to value friendly and supportive relationships.

## Changes in Interdepartmental Tension: 1970–73

Employees in the nineteen departments or units surveyed were asked to indicate the degree of tension they experienced in interactions with other departments at Baker. These responses were compared to those from the 1970 survey to determine changes in interdepartmental tension during the 1970-73 period. The major findings of this study were:

- There was no general increase in interdepartmental tension.

• There was a significant increase in tension between the medical staff and the rest of Baker Hospital.

• There was a significant increase in tension between the emergency room and the rest of Baker Hospital.

• There was a significant increase in tension between the pharmacy and the rest of Baker Hospital.

• There was a significant decrease in tension between the laboratory and the rest of Baker Hospital.

• There was a significant decrease in tension between radiology and the rest of Baker Hospital.

Although the case studies indicate that the increase in occupancy and introduction of team nursing, as well as Bureau activities, contributed to increases in individual stress and intradepartmental tension, our data indicate that there was no general increase in interdepartmental tension. On the contrary, there was a small though nonsignificant decrease in interdepartmental tension during the 1970-73 period. Of the five changes cited above, by far the largest change involved the medical staff. Eight departments reported significant increases in tension with the medical staff. Significant increases in tension with the emergency room and the pharmacy were reported by four and three departments, respectively. The number of significant decreases in tension between the laboratory and radiology and other departments at Baker was seven and six, respectively.

The increase in occupancy appears to explain the increases in tension between both the medical staff and the emergency room and the rest of Baker Hospital. A secondary factor can also be cited. During the 1970-73 period, about forty physicians were given privileges to practice at Baker. While there are no data available on the activity of these additional staff members, adding to the medical staff can be expected to account for some of the increased tension. Several changes may account for the increased tension with pharmacy. Ordering procedures were changed substantially, and a change was made in medical staff-pharmacy procedures to reduce errors. Baker is currently planning to change to a unit dose system, and this contemplated change may also have contributed to increased tensions with pharmacy. Although the Bureau worked extensively with radiology (a high impact department) and also had considerable activity with the laboratory (a moderate impact department), the decreases in tension between these departments and the rest of Baker Hospital do not appear to be related to any activity initiated by the Bureau. In candor, our data and our experience do not explain these decreases.

When the decreases in satisfaction with specific job characteristics and the decrease in intradepartmental problem solving are related to the interdepartmental tension findings, it would appear that changes in tension

**TABLE V.1.3**
Changes in intradepartmental activities at Baker Hospital: 1970–1973

| | *1970 sample size* | *1973 sample size* | *Changes in intra-departmental activities* | |
|---|---|---|---|---|
| | | | *Cooperation* | *Problem solving* |
| Total Baker Hospital | 388 | 436 | 0 | *DOWN* |
| High Bureau impact departments* | 150 | 163 | 0 | *DOWN* |
| Moderate Bureau impact departments* | 121 | 122 | *UP* | *UP* |
| Low Bureau impact departments* | 82 | 85 | 0 | 0 |
| High Bureau impact departments—nursing | 97 | 116 | up | *DOWN* |
| High Bureau impact departments—nonnursing | 54 | 47 | down | *DOWN* |

* High, moderate, and low impact departments less than total because several small departments were excluded.

*CAPS* — 95+% significance
Noncaps — 90–95% significance
(+) or (−) — direction of change, not significant
0 — no change

during the 1970-73 period were intradepartmental rather than interdepartmental. Since most hospital employees experience most of their interactions with members of their own units or departments, most of their tension (friction, strain, and/or conflict) can be expected to originate within their own departments. Consequently, the finding of no general increase in interdepartmental tension should be interpreted with this understanding.

### Interim Changes in Satisfaction among Nursing Personnel: 1970, 1971, 1973

As noted earlier, the responses of nurses and practical nurses were combined for this analysis because of their similar response pattern. The analysis studied only the direction and the pattern of change for the three questionnaire administrations—June 1970, February 1971, and May 1973. No tests of significance were made in this study. The results of the analysis are presented in table V.1.4. As the table indicates, the nurse-practical nurse group showed a general pattern of initial decline with a subsequent partial or complete recovery on four of the six satisfaction measures. One measure showed an initial decline and then remained at the same level; only one measure showed a double decline. The pattern of response for the nurse aides was very different; five of the six measures showed an overall decline for the three-year period. However, the interim pattern varied. Two measures showed a double decline, two measures were the same initially and then declined, and one measure showed an initial decline with a third response at the same level. Thus, the data indicate that nurses and practical nurses experienced their greatest dissatisfaction in 1971 while nurse aides experienced their greatest dissatisfaction in 1973.

This difference in the pattern of satisfaction between the nurse-practical nurse group and the nurse aides appears to be the result of difference in responses to both increased occupancy and the introduction of team nursing. The major occupancy increase occurred between the initial survey in August 1970 and the interim survey in February 1971, and this increase appeared to affect nurses and practical nurses more than aides. Both direct complaints and questionnaire comments indicated that the impact of this increase, both in greater patient responsibility and lesser ability to control admissions, was experienced most directly by the nurses. The increased occupancy appeared to have less effect on the work of the aides. This would explain why nurse aide satisfaction remained stable while nurse and practical nurse satisfaction decreased from 1970 to 1971. Subsequently, the introduction of team nursing appears to have affected aides more than nurses and practical nurses. Team nursing brought the aides into closer contact and under closer supervision than before, while it

**TABLE V.1.4**
Interim changes in satisfaction among nursing personnel at Baker Hospital: 1970, 1971, 1973

| | | *Informational feedback* | *Involvement in decision making* | *Interpersonal relations* | *Wages and working conditions* | *Career opportunities* | *Overall satisfaction* |
|---|---|---|---|---|---|---|---|
| RN and LPN* | *1970* | 4.48 | 4.30 | 4.37 | 4.59 | 4.51 | 4.67 |
| | *1971* | 4.08 | 3.73 | 4.13 | 4.02 | 4.06 | 3.78 |
| | *1973* | 4.32 | 3.87 | 3.73 | 4.56 | 4.06 | 4.23 |
| | *Change pattern* | 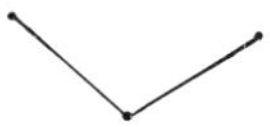 | 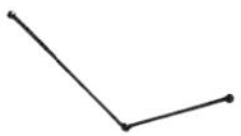 | 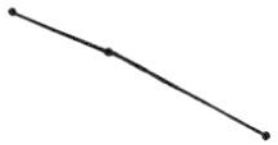 |  | 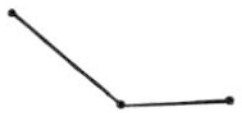 | 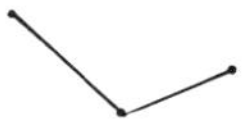 |
| Aides** | *1970* | 4.60 | 3.79 | 4.03 | 3.59 | 3.53 | 4.10 |
| | *1971* | 4.62 | 3.74 | 3.84 | 3.08 | 3.36 | 3.84 |
| | *1973* | 4.26 | 3.34 | 3.66 | 3.12 | 3.08 | 4.18 |
| | *Change pattern* | 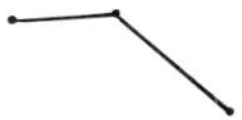 | 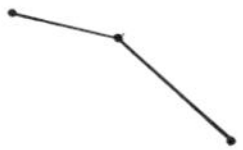 | 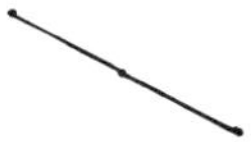 | 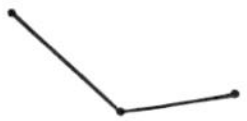 | 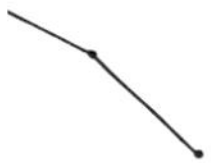 |  |

* Data are group means. 1970 N = 63; 1971 N = 51; 1973 N = 112.
** Data are group means. 1970 N = 90; 1971 N = 89; 1973 N = 68.

was favorably received by at least some of the nurses and practical nurses. We suspect, therefore, that team nursing explains the decrease in nurse aides' satisfaction, while the satisfaction of nurses and practical nurses increased as they began to adapt to increases in economy.

We must emphasize that the explanation above is consistent with our data, but is not proved by it. The pattern of rising satisfaction for nurses in the 1971-73 administrations gives some indication that the innovations introduced have at least not significantly reduced satisfaction. Nevertheless, to the exent that the Bureau has facilitated the maintenance of a high census we must also bear some responsibility for the general drop in satisfaction among high impact departments between 1970 and 1973.

## Conclusions

It seems safe to conclude that there was an improvement in the cost effectiveness of the management of Baker Hospital after January 1972. Table V.1.5 summarizes the more detailed discussion of cost, volume, and resource measures above.

**TABLE V.1.5**
Cost, volume, and resource measures

| *Indicator* | *Status* | *Significance* |
|---|---|---|
| Financial | | |
| Cost per patient day | Improved | Marginal |
| Nursing cost per patient day | Uncertain | Uncertain |
| Cost per patient stay | Not improved | High |
| Occupancy and volume (adult medical-surgical) | | |
| Census and occupancy | Improved | High |
| Discharges | Improved | Marginal |
| Length of stay | Improved | High |
| Manpower | | |
| FTE employees per bed | Improved | High |
| FTE employees per occupied bed | Improved | See text, p. 406 |
| Nursing hours per patient day | Improved | High |
| Medical-surgical nursing hours per patient day | Improved | High |

(Significance levels over 90% are noted as high; those where some of the tests were in the 70% to 90% range are noted as marginal. "Improved status" is a change in the direction of reduced cost, relative to earlier Baker Hospital status or comparison group status.)

The most striking exception, cost per stay, will apparently improve over time as length of stay is controlled and cost per patient day continues to improve. The more specific the indicator, the clearer the picture of improvement. While considerable uncertainty surrounds the financial indicators, the occupancy, volume, and manpower indicators generally reflect statistically significant improvement. In only one case in ten is there any inference of impairment of quality (medical-surgical nursing hours per patient day). This particular statistic was substantially below HAS medians. Even in that case there is room for argument, for the range of performance is wide and the relation to quality complex. Admittedly there are large problems with selection of indicators, validity of data, choice of comparison group, and permanence of change. Overall, however, we believe the data are sufficiently persuasive to warrant guarded acceptance of the hypothesis, at lease insofar as it applies to Baker Hospital.

The data on employee satisfaction also indicate areas for caution. It appears that changes in the operation are reflected in employee satisfaction, at least temporarily. Also, increased occupancy appears to decrease nursing satisfaction. Obviously, these effects should be monitored and attention should be given to ways to reduce them. At the same time, however, the overall stability of satisfaction is relatively high and there is little evidence that a well managed hospital will have serious problems.

The chains of events from increased occupancy to shortened stays to fewer personnel per bed to reduced cost per stay are by no means automatic, or even automatically desirable in every instance. If an improvement is made in occupancy, a potential savings in cost is incurred. A series of opportunities to use the savings is also created: more personnel in nursing and other services to handle higher patient loads, better wage and salary increases, more (or more expensive) supplies, higher expenditures on nonrelated areas (for example, more expenditures on industrial engineering), investment in new plant and equipment, and finally return to the patient through cost or charge reductions. The purpose of the systems described in this book is to permit the explicit and deliberate evaluation of all alternatives in this set. Even if they were perfect (and they certainly are not), the results probably would and should vary in each application. If the dominant overall goal is cost reduction, however, the most common result would be to pass the savings incurred to the patient.

It would be incorrect to say that the specific technologies described elsewhere in this book and implemented at Baker Hospistal caused the change in performance. The technologies are tools for skillful and well motivated administrators. The cause of improved performance can be likened to the cause of cutting down a tree. The cause may be the ax, the woodsman, or the lumber company which ordered the cutting. In the Baker Hospital case, the "company" was clearly interested in and supportive of efforts to control or reduce costs. The administrator had clear instructions and showed considerable skill at the task. The "ax"—the set of technologies employed—was sufficient. One might therefore assume that when these three elments are reassembled elsewhere, the same result will occur.

## NOTES

[1]D. H. Stimson and R. H. Stimson, *Operations Research in Hospitals: Diagnosis and Prognosis.* Chicago: Hospital Research and Educational Trust, 1971.

[2]C. P. Hardwick and H. Wolfe, "An Incentive Reimbursement/Industrial Engineering Experiment," DHEW Publication No. (HSM) 72-3003, 1971, pp. 22ff.

[3]J. R. Giffith, L. E. Weeks, and R. A. DeVries, "A Reappraisal of the McPherson Experiment in Progressive Patient Care," Research Report No. 2, Bureau of Hospital Administration, The University of Michigan, Ann Arbor, Michigan, 1970, p. 58.

[4]Hospital Administrative Services, American Hospital Association, Chicago, Illinois.

[5]Professional Activity Study, Commission on Professional and Hospital Activites, 1968 Green Road, Ann Arbor, Michigan 48105.

[6]RCCAC—Ratio of Beneficiary Charges to Total Charges Applied to Costs.

[7]J. R. Griffith, "Impact of Administrative and Cost Factors on Nurse Staffing," in *Research on Nurse Staffing in Hospitals*, DHEW Publication No. (NIH) 73-434, p. 87.

[8]Job assessment (satisfaction) items were adapted from Lyman Porter, "Job Attitudes in Management," *Journal of Applied Psychology*, December 1962, pp. 375-384, and April 1963, pp. 141-148. Influence and tension items were adapted from instruments developed in the Institute for Social Research, The University of Michigan, by Arnold Tannenbaum and others, and discussed in Basil Georgopoulos and Floyd Mann, *The Community General Hospital*, New York: Macmillan, 1962.

**TABLE V.1.6**
Trends in HAS per diem cost (RCCAC) and "adjusted per diem costs" (AHA)*

| Month | HAS Reports (RCCAC) | | | | AHA* |
|---|---|---|---|---|---|
| | *Baker* | *District* | *State (200–299 beds)* | *National (200–299 beds)* | *National Sample* |
| July 1970 | 82.47 | 89.56 | 82.55 | 69.11 | 83.00 |
| August | 85.83 | 92.58 | 84.43 | 72.38 | 81.00 |
| September | 80.85 | 95.56 | 90.18 | 74.22 | 82.00 |
| October | 77.72 | 97.79 | 87.72 | 74.32 | 80.00 |
| November | 82.26 | 94.60 | 87.70 | 74.20 | 83.00 |
| December | 89.13 | 98.06 | 87.93 | 74.38 | 88.00 |
| January 1971 | 80.28 | 94.30 | 90.04 | 75.67 | 79.00 |
| February | 75.03 | 93.47 | 85.86 | 75.88 | 83.00 |
| March | 77.78 | 93.89 | 88.30 | 77.49 | 83.00 |
| April | ** | ** | ** | ** | 84.00 |
| May | 80.79 | 99.77 | 90.05 | 77.40 | 86.00 |
| June | 100.94 | 102.40 | 94.25 | 78.46 | 88.00 |
| July | 96.75 | 103.20 | 93.75 | 80.12 | 89.00 |
| August | 91.19 | 105.42 | 89.67 | 81.06 | 92.00 |
| September | 101.19 | 102.60 | 92.12 | 84.71 | 93.00 |
| October | 86.98 | 105.55 | 92.28 | 83.37 | 89.00 |
| November | 94.26 | 105.44 | 91.22 | 83.22 | 90.00 |
| December | 104.75 | 104.72 | 94.34 | 82.70 | 101.00 |
| January 1972 | 106.41 | 106.54 | 96.53 | 84.12 | 88.00 |
| February | 85.26 | 108.63 | 94.92 | 84.33 | 92.00 |
| March | 86.31 | 112.19 | 98.32 | 85.41 | 94.00 |
| April | 83.93 | 108.78 | 91.80 | 82.99 | 95.00 |
| May | 89.22 | 110.68 | 91.45 | 85.87 | 95.00 |
| June | 97.39 | 109.90 | 92.05 | 85.28 | 100.00 |
| July | 107.98 | 129.44 | 110.13 | 98.95 | 101.00 |
| August | 104.11 | 111.96 | 100.94 | 87.64 | 101.00 |
| September | 100.85 | 116.81 | 99.89 | 92.19 | 101.00 |
| October | 95.87 | 113.69 | 99.69 | 89.49 | 100.00 |
| November | ** | ** | ** | ** | 101.00 |
| December | 102.76 | 114.55 | 103.85 | 89.81 | 108.00 |
| January 1973 | 100.59 | 120.85 | 105.30 | 91.86 | 96.00 |
| February | 100.92 | 114.25 | 103.03 | 91.38 | 100.00 |
| March | 105.82 | 119.23 | 101.40 | 91.47 | 101.00 |
| April | ** | 116.99 | 102.86 | 88.63 | 102.00 |
| May | ** | ** | ** | ** | 104.00 |
| June | 96.13 | 121.50 | 104.13 | 93.73 | 108.00 |

* *Hospitals, J.A.H.A.*, Indicators Adjusted by Source.
** Data not available.

**TABLE V.1.7**
Average total per diem cost reported to Michigan Blue Cross

| *Quarter Ending:* | *Baker Hospital* | *Category D M.B.C.** |
|---|---|---|
| March 1969 | 65.29 | 71.87 |
| June | 65.80 | 74.81 |
| September | 67.21 | 77.87 |
| December | 69.29 | 81.05 |
| March 1970 | 71.81 | 84.02 |
| June | 73.92 | 87.54 |
| September | 75.05 | 90.73 |
| December | 76.86 | 94.13 |
| March 1971 | 77.36 | 97.15 |
| June | 82.03 | 101.52 |
| September | 85.60 | 105.64 |
| December | 88.51 | 106.95 |
| March 1972 | 92.35 | 111.86 |
| June | 93.19 | 113.95 |
| September | 93.63 | 116.72 |
| December | 94.28 | 119.71** |
| March 1973 | 96.03 | 122.01** |
| June | 99.24 | 124.36** |

* Blue Cross Participating Hospitals in Southeast Michigan, over 149 beds.

** Less than 12 months audit. Adjustment for audit estimated by source.

Source: Michigan Blue Cross, "Report to Participating Hospitals," issued quarterly by M.B.C., Detroit. Adjusted by source for audits through 12 or 15 months except as noted.

**TABLE V.1.8**
Nursing direct cost per patient day

| | | HAS Reports | | |
|---|---|---|---|---|
| *Month* | *Baker* | *District* | *State* | *National* |
| July 1970 | 27.32 | 23.78 | 23.32 | 19.47 |
| August | 27.78 | 24.89 | 23.99 | 20.51 |
| September | 24.51 | 25.10 | 24.63 | 21.30 |
| October | 23.79 | 25.28 | 24.04 | 21.15 |
| November | 24.26 | 24.28 | 24.85 | 20.71 |
| December | 28.06 | 24.20 | 24.19 | 20.53 |
| January 1971 | 25.21 | 25.17 | 25.35 | 21.15 |
| February | 22.00 | 25.13 | 25.08 | 21.18 |
| March | 22.18 | 25.01 | 24.55 | 21.01 |
| April | * | * | * | * |
| May | 25.04 | 25.20 | 24.56 | 20.98 |
| June | 29.97 | 25.75 | 24.98 | 21.59 |
| July | 31.75 | 26.26 | 25.69 | 21.99 |
| August | 28.86 | 26.46 | 25.95 | 22.40 |
| September | 31.16 | 27.36 | 27.16 | 23.18 |
| October | 26.22 | 28.07 | 27.11 | 23.17 |
| November | 27.94 | 27.00 | 25.80 | 23.03 |
| December | 32.65 | 26.84 | 25.87 | 22.91 |
| January 1972 | 32.47 | 28.05 | 26.80 | 22.97 |
| February | 24.79 | 28.43 | 27.64 | 22.90 |
| March | 25.28 | 27.46 | 27.46 | 22.76 |
| April | 25.04 | 26.08 | 25.59 | 22.10 |
| May | 25.50 | 26.33 | 25.89 | 22.65 |
| June | 27.85 | 26.50 | 26.26 | 22.82 |
| July | 29.42 | 26.94 | 26.59 | 22.99 |
| August | 30.33 | 27.01 | 27.50 | 22.45 |
| September | 30.42 | 28.57 | 27.91 | 25.21 |
| October | 29.04 | 28.18 | 27.76 | 24.76 |
| November | * | * | * | * |
| December | 29.94 | 28.66 | 28.12 | 24.21 |
| January 1973 | 29.72 | 28.82 | 28.42 | 24.71 |
| February | 26.40 | 29.46 | 28.86 | 24.16 |
| March | 30.16 | 29.14 | 28.64 | 23.84 |
| April | * | 29.07 | 27.85 | 22.94 |
| May | * | * | * | * |
| June | 31.45 | 29.12 | 28.75 | 24.48 |

* Data not available.

**TABLE V.1.9**
Cost per patient stay (RCCAC)

| | HAS Reports | |
|---|---|---|
| *Month* | *Baker* | *State* |
| January 1972 | 798.08 | 611.55 |
| February | 655.03 | 626.57 |
| March | 655.96 | 647.41 |
| April | 679.83 | 645.66 |
| May | 678.07 | 673.38 |
| June | 749.90 | 643.01 |
| July | 842.24 | 688.75 |
| August | 770.04 | 623.12 |
| September | 726.12 | 672.99 |
| October | 687.30 | 681.02 |
| November | ** | ** |
| December | 801.53 | 646.38 |
| January 1973 | 764.48 | 704.57 |
| February | ** | 697.23 |
| March | 817.45 | 692.43 |
| April | 846.56 | 654.09 |
| May | ** | ** |
| June | 672.91 | 679.54 |

** Data not available for calculation.

**TABLE V.1.10**
Inpatient revenue as percentage of total

| | | *HAS Reports* | | |
|---|---|---|---|---|
| *Month* | *Baker* | *District* | *State* | *National* |
| July 1970 | 87.4 | 90.5 | 89.5 | 91.5 |
| August | 86.0 | 91.0 | 89.6 | 91.3 |
| September | 90.2 | 90.4 | 89.7 | 91.2 |
| October | 88.2 | 90.3 | 90.0 | 91.3 |
| November | 89.0 | 90.7 | 90.1 | 91.0 |
| December | 87.8 | 91.0 | 90.2 | 91.5 |
| January 1971 | 87.7 | 90.2 | 90.2 | 91.8 |
| February | 88.2 | 89.9 | 90.1 | 92.2 |
| March | 87.7 | 90.7 | 90.7 | 92.1 |
| April | * | * | * | * |
| May | 87.6 | 90.9 | 90.7 | 91.7 |
| June | 87.6 | 89.9 | 90.1 | 91.7 |
| July | 87.6 | 90.0 | 89.5 | 91.1 |
| August | 87.5 | 90.0 | 89.0 | 91.0 |
| September | 87.8 | 89.4 | 89.3 | 90.8 |
| October | 87.7 | 90.2 | 89.8 | 90.9 |
| November | 88.0 | 89.6 | 89.6 | 90.9 |
| December | 87.2 | 90.1 | 89.6 | 91.1 |
| January 1972 | 87.6 | 89.8 | 90.1 | 90.9 |
| February | 87.4 | 90.1 | 90.2 | 91.3 |
| March | 86.4 | 90.3 | 90.5 | 91.3 |
| April | 86.0 | 90.3 | 90.4 | 91.2 |
| May | 84.0 | 90.4 | 90.6 | 91.1 |
| June | 84.3 | 90.3 | 90.3 | 90.7 |
| July | 84.2 | 89.7 | 90.0 | 90.5 |
| August | 85.2 | 90.3 | 90.1 | 90.5 |
| September | 84.3 | 90.0 | 89.6 | 90.2 |
| October | * | * | * | * |
| November | * | * | * | * |
| December | 86.4 | 90.8 | 91.1 | 90.3 |
| January 1973 | 84.9 | 90.7 | 91.2 | 90.5 |
| February | 85.4 | 90.8 | 91.4 | 90.8 |
| March | 85.1 | 91.0 | 91.3 | 91.9 |
| April | 72.5 | 91.3 | 91.0 | 90.9 |
| May | * | * | * | * |
| June | 83.7 | 90.0 | 89.9 | 90.0 |

* Data not available.

**TABLE V.1.11**
Average daily census and occupancy by month, adult medical-surgical service excluding ICU/CCU, Baker Hospital

| *Month* | *Census* | *Occupancy* |
|---|---|---|
| July 1970 | 181.7 | 87.1 |
| August | 182.1 | 87.5 |
| September | 193.4 | 93.0 |
| October | 195.4 | 93.9 |
| November | 183.0 | 88.8 |
| December | 170.6 | 82.0 |
| January 1971 | 195.8 | 94.1 |
| February | 205.7 | 98.9 |
| March | 205.1 | 98.6 |
| April | 194.9 | 93.7 |
| May | 197.1 | 94.8 |
| June | 195.1 | 93.8 |
| July | 193.6 | 93.1 |
| August | 195.3 | 93.9 |
| September | 192.0 | 92.3 |
| October | 197.7 | 95.0 |
| November | 199.5 | 95.9 |
| December | 177.8 | 85.5 |
| January 1972 | 196.2 | 94.3 |
| February | 202.5 | 97.4 |
| March | 201.8 | 97.0 |
| April | 202.0 | 97.1 |
| May | 198.2 | 95.3 |
| June | 202.6 | 96.4 |
| Period 1 | 201.4 | 94.2 |
| 2 | 198.9 | 92.9 |
| 3 | 199.0 | 93.0 |
| 4 | 208.8 | 97.6 |
| 5 | 209.3 | 97.8 |
| 6 | 205.8 | 96.2 |
| 7 1973 | 177.0 | 82.7 |
| 8 | 207.9 | 97.1 |
| 9 | 205.4 | 96.0 |
| 10 | 203.5 | 95.1 |
| 11 | 195.6 | 91.4 |
| 12 | 195.2 | 91.2 |
| 13 | 199.7 | 93.3 |

Source: Hospital records. Occupancy based upon 208 beds July 1970–May 1972, 210 beds June 1972, 214 beds thereafter.

**TABLE V.1.12**
Adult medical-surgical patients discharged, Baker Hospital

| *Month* | *Discharges* |
|---|---|
| January 1971 | 643 |
| February | 659 |
| March | 701 |
| April | 692 |
| May | 764 |
| June | 710 |
| July | 753 |
| August | 721 |
| September | 667 |
| October | 781 |
| November | 707 |
| December | 678 |
| January 1972 | 692 |
| February | 703 |
| March | 797 |
| April | 683 |
| May | 715 |
| June | 718 |
| July | 709 |
| August | 770 |
| September | 703 |
| October | 732 |
| November | 736 |
| December | 722 |
| January 1973 | 668 |
| February | 672 |
| March | 790 |
| April | 752 |
| May | 801 |
| June | 812 |

Source: PAS, Form A.

**TABLE V.1.13**
Length of stay adjusted for case mix

| *Quarters* | *Average Stay* | *Average Stay-Matching Patients** | *Difference* | *Patient Difference Signifcnt.?* | *Average Stay-Matching Patients—All U.S.* |
|---|---|---|---|---|---|
| | | *Medicine* | | | |
| Oct.–Dec. 1970 | 11.8 | * | +1.6 | Yes | 10.2 |
| Jan.–Mar. 1971 | 12.2 | * | +1.7 | Yes | 10.5 |
| Apr.–June | 11.0 | * | +0.7 | Yes | 10.3 |
| July–Sept. | 11.2 | * | +0.6 | Yes | 10.6 |
| Oct.–Dec. | 11.4 | * | +0.9 | Yes | 10.2 |
| Jan.–Mar. 1972 | 12.2 | 10.9 | +1.3 | Yes | 10.6 |
| Apr.–June | 12.3 | 10.9 | +1.4 | Yes | 10.7 |
| July–Sept. | 11.6 | 10.9 | +0.7 | Yes | 10.6 |
| Oct.–Dec. | 11.9 | 10.9 | +1.0 | Yes | 10.6 |
| Jan.–Mar. 1973 | 11.8 | 10.5 | +1.3 | Yes | 10.2 |
| Apr.–June | 10.2 | 10.3 | −0.1 | — | 10.0 |
| | | *Surgery* | | | |
| Oct.–Dec. 1970 | 6.0 | * | −0.4 | — | 6.4 |
| Jan.–Mar. 1971 | 6.4 | * | 0.0 | — | 6.4 |
| Apr.–June | 6.1 | * | −0.3 | — | 6.4 |
| July–Sept. | 5.9 | * | −0.6 | — | 6.5 |
| Oct.–Dec. | 6.1 | * | −0.4 | — | 6.3 |
| Jan.–Mar. 1972 | 6.1 | 6.7 | −0.6 | — | 6.5 |
| Apr.–June | 6.6 | 6.8 | −0.2 | — | 6.7 |
| July–Sept. | 6.3 | 6.8 | −0.5 | — | 6.6 |
| Oct.–Dec. | 6.7 | 7.3 | −0.6 | — | 7.1 |
| Jan.–Mar. 1973 | 6.8 | 7.0 | −0.2 | — | 6.8 |
| Apr.–June | 6.3 | 7.1 | −0.8 | — | 6.9 |
| | | *Pediatric Medicine* | | | |
| Oct.–Dec. 1970 | 6.5 | * | +0.5 | Yes | 6.0 |
| Jan.–Mar. 1971 | 6.6 | * | +0.4 | Yes | 6.2 |
| Apr.–June | 5.9 | * | +0.2 | Yes | 5.7 |
| July–Sept. | 5.6 | * | −0.4 | — | 6.0 |
| Oct.–Dec. | 5.1 | * | −0.6 | — | 5.5 |
| Jan.–Mar. 1972 | 6.4 | 6.0 | +0.4 | Yes | 5.7 |
| Apr.–June | 6.1 | 5.9 | +0.2 | Yes | 5.7 |
| July–Sept. | 5.4 | 5.9 | −0.5 | — | 5.7 |
| Oct.–Dec. | 5.2 | 5.9 | −0.7 | — | 5.7 |
| Jan.–Mar. 1973 | 6.3 | 6.0 | +0.3 | Yes | 5.8 |
| Apr.–June | 6.0 | 5.6 | +0.4 | Yes | 5.4 |

**TABLE V.1.13** Cont.

| *Quarters* | *Average Stay* | *Average Stay-Matching Patients** | *Difference* | *Patient Difference Signifcnt.?* | *Average Stay-Matching Patients—All U.S.* |
|---|---|---|---|---|---|
| | | *Grand Total* | | | |
| Oct.–Dec. 1970 | 7.0 | * | +0.3 | Yes | 6.7 |
| Jan.–Mar. 1971 | 7.2 | * | +0.5 | Yes | 6.7 |
| Apr.–June | 7.0 | * | +0.1 | Yes | 6.7 |
| July–Sept. | 7.0 | * | 0.0 | — | 7.0 |
| Oct.–Dec. | 7.0 | * | +0.3 | Yes | 6.7 |
| Jan.–Mar. 1972 | 7.2 | 7.2 | 0.0 | — | 7.0 |
| Apr.–June | 7.6 | 7.3 | +0.3 | Yes | 7.1 |
| July–Sept. | 7.2 | 7.3 | −0.1 | — | 7.1 |
| Oct.–Dec. | 7.5 | 7.5 | 0.0 | — | 7.3 |
| Jan.–Mar. 1973 | 7.6 | 7.4 | +0.2 | Yes | 7.1 |
| Apr.–June | 6.8 | 7.3 | −0.5 | — | 7.0 |

* Regional data for Average Stay-Matching Patients—4th quarter 1970 to 4th quarter 1971 not available. National comparison used in Difference column. Regional and national data for Average Stay-Matching Patients—shown separately for 4th quarter 1971.

Source: PAS Form S.

**TABLE V.1.14**
Equivalent full time employees per bed

| | | HAS Reports | | |
|---|---|---|---|---|
| *Month* | *Baker* | *District* | *State* | *National* |
| July 1970 | 2.71 | 2.48 | 2.48 | 2.20 |
| August | 2.66 | 2.57 | 2.54 | 2.29 |
| September | 2.63 | 2.64 | 2.60 | 2.31 |
| October | 2.64 | 2.72 | 2.62 | 2.28 |
| November | 2.58 | 2.67 | 2.60 | 2.27 |
| December | 2.73 | 2.61 | 2.54 | 2.24 |
| January 1971 | 2.69 | 2.55 | 2.56 | 2.25 |
| February | 2.34 | 2.58 | 2.58 | 2.24 |
| March | 2.60 | 2.53 | 2.50 | 2.20 |
| April | * | * | * | * |
| May | 2.56 | 2.58 | 2.42 | 2.19 |
| June | 2.73 | 2.61 | 2.51 | 2.27 |
| July | 2.69 | 2.60 | 2.49 | 2.27 |
| August | 2.74 | 2.67 | 2.41 | 2.31 |
| September | 2.79 | 2.69 | 2.44 | 2.36 |
| October | 2.78 | 2.61 | 2.41 | 2.32 |
| November | 2.68 | 2.65 | 2.42 | 2.29 |
| December | 2.93 | 2.62 | 2.33 | 2.27 |
| January 1972 | 2.85 | 2.61 | 2.33 | 2.29 |
| February | 2.51 | 2.64 | 2.32 | 2.26 |
| March | 2.73 | 2.63 | 2.33 | 2.24 |
| April | 2.59 | 2.59 | 2.43 | 2.24 |
| May | 2.81 | 2.56 | 2.30 | 2.23 |
| June | 2.68 | 2.63 | 2.35 | 2.27 |
| July | 3.01 | 2.64 | 2.39 | 2.25 |
| August | 2.52 | 2.52 | 2.48 | 2.22 |
| September | 2.53 | 2.60 | 2.49 | 2.33 |
| October | 2.45 | 2.61 | 2.48 | 2.31 |
| November | * | * | * | * |
| December | 2.52 | 2.58 | 2.37 | 2.28 |
| January 1973 | 2.40 | 2.59 | 2.46 | 2.30 |
| February | 2.43 | 2.56 | 2.40 | 2.29 |
| March | 2.43 | 2.62 | 2.38 | 2.25 |
| April | 2.43 | 2.65 | 2.41 | 2.27 |
| May | * | * | * | * |
| June | 2.74 | 2.63 | 2.47 | 2.33 |

* Data not available.

**TABLE V.1.15**
Equivalent full time employees per occupied bed

| *Month* | *Baker* | *Comparison** |
|---|---|---|
| July 1970 | 3.32 | 2.75 |
| August | 3.44 | 2.84 |
| September | 2.88 | 2.96 |
| October | 2.88 | 2.99 |
| November | 2.88 | 2.93 |
| December | 3.42 | 2.89 |
| January 1971 | 2.92 | 3.02 |
| February | 2.41 | 2.96 |
| March | 2.70 | 2.82 |
| April | ** | ** |
| May | 2.84 | 2.68 |
| June | 3.03 | 2.85 |
| July | 3.19 | 2.85 |
| August | 3.11 | 2.86 |
| September | 3.28 | 2.96 |
| October | 2.90 | 2.96 |
| November | 2.89 | 2.97 |
| December | 3.53 | 2.89 |
| January 1972 | 3.27 | 2.88 |
| February | 2.44 | 2.84 |
| March | 2.70 | 2.84 |
| April | 2.54 | 2.86 |
| May | 2.77 | 2.69 |
| June | 2.60 | 2.71 |
| July | 3.24 | 2.78 |
| August | 2.86 | 2.95 |
| September | 2.75 | 3.05 |
| October | 2.60 | 3.06 |
| November | ** | ** |
| December | 2.71 | 2.78 |
| January 1973 | 2.53 | 2.92 |
| February | 2.35 | 2.83 |
| March | 2.69 | 2.75 |
| April | 2.69 | 2.65 |
| May | ** | ** |
| June | 3.03 | 2.79 |

* The Comparison group was constructed from table V.1.14, using HAS occupancy data after January 1972 when it was first reported and Region 4 AHA National Panel data for earlier months.

** Data not available.

**TABLE V.1.16**
Nursing manhours per patient day (all units)

| | HAS Reports | | | |
|---|---|---|---|---|
| *Month* | *Baker* | *District* | *State* | *National* |
| July 1970 | 5.98 | 5.48 | 5.54 | 5.18 |
| August | 5.89 | 5.69 | 5.74 | 5.37 |
| September | 6.16 | 5.81 | 5.83 | 5.40 |
| October | 5.89 | 5.78 | 5.82 | 5.38 |
| November | 5.83 | 5.61 | 5.82 | 5.34 |
| December | 6.15 | 5.65 | 5.63 | 5.26 |
| January 1971 | 6.03 | 5.60 | 5.68 | 5.32 |
| February | 5.56 | 5.73 | 5.79 | 5.30 |
| March | 5.66 | 5.71 | 5.80 | 5.38 |
| April | * | * | * | * |
| May | 5.73 | 5.65 | 5.79 | 5.32 |
| June | 6.34 | 5.69 | 5.68 | 5.32 |
| July | 6.10 | 5.69 | 5.63 | 5.28 |
| August | 6.14 | 5.72 | 5.41 | 5.41 |
| September | 6.53 | 5.86 | 5.75 | 5.53 |
| October | 6.02 | 5.75 | 5.65 | 5.39 |
| November | 6.10 | 5.58 | 5.56 | 5.34 |
| December | 6.36 | 5.60 | 5.39 | 5.26 |
| January 1972 | 5.51 | 5.08 | 4.98 | 4.79 |
| February | 5.37 | 5.11 | 5.02 | 4.79 |
| March | 5.26 | 5.01 | 4.93 | 4.73 |
| April | 5.21 | 5.02 | 4.85 | 4.74 |
| May | 5.39 | 5.00 | 4.75 | 4.67 |
| June | 5.16 | 5.04 | 4.86 | 4.74 |
| July | 5.94 | 5.05 | 4.74 | 4.69 |
| August | 4.87 | 4.67 | 4.85 | 4.37 |
| September | 5.12 | 5.33 | 5.13 | 4.91 |
| October | 4.71 | 5.31 | 5.14 | 4.84 |
| November | * | * | * | * |
| December | 5.97 | 5.93 | 6.11 | 6.01 |
| January 1973 | 5.60 | 6.16 | 6.45 | 6.13 |
| February | 5.12 | 6.04 | 5.92 | 6.02 |
| March | 5.90 | 6.03 | 5.83 | 5.86 |
| April | 5.70 | 5.81 | 5.73 | 5.73 |
| May | * | * | * | * |
| June | 5.87 | 6.06 | 6.03 | 5.93 |

* Data not available.

**TABLE V.1.17**
Nursing manhours per medical-surgical patient day

| | HAS Reports | | | |
|---|---|---|---|---|
| *Month* | *Baker* | *District* | *State* | *National* |
| July 1970 | 7.00 | 5.88 | 5.86 | 5.61 |
| August | 7.22 | 6.05 | 6.09 | 5.89 |
| September | 6.20 | 6.18 | 6.19 | 6.07 |
| October | 6.08 | 6.22 | 6.22 | 6.03 |
| November | 6.12 | 5.99 | 6.11 | 5.90 |
| December | 7.22 | 6.00 | 6.02 | 5.83 |
| January 1971 | 6.14 | 6.09 | 6.25 | 6.06 |
| February | 5.31 | 6.03 | 6.14 | 5.93 |
| March | 5.44 | 6.03 | 5.98 | 5.81 |
| April | * | * | * | * |
| May | 5.93 | 5.81 | 5.81 | 5.67 |
| June | 6.44 | 5.90 | 5.96 | 5.80 |
| July | 6.64 | 5.98 | 6.09 | 5.88 |
| August | 6.44 | 6.11 | 6.28 | 6.06 |
| September | 7.08 | 6.26 | 6.25 | 6.25 |
| October | 5.73 | 6.13 | 6.32 | 6.20 |
| November | 6.01 | 5.98 | 6.05 | 6.04 |
| December | 7.09 | 6.24 | 6.00 | 6.01 |
| January 1972 | 6.55 | 6.20 | 6.20 | 6.14 |
| February | 5.40 | 6.11 | 6.19 | 6.03 |
| March | 5.36 | 5.97 | 6.08 | 5.87 |
| April | 5.42 | 5.13 | 5.02 | 4.85 |
| May | 5.54 | 5.81 | 5.72 | 5.77 |
| June | 5.35 | 5.20 | 5.01 | 4.87 |
| July | 5.39 | 5.10 | 4.99 | 4.83 |
| August | 5.79 | 6.23 | 6.31 | 6.26 |
| September | 5.19 | 6.30 | 6.30 | 6.20 |
| October | 5.03 | 4.80 | 5.01 | 4.44 |
| November | * | * | * | * |
| December | 4.75 | 5.59 | 5.86 | 5.60 |
| January 1973 | 4.50 | 5.83 | 5.92 | 5.70 |
| February | 4.59 | 5.77 | 5.45 | 5.53 |
| March | 4.67 | 5.82 | 5.53 | 5.41 |
| April | 4.88 | 5.52 | 5.34 | 5.25 |
| May | * | * | * | * |
| June | 5.02 | 5.61 | 5.61 | 5.44 |

* Data not available.

# Index

*Compiled by Gene Regenstreif, A.M.L.S.*